POWER
FOOD

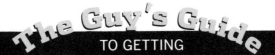

The Guy's Guide
TO GETTING

STRONGER · LEANER · SMARTER · HEALTHIER
· BETTER LOOKING · BETTER SEX
WITH FOOD!

POWER
FOOD

SUSAN M. KLEINER, PhD, RD, FACN, CNS, with **JEFF O'CONNELL**

RODALE

Notice

This book is intended as a reference volume only, not as a medical manual. The information given here is designed to help you make informed decisions about your health. It is not intended as a substitute for any treatment that may have been prescribed by your doctor. If you suspect that you have a medical problem, we urge you to seek competent medical help.

Mention of specific companies, organizations, or authorities in this book does not imply endorsement by the author or publisher, nor does mention of specific companies, organizations, or authorities imply that they endorse this book, its author, or the publisher.

Internet addresses and telephone numbers given in this book were accurate at the time it went to press.

© 2004 by Rodale Inc.

All rights reserved. No part of this publication may be reproduced or transmitted in any form or by any means, electronic or mechanical, including photocopying, recording, or any other information storage and retrieval system, without the written permission of the publisher.

Printed in the United States of America
Rodale Inc. makes every effort to use acid-free (∞), recycled paper ♻.

Book design by Christina Gaugler

Library of Congress Cataloging-in-Publication Data

Kleiner, Susan M.
    Power food : the guy's guide to getting stronger, leaner, smarter, healthier, better looking, better sex with food! / Susan M. Kleiner with Jeff O'Connell.
        p.   cm.
    Includes bibliographical references and index.
        ISBN 1–59486–002–5 hardcover
        1. Men—Health and hygiene.   2. Men—Nutrition.   I. O'Connell, Jeff.   II. Title.
    RA777.8.K545   2004
    613'.04234—dc22
                                                                                2004017042

2   4   6   8   10   9   7   5   3   hardcover

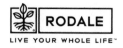
RODALE
LIVE YOUR WHOLE LIFE™

FOR MORE OF OUR PRODUCTS
WWW.RODALESTORE.COM
(800) 848-4735

To Jeff

Contents

Acknowledgments

This book has been a team effort. To Lou Schuler, thank you for your visionary concept and help in getting the project off the ground. To Jeff O'Connell, thank you for your humor and style—they have given the book a great voice. To Daniel Listwa, editor extraordinaire, and to Lois Hazel, thank you for being the champions of this project. Your support and attention to detail have been invaluable. Thank you to Karen Friedman-Kester for your creative menus and recipes, which helped turn the science into a tasty and practical diet. Many thanks to my agent, Al Zuckerman, for always giving me the right advice. Thank you to my numerous clients who contributed to this book by letting me tell your stories and by testing many versions of many diets over many years. To Jeff, Danielle, and Ilana, thank you for everything.

—SUSAN M. KLEINER

Introduction

Power Food is a guidebook to help you break out of your usual routine and challenge yourself to become more powerful in all areas of your life. The book breaks the usual mold for nutrition books.

First of all, it's aimed at men—not the usual nutrition book's target audience. But men have just as many, if not more reasons to eat right than women. I should know: my career in nutrition has always focused on men in one way or another. When I did my doctoral research, it was on male body builders. My clients, including many pro athletes, were almost all men until 1994, when I moved my practice to Seattle. Even today, about 60 percent of the work I do is with men. I, as well as anyone, know how badly men need healthy, practical eating advice. In this book, I look to do something about that. Also, rather than creating one diet that uses 10 chapters to explain how you can fit it into your life, I have created 20 different meal plans in 11 chapters dedicated to each of the different goals that you might want to excel in at some point in your life. You choose what you want to work on in your life, and when.

Generalized diets for the masses can get across the big do's and don'ts regarding health promotion, disease prevention, and basic body-weight management. I call them the Nutrition 101's of the diet world. But once you've got the basics down and you want to achieve more, you need to move on to sophisticated principles that draw on the cutting edge of nutrition science. I tell my clients that what I offer is a customized program based on their personal needs and goals. No one gets the same plan, and every consult is a graduate-level nutrition course based on you. That's how I wrote Power Food. It digs deeper and gives you more detail and practical guidance than the typical one-stop diet. Use Power Food right, and you can reach the levels of excellence that you strive to achieve, whether in the boardroom, the locker room, or the bedroom.

How to Use *Power Food*

Flip back to the Contents. You will see chapters on mood and brain power, weight loss, muscle building, athletic performance, daily health, longevity, appearance, sexual performance, and the Full-Power Meal Plan. Set your priorities. What do you want to work on first? If weight loss is your first goal, read chapter 1 and then turn to chapter 3. If you think that your body weight is just a symptom of mild depression, then go to chapter 2 first. Once you feel better, move on to chapter 3, and so forth.

Every chapter has one or more menus that incorporate the critical points addressed in the text. These diets are designed not just to stand alone, but to help you move from diet to diet as your needs change. If you start out working on weight loss in chapter 3, once you achieve your goals you'll be able to easily move to the muscle-building diet in chapter 4 without feeling overwhelmed with a completely different diet plan. You'll already be familiar with the basic food plan, so incorporating the new muscle-building elements should be easy.

It is the details that make the difference. Bill Belichik, head coach of the two-time winning Super Bowl champions, the New England Patriots, once told me that the difference between any athlete and a winner is attention to details. That's what I've incorporated into the *Power Food* diet plans: tweaks and details that will lift your body/mind above the realm of average men—changes that will give you championship-caliber results. You will know exactly what to eat and when to eat it, no matter what your personal goals.

Of course, once you've attained your specific goals, you'll want a meal plan that maintains your results and keeps you healthy for the rest of your life. Or perhaps your only goal is to have a healthier diet that really incorporates the latest information in nutrition. If so, turn to the Full-Power Meal Plan. It incorporates pretty much all of the health benefits in this book and delivers a 14-day nutrition plan designed to produce major results, fast. I firmly believe that it represents the best, most comprehensive diet for the vast majority of the men reading this book.

I'll keep this brief and end by saying that if you've ever taken food for granted, you won't after reading *Power Food*. The world of nutrition is complex—just as complex as the world of medicine, if not more so. The most celebrated experts in my field learning new ways to use food to benefit mankind every day, and will continue to do so until they retire. By reading this book, you're going to gain a new appreciation for the power of food. It's my hope that you'll take these lessons and put them to work to improve your entire life.

Good luck!

CHAPTER ONE

You, Only Better

TAKE CONTROL OF YOUR DIET
AND YOU'LL MAKE OVER YOUR LIFE

'm a dietitian by trade, not a writer or a preacher, so you'll have to forgive me for getting right to the meat of the matter.

Eating right can change your life.

The right foods can help you feel like a million bucks. They can give you dramatically more energy, and help you to look better than you ever have. Assuming your present diet leaves something to be desired—and the fact that you picked up this book suggests that it might—improving it can have a huge impact on your life. It will make a big difference.

All you need is the right knowledge. That's where *Power Food* comes in. What you hold in your hands is both bible and manual—an all-in-one guide to handling your dietary needs. It will help you to gain control over your eating and, in the process, make over your life.

Although I employ many strategies, there is only one overarching goal: to show men (or any women looking for a complete, no-nonsense guide to nutrition) how to use food to improve every aspect of their lives. This is more than a book about how to

lose weight or build bigger biceps (although those areas will be covered as thoroughly and truthfully as any book could cover them). It's about waking up refreshed and ready to start your day, enjoying sustained energy, saying goodbye to energy peaks and crashes, and having better workouts, better workdays, and better sex. It's about improving the condition of your body and the state of your mind.

Yes, you can have all of this simply by eating the right foods at the right times for the right effects.

We offer no gimmicks, no miracle nine-week makeovers, and no magical transformations from dud to stud. This is a book for the guy with a finely tuned B.S. detector—the one who knows that both his immediate goals and long-term health hinge largely on the food he eats.

Throughout these pages, you will find:

■ The latest science on muscle building, metabolism boosting, energy enhancing, and much, much more. We've pored over the latest research for you and boiled it all down into simple changes you can make for maximum impact. We don't hype or overstate the benefits of given foods. You'll find the truth—nothing less and nothing more.

■ Detailed meal plans and diet makeovers to help you put the science of nutrition to work in your life. It's one thing to know that some percentage of your calories should come from fat; it's quite another to actually put it into practice. These meal plans will help you do just that. Every chapter contains specific meal plans for boosting energy, heightening endurance, improving muscle building, and more. Once you successfully accomplish your targeted goal, you'll find a 14-day menu plan to keep you healthy for the rest of your life. No matter what your goals are, you'll find the meals and snacks you need—and advice on when to eat them.

■ Foods to minimize and foods to maximize in your diet. In each chapter, you'll find detailed lists of foods that benefit your sexual performance, appearance, weight, and so forth—as well as the foods to cut down on or avoid.

■ An insider's look at which industries are sabotaging your diet and which ones are not. In several chapters, you'll learn why you cannot always trust restaurants, food companies, gym chains, weight-loss centers, public and private schools, universities, the medical establishment—and, yes, even the U.S. government—to direct your food choices. For example, did you know that scientists discovered long ago that a common additive, used to extend the shelf life of processed foods, not only promotes weight gain but also may cause heart disease? This food additive— you'll soon learn more about it—is almost as dangerous for your health as cigarettes, yet the government hasn't required food manufacturers to place a warning label on their packaging, and only recently has required manufacturers to note that their products contain this ingredient.

We'll also take a close look at the medical establishment, the media, and even nutritionists, giving you the lowdown on who and what you should turn to for information.

■ The truth about supplements. From muscle-building protein powders to metabolism-boosting weight loss pills, you'll learn what works, what doesn't, what's dangerous, and what's a waste of your hard-earned cash.

It all starts now, in this chapter. You will soon take a 24-hour journey through a typical day in your stomach that will show you what you may be doing right and what you may be doing wrong. More important, you'll learn how it all affects your health, energy levels, mood, and physical and mental performance. There's a reason you pass out on your desk at 2:00 P.M. You'll soon learn how food plays a role in not only the mid-afternoon slump, but also insomnia, performance anxiety (at the office *and* in the bedroom), gastrointestinal upset, headaches, and more.

But first, let's take a look at what topics I'll be covering in chapters 2 through 10.

Chapter 2: Using food to improve mood. Do you find yourself daydreaming during your afternoon meetings? Are you angry all the time but not quite sure why? Your diet may be to blame. In this chapter, you'll learn the latest science on how foods influence your mood, energy levels, memory, mental sharpness, and stress levels. If your alertness takes a dive each afternoon, you'll also find a detailed meal plan to help turn things around.

Chapter 3: Using food to burn fat. Burning off those love handles requires more than simply eating fewer calories than you burn. You'll learn powerful ways to boost your metabolism so that you never feel hungry as the fat melts away.

Chapter4: Using food to build muscle. With our meal plans and advice, you'll finally be able to lay down some serious muscle. We've even included a special section for hardgainers—guys who struggle to build lean muscle. If you've been a skinny guy all your life, I've got some advice that really works.

Chapter 5: Using food to improve your athletic ability. Want to be a better athlete? You can shoot free throws until your arms fall off or run wind sprints until you faint, but if you aren't eating to fit your sport, you will never maximize your potential. In this chapter, you'll find the secret eating techniques that will take your strength and endurance to a new level.

Chapter 6: Using food to stay healthy. Want to have fewer colds? How about fewer stomach and intestinal problems? Are you looking for ways to recover faster after an injury? We've got the answers for you. Food can help heal your body in myriad ways, bolstering your overall health.

Chapter 7: Using food to live longer. Here's the chapter that can add decades to your life and keep you healthy while you live them. Find the most-current advice on using food to reduce your risk for heart disease, cancer, and diabetes.

Chapter 8: Using food to have better sex. I know, I know: That sounds vaguely dirty, but you get the point. Whether it's your first time or your five hundredth time, no one wants to be a lousy lover. Yet every day, guys shovel down food that stifles their sex drive and punishes their penises. In this chapter, you'll learn how to eat and drink so you can be a champ between the sheets.

Chapter 9: Using food to look better. Here I put the screws to the old saying "Beauty is only skin deep." It goes a lot deeper—all the way to the foods you eat and the fluids you drink. Here, you'll get the eating secrets for better skin, stronger hair, whiter teeth, and an assortment of other looks-related benefits. If you've ever been concerned about looking good—whether as a 20-year-old or as an 80-year-old—then you need the information in this chapter.

Chapter 10: The Full-Power Meal Plan. If you've read all the other chapters, you've learned how to eat for muscle. You know how to eat for weight loss. You know how to eat to avoid cancer, to feel energized, to have marathon sex. Now it's time to pull it all together. In this chapter, you'll find the one diet that packs enough all-around nutrition advice to be called the Full-Power Meal Plan.

If you need improvement in only a category or two, congratulations—you're ahead of the game. If you need help in all of the above, don't sweat it. You've finally come to the right place. There isn't a man alive who wouldn't benefit from the information contained herein.

You Are What You Eat

Along with death, taxes, and the haplessness of certain professional sports teams, the transforming power of nutrition should be added to the list of life's sure things. It's time that food received its due. The insiders—the models, trainers, and athletes who get paid to stay in shape—say that diet is 80 percent of the battle. But the masses often view it as a mere footnote to exercise. To illustrate that point, ask yourself the following two questions:

1. How many people do you know who've hired a personal trainer or taken some sort of exercise class taught by a fitness professional?
2. How many people do you know who've employed the services of a registered dietitian?

Although many people have hired personal trainers to help them go from bum to buff, very few have hired a registered dietitian. It should be the other way around. Don't get me wrong. Exercise *is* important. Exercise shapes and builds the muscles needed to bolster your metabolism and help you burn more calories. But exercise can take you only so far. For example, you'd need to run hard for more than 10 miles to burn off the number of calories in a typical fast-food meal. It's far easier to avoid the

Quarter Pounder with Cheese than it is to run 10 miles, don't you think?

Women know this already. That's why most of your girlfriends can name the top 10 best-selling diet books in rapid fire. They probably own them and have read them, too.

It's time for you to give diet the prominence it deserves. The right foods can do more than help you control your weight. They can also help im- prove the benefits you get from exercise. Eat the right foods after a workout and the iron you pumped will result in bigger biceps. Eat the wrong foods—or no food at all—and your biceps will always look like Popeye's arms *before* the spinach.

Once you've digested the information in this book, you'll see that you really *are* what you eat. (And drink, because the average guy's body is 60 to 65 percent water.) By consuming the best foods,

YOUR GENETIC HERITAGE

THE RIGHT DIET HAS ITS LIMITATIONS. Internally, your genetic makeup has hardwired many of your body's defining attributes: the good, the bad, and the ugly. But the bytes (no pun intended) of the program you're running over those circuits constitute your diet. Setting aside what goes on behind closed doors in your home, food and drink are the only things, other than the air you breathe, that enter your body (save a surgical implement, and I hope those insertions are infrequent). Every time you nourish your body, or choose not to, you and you alone are programming it.

Also, if your father and his father both suffered heart attacks before their fortieth birth- days, you may indeed be genetically predisposed to heart disease. Your doctor will certainly note that as he scans your personal information and, one would hope, watch vigilantly for high blood pressure, problematic cholesterol readings, and any of the other telltale signs that might foreshadow a similar fate befalling you.

To be predisposed, however, means to be susceptible to; it does not mean to be doomed by. If your doctor is better than merely competent, rather than looking for red flags he or she will encourage you to lift weights, do cardiovascular exercise, eat foods low in saturated fats, add fish to your diet, and employ other heart-saving strategies *before* something bad hap- pens. By doing so, you're likely to at least undermine or curtail the influence of any dangerous strands of genetic code, and you might be able to avoid them altogether.

On the other hand, if you avoid exercise and eat things that damage your cardiovas- cular system, your checkout time from Hotel Earth could be even earlier than that of your forefathers.

The bottom line is this: Although you can't control everything in your life, given the end- less number of variables involved, you can at least control your part of the equation. It's up to you whether the life you form and then project outward is more like a horror flick or more like an inspiring tale with a happy ending—or at least one with some dignity and redemption as the credits roll.

YOUR 24-HOUR MAKEOVER ■ 5

you can make yourself better than you could have imagined.

Your 24-Hour Makeover

To demonstrate how food can transform your life and how outside institutions conspire against you, let's take a look at a typical day in the life of an average guy's mouth and stomach. I'm not saying that what follows describes your diet to a T. I'm saying that, either partially or fully, this day echoes the experiences of a lot of guys a lot of the time.

What's important is that you learn how interdependent your dietary decisions are and how those decisions accumulate to influence and shape your life. Our journey starts at night, during those last few crucial hours before you hit the sack.

9:00 P.M.

The Coffee Cure

Relaxing in front of the tube or over a crossword puzzle, you slug down a cup of coffee. Normally at 9:00 P.M., a powerful substance called adenosine will signal your brain that it needs rest. Adenosine is what's called a *neuromodulator,* meaning it controls the rate at which nerve cells fire. In this case, adenosine is slowing down the activity of the brain's nerve cells. That makes you feel drowsy.

When you drink a cup of coffee, a cola, or any other caffeinated beverage, the caffeine binds to the receptors in your brain where adenosine would usually settle. But caffeine doesn't suppress nerve cells the way adenosine does. Therefore, because your brain doesn't "see" adenosine in its normal place, it doesn't slow down; on the contrary, things speed up. Instead of dilating, your blood vessels constrict. With your brain's electrical activity now resembling a shooting gallery, sleep is not an option. Instead, your adrenal glands release epinephrine, a.k.a.

adrenaline, which reverses many of the processes that normally precede sleep. Your respiration quickens, your heart pumps faster, your liver releases sugar into your bloodstream, and your muscles tighten.

While you're completing your crossword puzzle, this is all well and good. You *want* to feel alert. The problem is that the effect doesn't wear off on demand. As is the case with any stimulant, everyone's response to a dose of caffeine will fall somewhere along a bell curve. You could be clumped in the middle with most people, or you could fall on the periphery, meaning you'd have either a stronger- or weaker-than-average response to, say, a "grandé" Starbucks coffee.

Eventually, your liver will start breaking down the caffeine, making it less and less potent until, finally, you're no longer responding to it. The average half-life of coffee—meaning the length of time caffeine is active before wearing off—is $3\frac{1}{2}$ hours, but caffeine can stay in some people's systems for 6 hours or more. If you're one of them, and you drink coffee at 9:00 P.M., you may be up half the night or longer.

10:00 P.M.

A Man's Gotta Eat

Now you're hungry. You realize you've been working on your crossword puzzle so long that you forget to eat dinner. So you raid the fridge, make a Dagwood-style sandwich, wash it down with a Heineken, and finish everything off with a bowl of ice cream. That, too, will likely contribute to a restless night. While you sleep, your digestive system should be at least somewhat at rest. If you eat too late, a mess of hormones and enzymes will release into your bloodstream, and your body will think it should be waking up instead of falling asleep.

As if being tired weren't enough, late-night meals may be making you fatter. Conventional wisdom tells us that if you're sleepy, your body has slowed down; and if your body is slow, you're not burning a lot of calories. In truth, scientists aren't positive whether slowed metabolism at night is a big contributor to weight gain. But they are sure of this: Sleep is a crucial time for building muscle, and muscle, you'll learn, is one of the most important factors in burning fat. If you're not sleeping, your body won't release the hormones that build the muscle; and without the muscle, you're more prone to getting fat.

Finally, that Heineken you drank with dinner will hurt you several ways. First, it adds a bunch of calories to your meal. Alcohol contains 7 calories per gram, which means that the average alcoholic drink contains 105 calories. And it won't do your body any favors.

What's more, those calories lack nutritional value. A glass of milk, for example, also contributes calories, but at least it includes some protein, which helps synthesize new protein, which helps build muscle, which helps burn calories, and so on. Beer, in contrast, may taste great going down the hatch, but it contains nothing to help build muscle or otherwise improve your body.

Another downside to beer might explain why guys who drink it have stomachs the size of beach balls. Above and beyond the calories in alcohol, your body metabolizes it in a way that further promotes fat storage. To your body, alcohol is a toxin, so your liver, which neutralizes poisons in the blood, makes processing those calories a higher priority than, say, dealing with the Dagwood sandwich you washed down with it. The calories from the sandwich have to wait in line while the alcohol calories get "detoxed." While in a queue, those protein and carbohydrate calories run a high risk of being turned into triglycerides. Those can be stored in the liver as fat, which is why heavy drinkers often end up with a liver disease called *cirrhosis,* characterized by scar tissue replacing normal tissue in that organ, blocking the flow of blood through it. Each year, around 25,000 people die from that disease.

What's more, even though several drinks might knock you on your butt, alcohol doesn't promote quality sleep. In fact, it inhibits rapid-eye-movement (REM) sleep, when you do most of your dreaming, and lack of REM sleep leads to fatigue. Studies have shown that when people are automatically awakened every time they begin to enter a dream state, they become increasingly edgy over time.

Midnight

You Fall Asleep (Or at Least Try . . .)

So you *finally* figured out "28 across." You get into bed, close your eyes, and then . . . open your eyes. You try your left side; no good. You try your right side; still no good. You glance at the clock. You try your back.

Every cell in your body needs sleep, but you can't give them what they so desperately need. If you've ever had to go without sleep one night, you know exactly what I mean. You probably were irritable the next day, and you probably faded faster than usual as the day wore on, even if your cognitive skills weren't diminished.

Still, most people don't realize how critically important those 7 to 9 hours—the average amount needed by most adults—are. If you don't snooze, you lose, and you lose big.

7:00 A.M.

Alarming Developments

So 7:00 A.M. rolls around, the alarm clock rings, you roll over in bed, and the sheets, as if animated in some B movie, seem to reach out and pull you back. You prop yourself up on one elbow and steady your gaze on the alarm clock, trying to bring the LED readout into focus. Failing that, you surrender to the sheets and bury your head underneath the pillow in disgust.

This failure probably has less to do with your willpower than with how little sleep you got last night. You say you crashed at midnight, so waking at 7:00 A.M. should have been no problem? Well, maybe you hit the sack at 12:00, but you didn't actually doze off until quarter till 1:00, did you? What's more, instead of sleeping straight through till morning, your 9:00 P.M. coffee and 10:00 P.M. beer caused you to wake at least four times during the night.

And that means you missed your first round of slow-wave sleep. Still, a man's got to face the day. You eventually crawl out of bed. You've been fasting all night, and your metabolic mechanisms have slowed way, way down. To jump-start them, you need to get more oxygen moving through your system so that carbohydrate, blood glucose, and other nutrients can reach those cells. The energy-manufacturing centers that lie within those cells, called *mitochondria,* need these inputs to get humming again. They need the raw materials to crank up your metabolic rate.

If you're still having trouble picturing this internal dynamic, think of your body as a coal furnace for a moment. At night, before bed, it's as fired up as a bull rider on ephedrine, right? Then, slowly but surely through the night, things cool way down. When you wake up, some red embers still flicker in the fireplace, but the house is as cold as the North Pole. So you go down, throw some more coal in the furnace, and stoke it. Gradually, you prod the fire back to life, and the house starts warming up again.

Your body works exactly the same way.

Instead of getting up and fueling it properly, though, when you finally rise, feeling disoriented, you reach for the quick fix: another cup of coffee. There's nothing wrong with a cup of coffee in the morning, and I've discussed how it is a short-term pick-me-up, but it's not going to bring back much life to the smoldering embers of your downshifted metabolism. They might flicker for a few passing moments, but the fire will be short-lived. Unless

WAVES OF GAIN

LOSING JUST 3 HOURS OF SLEEP CAN CAUSE A 50 PERCENT REDUCTION IN IMMUNE FUNCTION, making someone who is sleep-deprived for an extended period of time far more disease-prone than someone who is sleeping sufficiently. Here's what happens in each sleep stage.

Sleep Stage	Brain Wave Type	Wave Speed	Bodily Reactions
Full wakefulness	Beta	20 cycles per second	You are awake and alert. Stimulants, such as caffeine, can produce this state.
Feeling sleepy	Alpha	10 cycles per second	The body is in a deeply relaxed state, with reduced input from the central nervous system.
Light sleep	Theta	3.5 to 7 cycles per second	Muscles relax completely, respiration slows, and blood pressure falls.
Deep sleep	Delta	3.5 cycles per second	Body builds and repairs muscles, replaces dead cells, bolsters the immune system, and restores internal systems.

you've got a boss who doesn't mind you taking a nice, long catnap in the middle of the workday—and don't we all work for employers like that?—you're probably going to hit the wall sometime this afternoon.

The most pressing problem you now face has less to do with that one cup of coffee than with the fluids and foods you haven't consumed. Your body doesn't have what it needs to get started—namely, carbohydrates (the energy packaged in bread, fruits, vegetables, oatmeal, and other sources of sugar, starch, and grains) and protein (the single most important nutrient required for building and repairing all the chemical messengers, cells, tissues, organs, and, of course, muscles in your body).

Without carbs, rather than propelling itself into the new day, your body is already backpedaling into catabolism—in other words, it's going to start breaking down its own tissues to get the protein and energy it needs to crank up the machinery that raises your metabolic rate. Though some of this may sound desirable (your body is eating up your fat stores, right?), it's not. Without the carbs, your body never revs up your metabolism to the level you would reach had you actually eaten breakfast. And without protein, you won't have the materials on hand that your body needs to build muscle later on in the day. In short, you must feed your body early in the day to put yourself in a muscle-building mode later.

9:30 A.M.

Doughnuts and Other Do-Nots

By the time you hit the office at 9:30 A.M., you want another cup of coffee—another pick-me-up. And because you don't have time to sit down for a good, healthy breakfast to go with it, you grab some fried fat and flour, also known as a doughnut with sprinkles. What the hell, right? You could use a little jolt of sugar.

The sugar on that doughnut actually enhances the absorption of the caffeine, so that this time it hits your system even faster and with a bigger wallop than that first cup. Plus the sugar itself gives you a righteous kick in the pants.

For the moment, anyway, you feel saved by this sudden surge of energy. That sugar is doing more than just giving you an energy boost, though; it's prompting your metabolic system to flood your bloodstream with insulin, whose marching orders are to transport that sugar into your cells. That may not be a problem for the moment, but come 11:30 or noon, you're in for a rude awakening. More on that later.

In the meantime, the doughnut is having other negative effects on your body, in large part because it's chock-full of partially hydrogenated fats. Now it's time for a little Chemistry 101. (Don't worry; this will be a short, painless lesson.) By adding hydrogen to otherwise benign unsaturated fats, food manufacturers create something called trans fats (a type of partially hydrogenated fat), which help extend the shelf life of baked goods and fried fast foods. Ever get a snack from a vending machine and have the sneaking suspicion that it's been housed there since the Clinton administration? Assuming that's true, you have trans fats to thank for its staying power.

If only trans fats had the same life-extending effect on your body. Instead, these fats introduce a nefarious kind of fatty acid into the bloodstream that raises levels of a type of cholesterol called low-density lipoproteins (LDL), which can elevate your risk of heart disease. In fact, many scientists contend that trans fats do more damage to arteries than saturated fats (the type found in prime rib and bacon).

Making matters worse, the Food and Drug Administration (FDA) has only recently required food manufacturers to list trans fats on food labels. On or before January 1, 2006, food labels must include a new entry for trans fats located directly under the line for saturated fat.

Will that single doughnut you just dunked in your coffee put you six feet under? Of course not—unless you choke to death on it. Will the hundreds, if not thousands, of doughnuts and other packaged baked goods that you've downed since elementary school do you in? Eventually, they just might make a big contribution to what would be an untimely end. As your arteries become lined with plaque, the by-product of years of elevated cholesterol, your body has to push harder and harder to deliver blood to the cells that depend on it for their—and your—survival.

This affects more than your heart. The difficulty you encountered satisfying your partner in bed a couple of nights ago? Your Johnson, like your heart, needs a constant, unimpeded supply of blood to rise to the occasion. You've been experiencing firsthand what happens when it doesn't receive it. Your ego isn't the only thing that's drooping these days.

10:00 A.M.

Crash Landing

The clock hits 10:00—time to attend your first meeting of the day, a session with marketing that promises to be about as much fun as a prostate exam. You reckon you'd better fortify yourself for this one, so you stop by the office kitchen to grab one more cup of coffee before heading to the conference room. Aside from hammering your already-shell-shocked central nervous system with yet another jolt of caffeine, you've now filled your stomach with enough acid to melt steel. You feel like you're on the verge of a heart attack as you take your seat at the conference table.

Like eating doughnuts day after day, drinking rivers of coffee may also be contributing to some longer-term health problems, although the latter isn't nearly as bad as the former. Scientists have studied the possible influence of coffee on blood pressure, heart disease, and numerous cancers, including those of the bladder and the urinary tract, and though fewer than three cups a day seems not to contribute to most of these maladies, the data get more equivocal when consumption rises above three cups daily. Keep in mind that you've already drunk that many, and it's only a few minutes past 10:00 A.M.

At the moment, though, as you sit in this meeting, dehydration poses the more pressing concern. We're not talking about the much-discussed diuretic effect of coffee, either, although if you drink enough java—say five or six cups a day—research shows that the drink can dehydrate you by an amount equal to 2 percent of your body weight. (Studies also show that if you're well hydrated to begin with, one or two cups of coffee will have virtually no dehydrating effect.)

No, you're dehydrated because of what you *haven't* been consuming—namely, water and other fluids. Dehydration is having any number of effects on you at this moment, none of them good. For one, because you're already dehydrated, you have a lower total blood volume, so the concentration of caffeine in your bloodstream from all that coffee you've drunk is higher than normal. In fact, the effect of any drug will become heightened in this state.

As the meeting heats up at 10:20, the absence of water is also affecting your mental acuity. Your brain is 80 percent water by weight. So if you're dehydrated, your brain doesn't have the available fluid needed for the transmission of electrical impulses from one neuron to the next. Nutrients aren't being transported to cells in the brain as effectively as they should be, nor are toxins being removed with maximum efficiency. Again, none of this is conducive to thinking quickly on your feet.

At 10:25, as you try to sit patiently listening to the presentations, all that caffeine you've consumed, accentuated by dehydration, is now coming back to haunt you. Remember how caffeine causes your blood vessels to become constricted, rather than dilated? That elevates your blood pressure and makes it harder for blood to flow unimpeded in and out of muscle tissue. You can feel your muscles clamping down on your frame. You're ready to be physically active, only you've got to sit still and listen to so-and-so ramble on about such-and-such. By 10:35, you're sitting there impatiently, grinding your teeth as you do a slow burn.

Makes a great impression on your colleagues, doesn't it?

11:15 A.M.

Calories Stat!

When the meeting ends, mercifully, at 11:15, you're not just fatigued, suddenly you're really hungry. Really, really hungry. In fact, you're feeling the kind of intense hunger pangs that make you fantasize about a 94-ounce sirloin steak, when you should be focused on finishing up the report that your employer wants on his desk by noon, or else.

These cravings point to one obvious problem: Your blood sugar (a.k.a. the amount of glucose in your blood) is too low.

How did this happen? Ideally, your blood sugar follows a rolling pattern throughout the day, rising steadily and falling steadily like hills and valleys. Keeping it this way is heavily dependent on the carbs you eat. Carbs are directly responsible for providing glucose to your body. When you consume carbs along with the other two macronutrients, proteins and fat, the carbs are absorbed by the digestive system and then time-released into the body as glucose. The glucose is then either used immediately for energy or transported, via insulin (a hormone we'll talk about in detail later), out of the bloodstream and into your muscles, where you'll be able to use it as fuel later.

But that carb-heavy doughnut you ate earlier has ensured the opposite: This morning, your blood sugar was peaking like a mountain. Now, it's dropped like the Grand Canyon. When you consume carbohydrates almost exclusively, they hit your bloodstream very fast. At first, this causes a major spike in blood sugar (the mountain)—thus, the sudden

surge of energy. But all that extra glucose is like a red flag to your body's insulin, which takes the extra sugar as a sign to work harder. The body over compensates, sending extra insulin to shuttle the glucose out of your blood. Pretty soon, your blood sugar has fallen precipitously, and you're left feeling fatigued and hungry. This is even more pronounced when your carbohydrates come in the form of sugars, which are simple carbs, rather than complex carbs.

To know why that's bad, you need to understand the glycemic index (GI), a scale that ranks a food according to how quickly it is converted to glucose in the bloodstream. Foods on the index are rated numerically, with pure glucose pegged at 100. The higher the number assigned to a food, the more quickly it converts to glucose. (For more on the glycemic index, see "Making Sense of the Glycemic Index," opposite.) So although taking in carbs in general causes the insulin levels to rise in blood, high-GI carbs are the real culprits when it comes to skyrocketing blood sugar.

Back to your hunger pangs. You don't have time to go to the local steak house—it's always crowded, anyway—but maybe, just maybe, you can make it to McDonald's and back and still have time to finish that report. So you hop into your car, speed down the street, and screech to a halt in front of a giant clown's head, into which you bark your order for a Quarter Pounder with Cheese, french fries, and a Coke. Your eyes are way bigger than your stomach now, so you decide to supersize it for good measure.

At this point, you feel your body heading for a crash landing. With few carbs in your system after a crummy night's sleep, you're heavily fatigued. Unless you poured some milk into one of those coffees, you've had virtually no protein since last night. That means you've ingested no L-tryptophan, the amino acid your body needs to synthesize the neurotransmitter serotonin. Along with playing important roles in facilitating blood clotting, stimulating a strong heartbeat, and helping you get good shut-eye, serotonin works to

MAKING SENSE OF THE GLYCEMIC INDEX

Foods ranked low on the glycemic index (GI) cause smaller fluctuations in blood glucose than more rapidly digested sugars would. Unfortunately, you have to either educate yourself about GI numbers or keep a reference guide handy because there's really little intuitive about these rankings. Oranges, bananas, apples, dried apricots, and pears are all low-GI carbs; watermelons and raisins are high. Go figure.

In general, foods high in fiber, protein, and fat digest more slowly and are often lower on the glycemic scale. To simplify matters, I've created a brief list (below) to use when trying to gauge the GI value of a given food. Because this is a new area of research, all foods have not been evaluated for their place on the glycemic index; that will take many years. Choose predominantly from the low and moderate GI columns, and sparingly from the high GI column. For more information, go to www.glycemicindex.com.

High Glycemic

BEVERAGES

Carbonated soft drinks	68
Gatorade	91

BREAD AND GRAIN PRODUCTS

Oatmeal	61
Grape Nuts cereal	67
Bread, whole wheat	69
Bread, white	70
Cream of wheat	70
Bagels	72
Bran flakes	74
Graham crackers	74
Puffed wheat	74
Cheerios	75
Breakfast bars	76
Total cereal	77
Corn flakes	84

FRUITS

Raisins	64
Watermelon	72
Honey	73

VEGETABLES

Potatoes, microwaved	82
Potatoes, baked	85

Moderate Glycemic

BREAD AND GRAIN PRODUCTS

Pasta	41
Pumpernickel bread	41
All Bran cereal	42
Muesli, toasted	43
Bulgur	47
Buckwheat (kasha)	54
Popcorn	55
Rice, brown	55
Special K	55
Rice, white	56
Mini-Wheats	58
Bran muffins	60

FRUITS

Apple juice, unsweetened	41
Oranges	43
Bananas, overripe	52
Orange juice	57

LEGUMES

Lentil soup	44
Baked beans	48

VEGETABLES

Peas	48
Sweet potatoes	54
Corn	55

Low Glycemic

BREAD AND GRAIN PRODUCTS

Barley	25
Power bar	30–35

DAIRY PRODUCTS

Whole milk	27
Skim milk	32
Yogurt, low-fat, fruit	33
Chocolate milk	34

FRUITS

Cherries	23
Grapefruit	25
Plums	25
Bananas, underripe	30
Peaches	30–40
Apricots, dried	31
Strawberries	32
Apples	36
Pears	36

LEGUMES

Soybeans	18
Kidney beans	27
Lentils	29
Black beans	30
Green beans	30
Soy milk	30
Lima beans	32
Split peas, yellow	32
Chickpeas	33
Pinto beans	39

VEGETABLES

All LGI (except those with starch)

combat feelings of depression. (Most drugs prescribed for depression treat it by elevating serotonin.)

What your body and mind want, then, is a quick high, some kind of big boost. One of your body's evolutionary adaptive mechanisms is now kicking in. Because your body thinks it's starving, its primal urge is to acquire fast and dense energy. And that means sugar and fat.

Before you've even made it back to the office, you've started swigging from that pony keg of a soda McDonald's handed you, which is flushing your body with a major influx of sugar. To put the size of this sweet onslaught into some perspective, a 12-ounce soft drink contains 10 teaspoons of sugar, equal to 160 calories. The soda you're drinking likely contains closer to 30 teaspoons of sugar and 480 calories. Those aren't misprints.

The supersize french fries you're washing down with that Coke as you pull back into the parking lot are even worse. They contain 610 calories, 260 from fat. Of their 29 fat grams, 5 are saturated, which is more than you'd find in a McDonald's hamburger. For good measure, you'll also be consuming 390 milligrams of sodium. On to your main course, sir, the Quarter Pounder with Cheese: 530 calories, 30 grams of fat, 13 grams of saturated fat, 95 milligrams of cholesterol, and 1,240 milligrams of sodium.

Totaled, that's 59 grams of fat, 30 teaspoons of sugar, 1,630 milligrams of sodium, and a grand total of 1,690 calories. Your server might as well have handed you an open-backed hospital gown along with your grease-stained paper bags.

2:00 P.M.

Fading Fast

The food from McDonald's sits in your stomach like a boulder and moves through your intestines about as fast as a circa 1987 computer. The rest of your afternoon isn't much more exciting. Just when you reach the home stretch at 4:30, you head off to the

---

Sugar Addiction

If sugar habitually plays a central role in your diet, you may be addicted to it. Sugar actually passes through the same neurotransmitter pathways that opiates do, so when you eat sweets repeatedly for a long period of time, the brain produces chemicals that identify this desirable sensation. This also triggers dopamine, which interacts with memory, which in turn tells your brain that it wants to have sweets again and again.

Studies with rats as subjects have shown that sugar addictions are real, complete with withdrawal symptoms when the sugar is taken away. (I know, they're rats, not humans. But rats have a remarkably similar brain physiology to ours. And recent human studies are showing similar brain activity as in the addicted rats. Extrapolating to humans, these studies suggest that the more frequently you eat sugar, the more likely you'll be to crave it. Couple these finely honed internal cues with external visual stimulation—for example, the sight of that lovely sugar doughnut sitting there when you first ordered your coffee, calling out your name—and resistance is futile, as they say.

---

restroom, hoping a trip there will help placate a digestive system in open revolt after having been bombarded all day with caffeine and sugar, with some saturated fat thrown in for good measure.

While there, you take a moment to look in the mirror and assess what your diet has done to your physical self. Sure, those bags under your bloodshot eyes can be chalked up to a bad night's sleep, but the love handles spilling over your belt attest to just how long you've been eating poorly, careening from one energy crash to another. You may be the most talented employee at your company, but you haven't received a promotion or even a glamorous gig for years now, and no wonder—you hardly look like someone anyone would entrust with major responsibilities. If you can't take care of yourself, why would anyone expect you to take care of something else?

5:30 P.M.

Death Takes a Jog

You've planned a workout for 5:30, so you slouch off to the gym. You hope to revive your tired body and salvage something from your otherwise thoroughly unproductive day. The fact that you've had a crummy one isn't a good reason to skip the gym, so kudos for at least getting in there and doing something.

(Momentary digression: In a worst-case scenario, if you're so totally out of it that you might accidentally drop a dumbbell on somebody's head, including your own, go for a walk instead. Live to fight another day, as they say. Don't kill yourself.)

As you step onto the treadmill, it's likely that you'll be able to train safely but not effectively. Your body looks for carbs right off the bat. It finds them readily available, a result of all the sugar you've had, so you shouldn't have too much trouble getting through a 20-minute jog of moderate intensity. Just as all of your systems are kicking in, with some fat beginning to be used as energy, you step off the machine. Still, so far, so good. Maybe you'll be able to salvage this workout after all.

On to the weights. At first, this goes okay, too. As you lift, you're still using carbs primarily, only now you're tapping into the carbs stored as glycogen in the very muscles you're training. You're relying on short, powerful bursts of energy, so when you're, say, bench-pressing, it doesn't matter how much glycogen you've got in your legs. You need the fuel where you're working it.

So if you did a heavy upper-body workout two days ago, and you're doing upper body again today, you haven't eaten well enough between then and now to replenish those localized glycogen stores. Just at the time you're gearing up for some closing supersets to finish off a particular muscle group, you feel the needle on your gas tank hitting empty. Even though you kicked ass for the first half of your workout, you're going to leave the gym feeling unfulfilled and unsatisfied.

6:30 P.M.

The Home Stretch

By this point, your diet has subjected your body to so many highs and lows that you're just really, really fatigued. You're still dehydrated, perhaps having lost up to 2 percent of your body weight in fluid.

Now you have an even bigger problem. The 28 grams you got from that Quarter Pounder with Cheese is all the protein you've consumed today, other than a few rogue grams cowering in your donut. Heading into the workout, sufficient protein would have allowed your body to limit the muscle breakdown during exercise. After the workout, you need even more protein and amino acids to rebuild the muscle tissue you just spent 45 minutes abusing. Too bad your body is running on empty—what it needs, you don't have.

Having thrown in the towel at the end of your disappointing workout, you head home, wanting nothing more than rest. Here, what you're not doing—eating and drinking—is sabotaging you further.

Consuming carbohydrates and protein here would boost your insulin levels and kick-start the muscle-building machinery inside your body. Given adequate nourishment within 2 hours post-workout, your body would refuel and repair your muscles. Because you're *not* topping off your tank when it's most receptive to being filled up, you're already undermining your next workout.

What You Should Have Done

The aforementioned 24 hours weren't a banner day by most people's standards. Yet no prescription or illegal drugs were taken. Only a moderate amount of alcohol and slightly more caffeine were consumed. And there was really no overeating, save that insane number of calories you ended up consuming from that McDonald's Value Meal when you supersized it. Nonetheless, perhaps you have a better understanding of how not doing certain things at critical times—and doing other things when you don't really need to—can turn your day into a train wreck.

Here's what you should do instead to stay on track.

Upon awakening. Drink several cups of fluid to replace what you lost overnight. When it comes to health, H_2O is liquid gold. It promotes the release of stored fat and maximizes metabolic efficiency. You didn't even get up to go to the bathroom, so

---

H_2Overnight

One thing you should consume before going to bed—but probably don't—is water. Think about it: If your growth hormone release is spiking at night, that will also be a peak time for protein metabolism in your cells. As I've already discussed, all of these proteins and enzymes are very active at night. And the whole machinery of protein manufacturing, muscle repair, and immune system bolstering occurs most effectively and efficiently during that time when it occurs within well-hydrated cells. Conversely, when a cell is not well hydrated—or *volumized* with water—that entire process becomes degraded. That's why you want to have sufficient water inside you 24/7, including while you sleep.

---

how much water could you have lost overnight? Quite a bit, actually. While sleeping, you still experience what are called "insensible" water losses from respiration, metabolic processes, and perspiration. You're still breathing and sweating and metabolizing things for those 8 hours or so that you're out cold, and water loss is one by-product. Water is the ideal replacement fluid here, but a glass of orange juice or even iced tea would also do the trick.

Another reason that guys often don't drink anything in the morning is that they're not thirsty. What they might not realize is that the human body's thirst mechanism is notoriously late. You can easily become fairly dehydrated before getting really thirsty.

Before leaving for work. Not too long afterward—maybe after you've taken your morning shower—eat breakfast. And I'm not talking about a bowl of Lucky Charms or a box of Hostess chocolate doughnuts, but real food that combines protein, carbohydrates, and healthful fats. One example is a bowl of whole-grain cereal and milk, maybe topped with a handful of raisins and a scoop of ground flaxseed that has already been cold-milled and vacuum-packed, like you'll find in a package at just about any supermarket or natural foods or supplement store.

Another great option is a smoothie, combining whey protein powder; milk; orange juice; some combination of frozen strawberries, papaya, and bananas; and a tablespoon of flaxseed oil. (If you hadn't guessed, I am a huge fan of flaxseed and flaxseed oil, a great source of essential fatty acids.) A couple of eggs and a slice of whole-grain toast would work, as would oatmeal topped with some sliced fresh fruit. Even a turkey sandwich would do the trick.

The options are nearly unlimited. Those just mentioned are all healthy and nutrition-packed, but the most important thing is to eat *something* before starting your day. A slice of cold pizza or leftover pasta and meatballs from the night before are way better than nothing.

Before the morning meeting. Before you lock horns with the marketing folks, have a healthy midmorning snack instead of another cup of coffee. Even if you eat a good breakfast, you'll still want to supply your body with another round of nourishment. If you feel like you're not hungry yet after eating a good

breakfast, have a midmorning snack anyway. Just as you should drink before you get thirsty, so should you eat before getting hungry—a state that would likely make you overeat. By the time you feel really hungry, your blood-sugar levels have already plummeted.

So what should you eat in this twilight zone of sorts between breakfast and lunch? Below, you'll find a number of great options.

CALORIES IN, CALORIES OUT

FOR YEARS, MANY, IF NOT MOST, nutritionists have dogmatically held that weight management is the difference between the calories you consume and the calories you expend. If the majority of calories are on the consumption side, you'll gain weight; if the balance is on the negative side, you'll lose it. Cut and dried. This approach to weight management has been a mantra for years.

The new research suggests that this "calories in, calories out" theory is simplistic to the point of being plain wrong. What the researchers are finding is that if your calorie deficit at any given time is up to 400 calories (300 for women), your metabolic rate—the rate at which you burn calories—doesn't decrease. Once the deficit exceeds 400 calories, though, your metabolism begins to downshift. What that means, theoretically, is the guy whose deficit is 400 calories could be losing more weight than a guy whose deficit is 500.

The same holds true in reverse. If you're an active person, you can probably safely eat 400 more calories each day than your body really needs. You won't gain weight, because your metabolism will burn up the excess.

What's more, calories in, calories out proponents have been equally dogmatic in insisting that the relevant time frame for the calorie variables to be entered into this equation is daily. In other words, if you consumed 3,000 calories and burned 2,750 on Tuesday, it wouldn't matter if all 3,000 were consumed at two sittings or dispersed across six or seven meals. At the end of the day, for the purposes of weight management, what matters is the sum total.

Or so they said. This, too, appears to be off the mark, according to this new research. It suggests that energy balance matters moment to moment, not just day to day. This suggests that eating smaller meals more frequently is the way to go for weight gain and weight loss. It's also much better for preventing that daily energy roller coaster ride I've talked about, and the positive effect of that smoothing-out process on mood and other things will be discussed in subsequent chapters. This new view on calories is consistent with observations of many of us in the trenches, but for the first time, hard data support that view.

■ A piece of fruit or nuts with some cheese

■ Natural peanut butter on whole-grain bread

■ Low-fat cream cheese on a bagel

■ Protein powder mixed with orange juice

■ Low-fat cottage cheese with fruit

One of the primary goals here is to avoid a big spike in your blood sugar, which is why I recommend protein-rich foods mixed with low-GI carbs, especially fruits. Along with being sweet and tasty (thanks to fructose, the main sugar in fruits), fruits are packed with all sorts of things that boost your health. Citrus fruits are an awesome source of vitamin C, but other good sources are kiwifruit, papaya, and strawberries. Also found abundantly in fruits are beta-carotene, folate, vitamin E, potassium, and magnesium, all of which have been tar-geted for research concerning their possible roles in preventing and fighting disease. Fruits also contain loads of fiber and something called phytochemicals, which are receiving much attention for their possible roles in reducing the incidence of chronic diseases like cancer, heart disease, and diabetes.

The average fruit serving is only 60 calories with virtually no fat. The water content of fruits—greater than 70 percent—allows them to be crisp and juicy.

Manufactured foods, such as energy bars, aren't a good call for your midmorning snack (see "The Bar Crawl," below). Still, they're better than eating nothing or hitting the vending machine. The one exception is for guys who're extremely active. If you're one of them, you may need a convenient way to re-

THE BAR CRAWL

ENERGY-BAR LABELS CAN BE INCOMPLETE AT BEST, and misleading at worst. A bar advertised as "high-protein" and/or "low-carb" may not include certain ingredients in its list of carbohydrates because the ingredients are considered "non-impact," meaning they don't have the same carbohydrate-like effects on your blood sugar levels as ordinary sugars or starches. A term such as "net carbs" subtracts dietary fiber and sugar alcohol from the total, with the intent to indicate that the "effective carbohydrate" amount (starch and sugar) is lower than the "total carbohydrate" listed. These include glycerine and sugar alcohols. In the latter category are polydextrose, maltitol, xylitol, and others.

Glycerine, a.k.a. glycerol, is the chemical backbone of fatty acids. Manufacturers use it to trap water within the bar, keeping it soft. Glycerine provides calories similar to those of sugar and can be converted into sugar in the body. Apparently, because glycerine does not start out as sugar, the low-carb food industry does not count it as an "effective carb." Sugar alcohols are used in place of sucrose, fructose, or glucose as sweetening agents. Contrary to the impression left by the advertising, they *do* raise blood sugar levels but less so than ordinary sugar or starches.

Currently, no carbohydrate claims are approved by the U.S. Food and Drug Administration. These creative approaches to labeling are certain to undergo federal scrutiny that will lead to consistent standards based on science.

plenish the nutrients you're expending. Otherwise, avoid them.

If you simply don't have access to whole foods, a better alternative is a meal-replacement product (MRP) mixed into a shake along with some fruit. The first MRP—MET-Rx, a proprietary blend of protein, vitamins, and carbs—came along in 1991. MRPs went on to become the most popular and successful type of protein-based supplement ever developed. (They became hip thanks in part to director Quentin Tarantino, whose movie *Jackie Brown* showed Bridget Fonda offering to blend one for a thoroughly wasted Robert DeNiro; it was one of the all-time great examples of cinematic product placement.)

Saying that these powders replace meals is a bit of a stretch, given that they provide you with only 250 to 300 calories per individual serving. But with 40 or so grams of (usually) high-quality protein and 25 grams of carbs, they can play a really important role when you're eating smaller meals more frequently than before. And they are convenient. No complicated shopping, cooking, or storage problems—simply open a packet, pour it into a blender, add water, mix, and drink. Even easier are the RTDs (ready to drinks) that require only a flip of the top of a can. That makes them great post-workout, which I'll discuss later.

At lunch. You have any number of good choices. Just make it light. Maybe you get the deli to send over a turkey or chicken sandwich on whole-wheat bread, with lettuce, tomato, and mustard. Add an orange and maybe a few peanuts, and you have a lunch that helps you stay focused and energized for the rest of the afternoon.

If you decide to go out, think United Nations: Chinese, Thai, Japanese, Indian, Vietnamese—anything ethnic is probably a good call for you here. The advantage with these cuisines is that you're likely to get more vegetables than you would with conventional American fare, where vegetables often amount to a slice of tomato plopped on top of a greasy cheeseburger. Some of the dishes in ethnic restaurants are high in fat, but it's rarely the dangerous, saturated kind. The fat is usually from peanut oil or some other unsaturated source.

Another safe choice is Subway, where a 6-inch submarine sandwich may have fewer than 6 grams of fat. Stack the sandwich with all the vegetables that look good to you—olives, onions, lettuce, tomato, and green peppers. Choose a fat-free condiment like honey-mustard sauce instead of mayonnaise.

If you end up shouting your order into a video screen or clown's head, think damage control. You can still go to Wendy's, but opt for something like a chicken breast without the fried coating, watch the dressing when you get a salad, and replace soda with milk or plain water. The chili is another safe choice.

In the late afternoon. Having cruised through your afternoon tasks feeling energetic and alert, you should then have another nutritious snack come 4:00 P.M. The value of a small meal at this time of day is twofold. First, eating now will keep your body's gas tank full and your metabolism humming. Second, it primes your body for the workout to come, with carbohydrates for energy and protein to give your muscles a jump-start on the building process.

This is the third meal you've eaten since you finished breakfast and left for work. You can't do this successfully without some preparation. That means bringing food from home. You may feel self-conscious at first, but I know plenty of successful businessmen who don't leave home without snacks in Tupperware in the backpack or briefcase. Other guys I know keep MRP packets in their desk drawers, along with packages of cashews or beef jerky. (Not exotic enough for you? How about *tuna* jerky, available at www.tunatuna.com.)

Now you can even refrigerate items at your desk using small plug-in refrigerators, available at stores like Restoration Hardware, that are big enough to house a lunch bag. If you're a sales rep glued to the phone 9-to-5 but a serious athlete on the side, these things were made for you. Take advantage of them.

If you're planning to lift weights, your pre-workout meal should include both protein and carbohydrates. About 50 to 75 calories of your 200- to 300-calorie snack should come from protein and the rest from carbohydrates. That translates to 13 to 20 grams of protein and 30 to 50 grams of carbohydrates. Below you'll find some snacks that meet these requirements.

- ½ cup Shredded Wheat, ½ cup blueberries, 1 cup nonfat milk
- Low-fat or fat-free vanilla or coffee yogurt, ½ cup strawberries
- 1 cup fat-free milk, ½ cup orange juice, 1 cup strawberries, 15 grams milk/egg protein powder
- 1 ounce turkey jerky, 1 medium apple, 1 cup nonfat milk
- Turkey sandwich with 4 ounces turkey
- Myoplex Lite energy bar, 1 cup nonfat milk
- Medium apple, 2 tablespoons peanut butter, 1 cup nonfat milk

Soy Wonder

Edamame (also known as soybeans) are a great healthy snack for late afternoon or early evening. Think of them as a super-utility infielder: They're convenient, they taste great, and they're filled with phytochemicals, fiber, and protein. Buy them frozen in a bag, and all you have to do is boil them in water for 5 minutes. When the timer dings, throw the edamame in a colander, spray with cool water, and sprinkle with a bit of salt. Once you start popping the shells open, you'll feel like you're eating popcorn or peanuts, except that these are much better for you. Or you can pack them to go.

In the early evening. Driving to the gym after work is a great time to pour more water into your system. Again, preparation is key here. If the weather's mild (neither boiling hot nor freezing cold), you can keep a bottle of water in your car. Otherwise, you can lug a bottle with you (hey, the weight adds a little more exercise to your day), refilling it whenever you see a drinking fountain. During the workout itself, you should drink 4 to 6 ounces of water every 15 to 20 minutes. Muscle contractions involve complex interactions among minerals, and dehydration can throw them out of whack. That leads to muscle cramps. Afterward, you want to take in at least 2 to 3 more cups of fluid for every pound of body weight lost.

Within an hour of training, you want to take in 250 to 700 calories, depending on how big you are and how hard you train. The ideal mix is 40 to 120 grams of carbohydrates and 20 to 40 grams of protein. Consumed post-workout, protein not only assists with muscle building and repair but also makes a dramatic difference in how efficiently the body can store carbs in muscle as glycogen, according to a study published in the *Journal of Applied Physiology*.

Time is muscle after your workout; if you blow the window of opportunity to feed your muscles, you make smaller gains (if you gain at all). That's why you don't have to worry about sitting down to a meal here. A post-workout shake will work just as well, if not better. (Liquid nutrition will move out of your stomach and into your bloodstream faster than solid food.)

Because of the time factor, you may not be able to sit down for a balanced meal of whole foods within this window. In fact, the idea of taking in a bunch of food might seem unappealing. If that's the case, mix a smoothie instead. If a blender isn't available, drink something premade, such as Countdown.

Once again, I'll preach preparedness. Blend a shake beforehand and take it with you. Companies now make throwaway plastic containers with lids, and you can fill three or four of them out of one blender mix. Throw them into the freezer, and then if you have a workout that day, pull one out and take it with you. By the time you finish your late-afternoon or early-evening workout, it'll be melted and ready to drink.

At dinner. Two hours or so after your post-workout meal or shake, enjoy a nice, healthy dinner. But not a *big* dinner. One of your goals is to consume the majority of your calories earlier in the day. As you approach day's end, taper down on volume. Dinner should be a relatively small meal and certainly not your biggest of the day. (In a perfect world, that distinction would go to breakfast.) If you're treating dinner as your major meal of the day, you're probably setting yourself up for the disrupted sleep cycle I've already discussed.

For this meal, I strongly recommend fish; in fact, I'd love for you to have it five times a week. Why would I suggest that you eat the same thing so frequently? Well, for one, fish offers some incredibly important nutritional benefits. It's a great source of omega-3 fatty acids, which are important for heart health and also for maintaining healthy fat metabolism, which in turn is important for decreasing abdominal fat. What's more, fish plays an important role in muscle growth and repair, as well as helping to keep your hormones working at peak efficiency. There's also some intriguing research suggesting that the protein in fish has specific benefits for people on weight-loss diets. When it comes to fish, it's all good, as far as I'm concerned.

There's an incredible range of fresh fish and seafood available now to consumers, appealing to every imaginable palate. Great fatty fish like salmon, black cod, and halibut are available nationwide. If you live in the landlocked Midwest, you're no longer limited to eating fresh fish only in summer, when it can be rescued from Lake Erie. It's flown in from all over. And just about anywhere you

---

Vegetable Heaven

Vegetables are easy to dress up without adding buckets of calorie-dense sauces. A light ranch dressing works; better still is mustard. Experiment with the different types of mustards in your market until you find one that works best with your vegetables of choice. Our two favorites are Westbrae mustard, with tamari and wasabe; and lemon-dill mustard.

Even the most boring vegetables can be made more palatable with just a bit of prep. Take cauliflower, which you probably haven't even considered eating since your grandmother stopped force-feeding it to you. Try this: Steam it lightly; add some plain yogurt and bread crumbs; and then stick it under the broiler.

---

live, you can find frozen shrimp in your supermarket freezer.

A post-workout dinner is also a great time to load up on antioxidant-rich vegetables, such as dark, leafy greens. Root vegetables are also good choices, although for most people that means a white potato. But you can do a lot better than that. Try a yam or sweet potato instead. Preparing the latter can be as simple as popping it into a microwave oven. Winter squash can also be nuked quickly and conveniently: Poke it with a fork four or five times, stick it into the microwave, and cook as you would a baked potato. Then cut it in half, scoop out the seeds, and put a teaspoon of honey or maple syrup on top if it's not already sweet enough for you.

Broccoli is easier still. Cut it up and either eat it raw or add it to a salad. If you don't have the time or the inclination to cut vegetables, buy them precut in the supermarket. And remember that frozen vegetables are generally as good as fresh. Sometimes they're better, because they were probably frozen before they sat around for days, as they would in a store and your crisper.

Dinner is also a great time to experiment with different kinds of grains, rather than having just white rice or a few slices of white bread. U.S. consumers tend to eat wheat and rice, and maybe some corn during the summer, but that's only a fraction of the good stuff available. You can try wild rice (which actually consists of seeds rather than grains). Or make buckwheat, which has a nutty flavor and prepares easily. Untasted by many Americans, kasha is absolutely delicious.

Triticale also tastes great and has an above-average amount of protein for a grain. The same goes for quinoa. Multigrain breads are always a good call, too.

This is also a great time to include something tomato-derived in your diet. You could drink vegetable juice or have tomato sauce atop pasta. Your goal is to ingest a phytonutrient called lycopene, which studies have shown reduces the incidence of prostate cancer. Tomatoes themselves are great vegetables, and I would never discourage you from eating them. But as lycopene dispensers, they're ac-

WHO CAN YOU TRUST?

Not the health care industry

PHYSICIANS AND HOSPITALS DO WONDERFUL, MIRACULOUS THINGS every hour of every day, and a lot of people walking the streets today can thank them for not only their health but also their life.

I will also say this: Particularly in the age of managed care, with all the time constraints hamstringing physicians, the U.S. health care industry as a whole fails, sometimes miserably, at educating patients on the profound influence food has on health, good and bad. It doesn't warn you sufficiently about the damage bad eating can do, nor does it enlighten you as to how food can help prevent disease—and help cure it once it occurs. Put it this way: The time to counsel you about the cancer-fighting properties of fruits and vegetables isn't after you've been diagnosed with a malignant tumor—it's 5 or 10 years earlier, before the illness strikes. Too often, the opposite is true.

A classic example is the guy who goes in for coronary-bypass surgery and is then served eggs and bacon when he wakes up in a hospital bed the next day. That's why "health insurance" is really a misnomer. It's sickness insurance. Health insurance is eating right, exercising, and getting your rest.

In a word, prevention.

In contrast, physicians need to bill you for something. Taking something out of your body or prescribing a medication is usually right up their alley. Spending 10 minutes to explain how dietary changes you make now will spare you a heart attack in 20 years? Well . . . come back in 20 years, basically. Our entire health care system is set up to treat sick people.

Before I became a nutritionist, I actually had my heart set on attending medical school. A vegetarian then, I was very interested in health and fitness—I had been a modern dancer—

tually not as effective as more-concentrated forms, such as juices, sauces, and soups.

Moving Forward

Now that you've caught a glimpse of how profoundly nutrition influences your day and how much better that day could be if you ate differently, you're ready to move on to a series of chapters that will show you how to target specific areas of your life. If there's a take-home lesson from this chapter, it's that you need to take responsibility for your diet and your life, rather than treating it as something outside your control.

If you don't, you're going to continue making or settling for bad choices because those are the ones that are marketed and sold to you—you're not going to see commercials for whole grains or most of the rest of what I recommend here. (Maybe the ketchup and pasta sauces, but that's only because they're packed with sugar as well as prostate-protecting lycopene.) Nutrition as practiced and preached in the broader culture is the antithesis of healthy eating. And if you don't look out for yourself, nobody will.

and I sort of viewed nutrition as a hobby. I went to Hiram College, a small liberal arts school in rural Ohio, for my undergraduate studies, and I actually grew my own vegetables on some fallow farmland nearby.

So after taking the exam to get into medical school, I went to speak with the dean of admissions at Case Western Reserve University School of Medicine, who was the father of a good friend of mine. He knew me well, and I had a long talk, and he said, "Susan, I'd love to have you in our medical school, but the fact is that you would go through 4 years and not learn anything about what you're interested in: health. We teach people how to treat disease. Go talk to the department of nutrition instead."

His advice changed my life. He told me the truth: that the medical establishment is set up to treat disease. When they survey first-year medical students and ask them to rank their priorities, nutrition is usually among the top five. When they're surveyed upon graduation, it's not even on the list because it hasn't been emphasized. Even to this day, it's unusual for medical students to get more than a few hours of nutrition education throughout their entire degree. And if they do, it's because they're in an unusual place or they made a personal effort. When there's so little taught about nutrition, why should they think it's important?

No wonder health care costs are so out of control in the United States that it poses a significant threat to the nation's economy. The whole system is backward. We certainly need sickness insurance, but we also need real health insurance—and you're the person who provides it to yourself through the decisions you make, particularly when it comes to exercise and nutrition.

CHAPTER TWO

Food, Mood, and Brain Power

SIMPLE STRATEGIES THAT WILL HAVE YOU FEELING GOOD AND THINKING CLEARLY

Men refer to it a number of ways—"energy," "mood," "stamina," "temper," "consistency," "focus." But all these words circle around one issue: Everyone wants to feel good throughout the day. No one wants to peak and crash multiple times. For many of us, the ability to focus on demand isn't just nice; it's essential to our livelihoods.

Feeling good is apparently a tricky thing. Americans spend billions of dollars annually on pills like Prozac, Paxil, and other calm-inducing remedies. We exercise. Some of us get regular massages or even take breaks to meditate or pray. When all else fails, we watch sports or go shopping. And yet, for all that firepower, who among us doesn't feel crappy from time to time? We get annoyed or anxious during the day. Our attention begins to wane when we need to be sharp. Have you ever taken a nap at your desk against your better judgment? If so, you know what I'm talking about.

Here's a suggestion: The next time you're feeling down or sluggish, look at what you've been eating. It could be that your diet is hurting your mood or sapping your ability to concentrate. We all have ideal chemical balances in our bodies, and food plays a big role in controlling them. Eat junk and you'll probably feel like junk. Eat the right stuff, and you'll sail through the day alert and enthusiastic.

And I'm not just talking about the easy days. Food can get you through the tough times, too. For example, research published in the journal *Appetite* suggests that stress-prone individuals who find themselves in stressful situations can increase personal control by eating meals rich in carbohydrates and light on protein.

Scientists are making more and more discoveries like these—ones you can harness for optimum brainpower. Although some of this nutritional science is still murky, much of it is very well studied, providing some hard-and-fast rules you can use to boost your mood, energy levels, and mental performance.

The Food-Mood Connection

You didn't buy this book for a course on human biology, and I know you're eager to get to the good stuff.

But there are things you should know first to help you understand how and why foods affect your mood.

Scientists like to compare the human body to a car. Your stomach is the gas tank, and food is the gas. But that metaphor is incomplete—your body is far more complicated than a car, and the range of fuels you need (carbs, protein, etc.) is far more varied and complicated than gasoline. I prefer a different metaphor: the body as a chemistry set. If you are like a lot of guys, you owned one of these while growing up. Remember how carefully you needed to measure various powders and liquids to get the right result? Your body is the same way: Every time you eat, you're setting off a chemical reaction. To get the desired chemical effects, you need to eat the right way.

The best example of this is the tricky relationship in your body between serotonin, blood sugar, and tryptophan.

Picture your brain: a collection of circuits, structures, and chemicals that control everything in your body, including your mood. Among these parts is the system responsible for creating the neurotransmitter serotonin, a highly talked-about chemical in your brain and one of the most significant factors in mood and the development of mood disorders.

How you eat—specifically, the ratio of protein to carbohydrate in what you eat—plays a big role in your serotonin levels. At the heart of this tricky chemical process is tryptophan, a dietary amino acid found predominantly in proteins. When there is more tryptophan in your brain, you create more serotonin and feel good. When tryptophan levels are low, your serotonin levels will stay low and you'll feel crappy.

This begs the question: How do you get more tryptophan? The answer is not as easy as scientists once thought. For years, scientists pointed their patients toward meals heavy in protein, arguing that if something is high in tryptophan and you ingest it, you process more tryptophan. But research now shows that getting tryptophan into your brain is harder than just feasting on meats. Unless the protein you're eating is very heavy in tryptophan and light on other amino acids (think dairy products and turkey), consuming a high-protein diet doesn't crank up your body's serotonin production at all. In fact, because tryptophan competes with so many other amino acids for the same brain receptors, a high-protein diet can essentially shut out tryptophan.

On the other hand, when you consume a meal lower in protein and higher in carbs, the tryptophan available has a greater chance of attaching itself to these receptors and raising serotonin levels. What's more, elevated levels of blood sugar—caused by carbs—leads to a rise in insulin. And insulin, as luck would have it, is a natural springboard for tryptophan, launching it into the brain. At the same time, insulin locks out other amino acids.

Conversely, when you eat a meal high in protein and low in carbs, blood glucose levels fall and insulin levels drop, leading to a rise in another hormone, cortisol. Cortisol's job is to break down proteins. Broken-down proteins mean more amino acids in the blood. More amino acids mean less room for tryptophan to get the brain's attention. Serotonin levels fall, and so does mood.

So what does this mean for the food-mood connection? That contrary to popular belief, it's not a high-protein meal that elevates your mood, it's a meal a little higher in carbohydrates and a little lower in protein. That's why all those people on high-protein diets are so crabby. The best combination of foods to elevate mood is a small amount of dairy and turkey (both high in tryptophan) combined with one to three servings of low- to moderate-GI carbohydrate sources like whole grains, rice, starchy vegetables, beans, fruits, and milk (see the discussion of dietary sugar on page 24 for more on low- versus high-glycemic carbs). This meal will cause a moderate rise in insulin levels that will promote the cascade of events leading to elevated levels of serotonin in your brain: It will put a smile on your face.

There are plenty of other ways in which food affects happiness, but two others that are extremely important to remember are:

1. How good fats lead to happiness
2. How dietary sugar can sour your mood

Just the (Good) Fats, Ma'am

No, I'm not about to tell you that the key to happiness is getting fat. Actually, the key to happiness is fish. If you're like me, you grew up hearing that fish is "brain food." In a way, it's true—fish can help your brain work at peak levels. But it might be more accurate to call fish "mood food."

A while back, scientists began noticing that the countries with the highest fish consumption per capita also had the lowest levels of depression. Curious, researchers at the National Institutes of Health conducted a series of studies, using piglets as subjects, to observe the effect of fish consumption on mood.

The results? Let's just say there are few creatures perkier than a fish-fed pig. Based on this study and others that followed, scientists determined that fish oils containing omega-3 fatty acids—polyunsaturated fats, which the body can't produce and therefore must get from your diet—produce effects similar to those of Prozac and other antidepressant drugs. Other experiments, including ones that study the omega-3s found in flaxseed oil and hempseed oil, have only strengthened the theory.

How do the fats work? Like those drugs, they raise levels of serotonin in the frontal cortex of your brain, where depression and impulsivity are modulated. The pig-studying scientists found that their livestock's serotonin *doubled* after 18 days of eating fish.

The human research on omega-3 fatty acids has been pretty convincing, too. Here's one of my favorites: A researcher at Sheffield University in England studied 70 depressed patients—none of whom had responded to antidepressant drugs—who were admin-istered omega-3 fatty acids for 12 weeks. Sixty-nine percent of them showed marked improvement, compared with only 25 percent of those who received placebos.

Overall, fat is the most underrated of the three macronutrients when it comes to determining whether you're headstrong or a head case. (Fats constitute as much as 60 percent of your brain's structure, and fatty compounds make up the inner and outer membranes of cells.) These compounds play a key role in how well brain cells interact and communicate with each other, as well as how smoothly and efficiently chemical messages move from one neuron to another. (This may explain why the omega-3s found in fish oil seem to improve cognitive skills as well as mood.)

Moreover, nerve fibers that travel from the brain to the spinal cord and then snake through the rest of the body, enervating it, are wrapped in a white-colored fatty substance called myelin. If you stopped eating fat, you'd stop nourishing and replenishing these and other fat stores. Maybe that would make your body look fabulous, but it would also impair your brain's ability to perform key functions.

Don't Let Sugar Get You Down

On the other end of the spectrum from good fats is sugar. Perhaps no single food affects stress hormones, mood regulators, and appetite signalers as negatively as excess sugar. Learn to control sugar, and you'll go a long way toward controlling how you feel throughout the day.

To understand why sugar is more problematic than other forms of carbs, consider where it falls in the carbohydrate spectrum. Whole, unrefined carbohydrate sources such as whole grains, beans, nuts, seeds, vegetables, and fruits are packed with nutrients, dietary fiber, and phytochemicals—most with a long list of impressive health benefits to their name. They are also credited with helping you maintain steady blood-sugar levels. When your blood sugar stays consistent, your mood is elevated, and you don't feel terribly hungry. In other words, you feel good.

But sugar is at the very top of the GI scale, and foods containing large amounts of sugar are right up there with it. These foods often offer virtually no nutrients along with the calories. What's worse, they often cause a rapid rise in blood glucose, which then causes a fast peak in insulin levels. Brain tryptophan rises and you feel energized for a bit, but the insulin moves blood sugar out of your system so fast that blood-sugar levels quickly fall, followed by lowering insulin levels. This roller coaster ride often leaves people feeling drained, in a foul mood, and, usually, uncomfortably hungry.

When you factor in all the other ways sugar can hurt you—excessive sugar consumption has been associated with tooth decay, obesity, cardiovascular disease, and blood-sugar metabolism disorders such as diabetes and hypoglycemia—you have to wonder why our bodies crave it so much. The answer lies in our evolutionary past. For thousands of years, *Homo sapiens* evolved to seek out sweet-tasting foods instinctively as a means of survival. Depending on the time of year and where they lived, people would scavenge for foods that were dense in energy and loaded with nutrients. Fresh ripe fruits on trees and vines, honey from combs, and sweet saps from trees and plants—all of which contain natural sugars—became the prehistoric chow of choice.

HOW MUCH SUGAR IS IN YOUR FOOD?

THE U.S. DEPARTMENT OF AGRICULTURE RECOMMENDS THAT THE AVERAGE PERSON EAT no more than 6 to 10 teaspoons of added sugar per day, depending on your calorie level. That's equal to 24 to 40 grams or 96 to 160 calories per day. Even without knowing the amount of added sugar specifically, you can use this guideline for setting your total sugar goal, and then determine how much total sugar you are eating by reading food labels and counting sugar grams.

Food	Teaspoons of Added Sugar	Food	Teaspoons of Added Sugar
1 serving coleslaw dressing	2½	½ cup gelatin dessert	5
1 package hot cocoa mix	2½	5 ounces pudding	5
1 serving vegetarian baked beans	2½	2.1-ounce Snickers bar	5½
1 serving canned creamy tomato soup	3	1 cup fruit yogurt	7½
6 ounces powdered drink mix	4	12-ounce soft drink	10
1 Power Bar	4	12-ounce fruit drink or fruit-ade	10
½ cup sugar-sweetened cereal	4	10-ounce McDonald's Vanilla Shake	12
1 serving flavored milk	4½	20-ounce Strawberry Passion Awareness Fruitopia	17½
1.2-ounce chocolate bar	4½	32-ounce Dairy Queen Mr. Misty Slush	28
1 cupcake	5		

Sources: Center for Science in the Public Interest, August 1999; *Eating Well*, Fall 2002; University of Connecticut Cooperative Extension System College of Agriculture and Natural Resources.

As an adaptive mechanism, sweet tastes triggered the brain to produce the chemical messengers I've already discussed that affect our brain function, memory, and behavior patterns. When a person eats food, the brain produces *opioids,* neurotransmitters that identify desirable sensations—in this case, sweet taste. Simultaneously, it triggers the production of dopamine, the neurotransmitter that helps you remember what brought on that desirable sensation, leaving you with the urge to feel it again in the future.

So the human sweet tooth became a kind of self-perpetuating phenomenon. Through memory and visual cues, neurotransmitters drove people to seek out sweet tastes, and once such food was eaten, the same neurotransmitters encouraged them to keep eating it. During times of famine, this calorie-hoarding strategy could be a lifesaver, and for hunter-gatherer types, it was a sensible strategy even when they weren't in such dire dietary straits. It made sense to feast, even binge on huge amounts of sweet foods while they were in season in order to store up energy for the leaner times caused by natural seasonal variations in food availability.

That makes much less sense today. Food-processing technology has outrun natural selection. Most people in the United States, at least, have access to as much food as they want 24/7, eliminating the need for this adaptive survival instinct. But your body isn't very time-savvy, and the desire for sugar is hardwired. For example, babies tested at birth still prefer a sweet taste to alternatives—and probably will for a long time to come.

To keep both your mood and your energy as bal-

THE SUGAR JONES

RECENT STUDIES SUGGEST THAT SUGAR MAY BE ABLE TO TURN SOME FOLKS INTO JUNKIES pretty easily. Researchers in the psychology department at Princeton University gave rats a steady diet of sugar and then observed the physical symptoms and changes in brain chemistry induced by chemical dependence. Subsequently, once sugar was eliminated from their diets, the rodents had the shakes: chattering teeth, forepaw and head tremors, and increased anxiety during maze tests.

Researchers now believe that the similarities are because the same chemical reactions that get us hooked to drugs take place when we have too much sugar.

Some guys are more prone than others to addictions, and that certainly applies to sugar as well. To find out whether you are addicted, ask yourself the following questions:

1. Do you crave sugar daily? If you feel satisfied after eating something sweet when nothing else will do the trick, or you get a headache or become crabby or shaky when you can't get your sugar fix, you might be addicted.

2. How many teaspoons of added sugar do you eat in a day? If it's more than 8 to 10 teaspoons, and you're not using sugar specifically for training (see chapter 4), you may have a sugar problem. (One teaspoon equals 4 grams of simple carbohydrate.)

3. Can you cut your daily sugar consumption in half without feeling sluggish, jittery, and shaky? If not, you might be addicted.

anced as possible—and to keep from getting fat—it's imperative that you limit your sugar intake. It's not easy: Today's processed food supply is bursting with sugar-laden foods. From hamburger buns to pasta sauces, most processed foods include added sugar. Food manufacturers certainly realize how addictive sugar can be, so they add it to just about everything, knowing that sweeter products often outsell less-sweet alternatives.

So how do you satisfy your body's desire for the sweet stuff without throwing your mood out of whack? My suggestion: Lay off the heavily processed foods and, when you have a craving, return to the sugars that our ancestors ate. Replace those candy bars and cakes with fruits and natural sugars, like honey. Over time, your mood—not to mention the rest of your body—will benefit from it.

Additional Mood Elevators and Depressors

Beyond fats and sugars, there are infinite smaller ways that food can affect your mood. Here is the best advice I can give on which foods to eat—and which to avoid—in order to boost your spirits.

Eat more vitamin D–rich foods. Vitamin D boosts serotonin levels, which is one reason that most people feel happier and calmer on sunny days. Your skin absorbs ultraviolet energy from the sun, which your body converts into vitamin D. Fifteen minutes outdoors without sunscreen will give your body all the vitamin D it needs. Yet recent research shows that many people, particularly those who live in northern areas, don't get enough sunlight to meet their vitamin D needs. Vitamin D is also found in a handful of foods, including oily fish (such as salmon and mackerel), and vitamin D–fortified foods (such as fortified milk). To boost your mood, eat fish five times a week and drink 3 to 4 cups of low-fat milk daily.

Consume caffeine with intelligence. Anyone who has traveled in the morning with a grump who

---

> ### Mood Depressors
>
> The following foods can make you feel depressed:
>
> Alcohol
>
> Caffeine (large doses)
>
> Fatty meats
>
> Fatty snack foods
>
> Fried foods
>
> Refined sugars and starches

---

comes to life only after his first cup of Joe can probably vouch for caffeine's ability to boost mood as well as stimulate the central nervous system. Caffeine increases levels of the neurotransmitter dopamine in the same way that amphetamines do, by activating the brain's so-called pleasure center. Caffeine's effect doesn't compare with that of heroin, but the same mechanism is at work. The dopamine also explains why caffeine might be physically addictive.

If you keep in mind that caffeine is a drug, you can learn how to use it to your advantage without falling victim to addiction or negative side effects. If you wake up on the wrong side of the bed, it's perfectly fine to drink a cup of coffee or green tea. If it's time for your evening workout and you need a kick in the pants to get yourself to the gym, have a fat-free latte, which will provide both caffeine and whey protein (also good for mood). As long as you keep your caffeine consumption sporadic and deliberate, you can use it to your advantage. As soon as you begin to turn to it several times a day, however, caffeine will begin to get the best of you.

Eat a little chocolate. Europeans living in the 17th century viewed this dark, sweet substance as a healing food—which may explain why men and women alike seem to reach for it when they're hitting rock bottom. Given that connection, chocolate's possible effect on mood is hard to ignore. Might it actually contain some magical chemical components capable of chasing the blues away?

To test that theory, researchers at the University of Pennsylvania divided students into three groups. One group was given milk chocolate; the second, white chocolate, which contains no cocoa, just cocoa butter and flavoring; and the third, a pill containing

LABEL FABLES

READING THE LABELS ATTACHED TO PROCESSED FOODS doesn't always give you an accurate idea of their sugar content. Even though new food label laws require that "total sugars" be listed in the nutrient contents, added sugars aren't broken out and listed separately. There's no way to tell how much sugar nature placed in the food and how much of it entered the mix during processing.

Combine all of these phenomena, and there's a high probability that you're consuming more sugar than you think. Check that—way more. Foods that aren't traditionally thought of as containing sugar (including breads, pasta sauces, and canned soups) now often contain it. The number-one source of sugar in the American diet is soft drinks, but you wouldn't know it from looking at their labels. What you'll see instead is something called "high-fructose corn syrup." To get a handle on the various names sugar masquerades as on labels, see below.

Fructose. A simple sugar refined from fruit; the sweetest sugar of all.

Sugar (sucrose). Refined crystallized sap of the sugar cane or sugar beet; a combination of fructose and dextrose; less sweet than fructose.

Dextrose (glucose). A simpler sugar than fructose or sucrose.

Maltose. A simple sugar made from starch; less sweet than fructose or sucrose.

Maltodextrin. A manufactured sugar made from dextrose and maltose.

Lactose. A simple sugar from milk; less sweet than fructose, sucrose, or maltose.

Brown sugar. A refined sugar coated with molasses. The minerals calcium, iron, and potassium are present in this sugar from the molasses.

Raw sugar. A less refined sugar that still has some natural molasses coating.

Molasses. The syrup separated from sugar crystals during the refining process. Blackstrap molasses is a good source of calcium, iron, and potassium.

Honey. A concentrated solution of fructose and dextrose (80 percent) and some sucrose.

Maple syrup. A concentrated sap from sugar maple trees; predominantly fructose.

Corn syrup. A manufactured syrup from cornstarch, containing varying proportions of dextrose and maltose.

High-fructose corn syrup. A highly concentrated engineered syrup of predominantly fructose.

White grape juice. A highly purified fructose solution; virtually no other nutrients are present.

Adapted with permission from Kleiner, S., and Greenwood-Robinson, M. *High-Performance Nutrition.* John Wiley and Sons, Inc., New York, NY, 1996.

many of the stimulants commonly found in chocolate. The pill didn't do the trick, but both the white and milk chocolates satisfied the students. This suggests that it's not some secret ingredient in chocolate that boosts mood and imparts a sense of satisfaction, but something else—perhaps the calories, the saturated fat, or the sensory experience of the taste, smoothness, or aroma.

Chocolate does contain mood-enhancing chemicals—anandamides, cannabinoid-like fatty acids, and phenylethylamine among them—but it probably doesn't contain enough of them to affect your brain chemistry much. If you love chocolate and it makes you feel good, plan for it in your menu so you can indulge guiltlessly.

Note: Indulging your taste for chocolate does not mean overindulging. Remember, most chocolate is heavily caloric and has refined sugars in it, which will bring you down if you have too much. Choose small, controllable portions, such as individually foil-wrapped pieces or mini frozen treats.

Eat carbs late in the day. You want to get some carbohydrates into your system at day's end. As explained above, carbs will lift your spirits by prompting secretion of serotonin, which will help you sleep soundly as well. Research has shown that high-carb meals are more effective than high-protein meals for elevating mood, and that protein-only meals make people more sluggish.

Keep in mind that carbs also trigger an insulin response—a good thing in small doses but counterproductive and possibly fattening if you have too much. You'll generally want to mix in some protein with your carbs to keep insulin levels steady. Especially if you're going to be working late or studying into the midnight hour or beyond, make sure any carbs you eat are balanced by protein, or you'll fade fast.

Shoot for the whole. Use your head when it comes to putting things into your stomach. When you shop, read food labels—including the fine print. Make sure that you know what you're buying and

---

Mood Elevators

The following foods can elevate your mood:

Air-popped popcorn	Lean pork
Bananas	Low-fat and fat-free milk and milk products
Beans	
Blueberries	
Broccoli	Mangoes
Caffeine-containing beverages (1 to 2 servings)	Nuts
	Olives and olive oil
	Oranges
Chocolate (small amounts)	Romaine and other dark green lettuces
Edamame and other soy products	Spinach
	Strawberries
Fish and seafood (salmon, black cod, halibut, flounder, crab, shrimp)	Sunflower seeds
	Turkey
	Water
Flaxseed	Whole grains

---

what you're eating. If sugar is potentially as addictive as a narcotic, don't fall prey to its pushers.

Instead, make whole, unprocessed foods the foundation of your menu. Gradually eliminate sugar-sweetened soft drinks and fruit-ades to avoid any possibility of withdrawal symptoms and rebound sugar fixes. This will remove the majority of added sugar in your diet but still leave room for some splurging here and there to keep your natural instincts satisfied.

Get into good food habits. How you eat influences how you look, a subject that will be explored repeatedly in this book. For many guys, appearance has a huge effect on self-image, and self-esteem affects mood. If you eat badly, you won't look good, you won't feel in control, and you'll feel depressed as a result. The act of eating can also affect mood. If you eat a huge portion of high-fat food for lunch, you'll feel sluggish afterward, not to mention guilty for having pigged out.

You can reverse this vicious cycle, turning small failures into small successes and enjoying the cumulative effect in reverse. Even a simple task like drinking enough water is something you can control and build upon. Make daily and weekly goals; when you experience success repeatedly, you'll feel emboldened and better suited to handle other challenges.

Mental Acuity and Memory

Call me a science geek, but I love attending conferences and symposiums on nutrition. There is almost always a brilliant speaker or two delivering news of a successful breakthrough or a revolutionary discovery. Perhaps my most memorable experience at a conference, however, was a lecture I can't remember at all.

I was in Denver for a meeting of the American Dietetic Association and was primed to hear a lecture by one of the most distinguished scientists in my field. Obviously, I wasn't alone: I entered the auditorium to find that several hundreds of other experts had shown up for the event. I settled into a chair as the lights dimmed and the speaker began. About 15 minutes in, I remember thinking, "I'm feeling a bit drowsy."

Twenty minutes later, I awoke to the sound of applause and the light trickle of drool on my chin. I had come nearly 1,000 miles to hear this man I admired, and I had slept through the entire thing!

Thinking back, I realize I couldn't stay awake or focused that day for several reasons. I wasn't used to the thin mountain air; I was in a hot, dark room; I had been traveling. But perhaps most important, I hadn't been eating right. As a nutrition expert, I have an entire arsenal of dietary tricks to keep me alert and awake. But my travel schedule sometimes keeps me from eating the way I know I should (sound familiar?), and I forgot to plan ahead. I re-member celebrating with friends late the night before: a little too much food, a few glasses of champagne, and a disturbed night's sleep. The next morning, I found myself without a water bottle, and I was left dehydrated that day—not ideal if you want to keep an active mind.

This section will help you avoid gaffes like my Denver nap. Aside from adequate rest—you should be getting about 8 hours nightly—and exercise, food is your best weapon for fighting mental fatigue and memory lapses. When you sit down to feed your body, you're feeding your brain as well. If you don't consider the special needs of your head as well as the rest of your body, you can't operate at peak levels.

Just like any organ in your body, your brain requires fuel to run. Brain cells are a little pickier about their fuel source than most of the rest of the cells in your body—brain cells use only glucose for fuel, so the easiest and fastest way to boost brainpower is by eating carbohydrates. But over the long haul, you'll want to feed it the way I've been telling you so far: plenty of low- to moderate-GI carbs, with some protein and a little fat to help slow digestion and absorption. That way, your blood sugar will stay well balanced and your brain will get its energy in a constant, time-released manner. You'll stay alert and active.

There are tricks to getting your brain to work better. For instance, be careful of how much food you eat. A big meal is a signal to pool your body's resources around your stomach, rather than around your brain. High-fat meals will do the same, and fatigue will set in fast. Instead, you should be eating small, nutrient-packed, well-balanced meals throughout the day. Ideally, each of those five or six meals should contain 300 to 600 calories, emphasizing lean protein and unrefined, complex carbs over simple sugars and saturated fat.

Here are a few more big tips to get your brain in gear.

1. Eat lots of fish rich in omega-3 fatty acids.
2. Make water a constant presence in your daily life.
3. Remember breakfast, and you'll remember other stuff.

We've already talked about the fish (the benefits are pretty similar), so let's look at how water and scheduling, as well as other changes, can help your brain manipulate information like a Cray supercomputer instead of a creaky file cabinet.

Make water a mainstay. I'm going to bring up water a lot in this book. In my years of research, I've learned many inarguable facts, and your body's dependence on water to do just about everything is one of them. You probably know that your body is two-thirds water, but did you know that if your water weight drops just a little bit, it has far-reaching effects on the body? Water fills virtually every space in cells and between them. Without water, all the small biochemical reactions that run your body would shut down. You wouldn't be able to create energy. Even if you could, your joints wouldn't have any lubrication to move. And forget about reproduction or waste removal: Without enough water, it would be impossible.

Your mind is no exception to the rule. In one study from India, scientists tested the mental abilities of subjects after heat-induced dehydration. As they became more dehydrated, the subjects' ability to solve math problems decreased, as did their short-term memory and eye-hand coordination. As it turns out, the level of dehydration among the people studied—about a 2 percent drop in body weight due to fluid loss—is the state most of us are in daily. The next time you are in the office, look around at your co-workers. Are many of them drinking water? Chances are, they aren't performing much better than those guys in the India study.

How do you know if you need more water? This may surprise you, but thirst isn't the best indicator of adequate hydration. By the time you are thirsty, you are already dehydrated. The thirst mechanism doesn't kick in until you've lost 1 to 2 percent of your body weight in fluid. If you're exercising or if you're older, you have an even steeper disadvantage because age and exercise may decrease your ability to judge how much water you need.

The most dependable gauge is the color of your urine, and a self-check is simple. Monitor your urine every 2 to 4 hours. If you're adequately hydrated, it should be pale yellow or almost clear. If you're dehydrated, it'll be dark yellow and have a strong odor. Other indicators of possible dehydration include dark circles under the eyes, dry mouth, dry eyes, burning stomach, headache, calf cramping after an intense workout, and extreme fatigue.

As a rule, consume at least 9 to 11 eight-ounce cups of fluid each day, and make at least 5 of those cups water. If you drink more than 2 or 3 cups of caffeinated beverages each day, replace each cup above the third one with $1/2$ to 1 cup of a noncaffeinated beverage. Because alcohol is also naturally dehydrating, replace each alcoholic beverage with $1/2$ to 1 cup of a nonalcoholic, noncaffeinated beverage.

Get your breakfast. For both body and mind, the most important meal of the day is breakfast. Although the brain has been working all night, when you awaken your fuel stores are low. Your brain function will diminish quickly without fuel. Numerous studies have shown that children perform markedly better on tests when they've eaten breakfast. So refueling ASAP is the goal.

Breakfast should include unrefined complex carbs like those found in oatmeal, which help stabilize blood glucose levels and provide a steady energy supply. Adding some protein and healthy fat helps support the stabilization of blood glucose levels and helps with endorphin release to improve your mood. Pour some milk and a tablespoon of ground flaxseed on that oatmeal, or sprinkle on some almonds and heat up a few turkey sausage links.

Limit alcohol. We don't expect you to be a teetotaler, but you're going to have to control alcohol, rather than vice versa, to implement most of the strategies in this book. As for its effects on cognition and memory, just recall the last time you got hammered at a club and ended up dancing with a chair into the wee hours. What's that, you don't remember? 'Nuff said. Hold yourself to no more than two drinks a day. One alcoholic serving equals 5 ounces of wine, 1 ounce of liquor, or 12 ounces of beer.

Use caffeine only for emergencies. Because caffeine blocks adenosine reception, making you feel more alert for a short period of time, it likely has some positive—albeit transitory—effect on mental performance. You've probably experienced it firsthand in a business meeting, where, after a few sips of Joe, you're a little faster on the draw when it comes to idea generation.

Be careful, though. Caffeine is hiding in numerous foods and beverages—even some aspirin products contain it—and consumption can add up quickly. Too much caffeine can actually impair performance by overstimulating your central nervous system, reducing your ability to focus on the task or competition at hand. How much is too much depends on you. Pay attention to how you feel after you consume caffeine. If you feel jittery and nervous rather than alert and ready to tackle the world, it's probably time to cut back.

Physical Energy

The most basic rule of having enough energy is to eat. A smart man knows how many calories he needs and makes sure he puts enough into his body. Without enough calories, you run out of gas—plain and simple. You won't be able to think fast, work out very hard, grow muscle, or deal with the emotional turmoil in life.

Energy is surprisingly like mood: Just eating enough calories isn't the whole answer. If it were, you could sit down in front of the tube at midnight, eat all of your 2,400 calories out of a Häagen-Dazs carton, and be done with it. Instead, for maximum

---

Energy Busters

The following foods can make you feel like a giant slug:

Alcohol	Fried foods
Cake	Fatty meats
Candy	Fatty snack foods
Cookies	Refined sugars and
Doughnuts	starches

---

impact, your calories need to come in at the right times and in the right combinations. Regarding the form those calories should take, below are some basic guidelines for consuming the three macronutrients—carbohydrates, protein, and fats—to maximize your energy.

CARBS. Carbohydrates are your body's primary energy source. They're the easiest of the macronutrients for your body to burn and, gram for gram, the most efficient source of energy. I'd suggest eating carbs to the tune of 2 to 3 grams per pound of body weight per day. (To calculate your needs, use the menus at the end of the chapter.) This should be enough to fuel your daily activities, as well as your workouts, muscle repair, and the muscle growth that follows.

When choosing carbs, the choice is simple: The unrefined complex carbs found in whole foods like fruits, vegetables, and whole grains are far superior to refined carbs, which appear most obviously in crackers and cookies but can also lurk in places you wouldn't expect. If you doubt me, check the label of certain ready-to-eat boxed cereals. First, look at the sugar content of whole-grain Shredded Wheat: It's zero. Now look at the sugar content of just about any other cereal. It starts at about 9 grams per serving and goes up from there. That's all added sugar; none of it is there naturally. Shredded Wheat has 6 grams of protein and 6 grams of fiber in one serving. There are a "whopping" 1 to 2 grams of protein and 0 to 2 grams of fiber in most other cereals. All the good stuff has been stripped from the grain. The differences are pretty obvious.

Also, just as sugar has a huge impact on mood, it exerts a greater effect on your energy levels than anything else you put into your body during a given day. Why? When you consume lots of sugar, your blood-sugar levels spike dramatically as your body attempts to accommodate the influx. This produces a lightning-bolt energy rush.

Alas, it's short-lived because your body over-compensates. It wants to take all of that glucose in your bloodstream and shuttle it into the cells, so it secretes a heavy flow of insulin. Suddenly, your blood-sugar levels drop just as dramatically as they rose. Eat sugar throughout the day, and the highs and lows are strung together roller-coaster style. Along with making you hungry again and slowing down your brain, these drops make you chronically tired.

PROTEIN. Protein on its own isn't terribly good for boosting energy, but eaten with carbs it can do wonders. First off, it helps transport glucose, which carries fuel from the blood into muscle cells. It also manufactures all of the enzymes and hormones needed for energy metabolism. If you eat a lot of carbs without protein, your body can't access as much energy as it would if you combine them.

And in the same way that protein helps regulate the release of energy to the brain, it helps

UNCOMMON GROUNDS

BELOW YOU'LL FIND THE CAFFEINE CONTENT OF VARIOUS PRODUCTS, rounded to the nearest 5 milligrams.

Product	Caffeine (mg)	Product	Caffeine (mg)
Coffee, grandé (16 ounces), Starbucks	550	Caffe Latte or Cappuccino, grandé (16 ounces), Starbucks	70
Coffee, tall (12 ounces), Starbucks	375	Caffe Mocha, grandé (16 ounces), Starbucks	70
Coffee, short (8 ounces), Starbucks	250	Anacin (2)	65
NoDoz, Maximum Strength (1), or Vivarin (1)	200	Cola (20 ounces)	60*
7-Eleven Big Gulp cola (64 ounces)	190	Tea, leaf or bag (8 ounces)	50
Excedrin (2)	130	Cola (12 ounces)	35*
Coffee (8 ounces), Maxwell House	110	Espresso (1 ounce), Starbucks	35
Caffe Americano, grandé (16 ounces), Starbucks	105	Chocolate, dark, bittersweet, or semisweet (1 ounce)	20*
NoDoz, Regular Strength (1)	100	Coffee, decaf, short (8 ounces) or tall (12 ounces), Starbucks	10
Coffee, instant (8 ounces)	95	Cocoa or hot chocolate (8 ounces)	5*

*Estimate

Sources: National Coffee Association; National Soft Drink Association; Tea Council of the USA; Starbucks Coffee Company, package labels; Center for Science in the Public Interest.

Caffeine's Wake-Up Call

Despite the growing popularity of herbs purported to boost mental acuity, their combined consumption is merely a drop compared with the torrent of caffeine Americans consume, usually in the form of coffee or soda. Used in moderation, caffeine is a safe stimulant, and although it doesn't enhance memory or learning per se, it can boost concentration and fight fatigue. Some experts speculate that caffeine speeds reaction time and helps with routine processing skills, such as arithmetic and proofreading, but that it hinders the performance of more-complicated intellectual tasks.

Although most people can comfortably handle more, as little as 200 milligrams of caffeine can prompt nervousness and anxiety in some people. A typical cup of coffee contains 100 to 150 milligrams of caffeine, but two grandé (16-ounce) cups of Starbucks coffee, for example, contain 1,100—enough to leave even a veteran coffee drinker pretty wired. Usually that sort of buzz is no big deal, but stimulating your central nervous system to the point of distraction can be counterproductive before an exam or an oral presentation.

regulate your body's use of energy. When protein mixes with carbohydrates in your stomach and intestines, you can't digest or metabolize the carbs as quickly. Thus, you can't absorb the carbohydrates as quickly into your bloodstream, which helps balance blood-sugar levels and energy throughout the day.

Ideally, you'll consume between 0.8 and 1 gram of protein per pound of body weight per day. That's about double what Uncle Sam recommends, but if you learn anything from this book, it's that his nutritional advice probably doesn't meet the needs of active people since the 1950s. For an idea of how much 0.8 to 1 gram per pound of body weight comes to in real food, see "The All-Day-Energy Meal Plan" on page 40.

FATS. We mentioned earlier that certain fats can help enhance your mood, which helps boost your energy. Your body also needs fat to produce certain hormones, including testosterone. More testosterone equals more energy and perceived strength. Fat should constitute about 25 percent of your total calories. That comes to about five servings of fat a day. Feast on salmon, nuts, seeds, and other foods that contain significant amounts of essential fatty acids.

Additional Energy Boosters and Plungers

In addition to eating a healthful balance of carbohydrates, protein, and fats, follow these tips for optimal energy and alertness.

Trade soda for water. By the time you're finished with this book, you'll never forget that water influences virtually every aspect of your health and well-being. If you're not drinking enough H_2O, you'll run out of gas soon enough. Trust us. This is especially true when you're replacing cola: It contains boatloads of sugar that may give you a temporary energy spike due to increased insulin in your blood, but in the end it will wear you out.

Cut back on caffeine. Just as caffeine can affect your mood, too much of it can affect your energy. In the short term, you'll *feel* like you have more juice, but it's an illusory, fleeting sensation caused by increased neuron firing in your brain, owing to the adenosine receptors being tricked by the similar chemical structures of caffeine. Sure, it'll cause adrenaline to be injected into your system, and yes, your heart will start to beat faster. But as I've already indicated, the feeling won't last. Caffeine doesn't

Energy Boosters

The following foods can help boost your energy:

Apples	Mushrooms
Asparagus	Nuts
Baked beans	Oranges
Beans	Peanut-butter-and-
Corn	jelly sandwiches
Corn bread	Pears
Dried apricots	Popcorn
Edamame	Soy nuts
Grapefruit	Sweet potatoes/yams
Lean meat	Water
Low-fat cheese	Yogurt
Milk (white or	
chocolate)	

body. One German study showed that subjects who drank the equivalent of 6 cups of coffee (equal to 642 milligrams of caffeine) in a day became dehydrated. But recent studies have shown that moderate coffee drinkers (those who drink 1 to 3 cups of coffee daily, consuming 114 to 253 grams of caffeine) didn't face dehydration.

Stress

Despite how well you are eating, stress can wreak havoc on every aspect of mental well-being, including mood, memory, and energy. During periods of high stress, you may feel as if the gears upstairs need a squirt of WD-40, even if you're eating well and are sleeping enough. Stressors don't have to be extreme to take their toll. They can be as subtle and insidious as environmental toxins, which take their toll on brain function over time through inflammation, free-radical damage, and general wear and tear in the spaces between neurons, where brain cell communication occurs. You don't have to spend your days mining coal for this to happen, either. It's a reality of the increasingly urbanized world in which many of us live.

solve any of your energy problems in the way that, say, a helping of complex carbs would.

But it's not just that caffeine's effects fade fast. The real problem is the longer-term effects that caffeine has on energy when it's constantly used as a substitute for eating well and resting enough. Once the caffeine-induced adrenaline surge wanes, the fatigue that it masked will reassert itself with a vengeance. The typical response is to consume even more caffeine to recapture that feeling you just lost. Next thing you know, you're in a vicious cycle that can leave you jumpy, irritable, unfocused, and unproductive. And because caffeine is physically addictive, stopping cold turkey will make you feel like someone just unplugged your body.

You probably think I'm also worried about the dehydrating effects of caffeine, which many people accept as gospel. I'm not. It is true that caffeine can speed up the mechanisms that flush water from your

If you're feeling stressed out, you may be drinking too much caffeine, eating too much sugar and refined foods, and not eating enough fruits and vegetables. To calm down, increase your consumption of whey protein and dairy, consume more carbs during the day to stimulate serotonin release, stick with carbs that have a low to moderate GI, avoid caffeine, and increase your consumption of antioxidants (like blueberries, strawberries, spinach, B vitamins, nuts, and nut butters).

No matter the cause of your stress, certain herbal-based dietary supplements on the market might help you improve your mood, cognition, and memory. The margin of improvement could be small. If you think about it, though, in this day and age, where guys with 4.2 GPAs get turned away from good universities, or you compete with 10 other qualified candidates for one promotion, the smallest of margins can be the difference between success and failure. (If you're even possibly at risk of some sort of clinical disorder, or the stress you're experiencing is making you dysfunctional, see a health professional.)

Another useful way to look at some of these supplements is as a defense of sorts. If you know ahead of time that you're going to be really, really stressed out for a couple of months and that impending stress is unavoidable, some of these supplements may be worth trying.

As you read through the summaries of each, you'll notice that many of the recommendations are speculative and conditional. To some extent, that's the nature of the beast when you're dealing with

herbs exerting an effect on something as complicated and quixotic as the human brain and central nervous system. A lot of variables are at play under any circumstance, and it's understandably difficult for researchers to tease out the precise effect that an herb or an herb-based pill is having on someone's cognitive skills or mood.

Because researchers want to show some sort of measurable change over time, many study individuals who already have some sort of pathology, such as Alzheimer's or Parkinson's disease. Those results then have to be extrapolated to subjects who are neither old nor infirm, and for whom no—or minimal—clinical data exist. Those extrapolations, therefore, should be taken with a grain of salt.

Another reason that research surrounding these

WHO CAN YOU TRUST?

The media? Not necessarily...

MUCH OF WHAT YOU HEAR ON THE NEWS IS USEFUL, but a lot of it is crapola, and it's sometimes hard to tell the difference. The emergence of the Internet as a primary information source for many guys has only made matters worse—there's enough junk on the Web to fill the Hoover Dam.

The most commonly heard complaint among consumers is that much of what they read, see, and hear about nutrition seems contradictory. Part of that is a result of the evolution of scientific meetings, where many of the studies that will end up in mainstream media outlets are first presented by researchers. Once upon a time, such meetings were closed to the media. When the results of a study were first presented in the form of an abstract, participants would thoroughly discuss its contents and debate its merits, seeking to punch holes in arguments wherever possible. At the next meeting, another study or couple of studies undertaken on the same or similar subjects would surface—until eventually, a decade or so of research would accumulate on one subject. The conference would then release a consensus statement. Twenty years of solid research could predate a consensus statement that was released in the 1970s; but when it finally came out, the public received a clear, unambiguous message.

A lot has changed since then, including the quality, quantity, and availability of research. Today, studies are available for media reporting often before they are published in a journal. Although this allows a great amount of new and wonderful research to gain a venue for presenta-

supplements needs to be evaluated carefully is that often, the dosages used in a particular clinical study aren't the same amounts in the products sold in stores. When marketing a supplement, companies strive to find the price point at which consumers will buy it, while leaving an acceptable profit margin once the raw materials have been procured and the product has been manufactured and marketed. That's not to say that companies pick doses out of the air, but the dose has to make economic sense or the product won't make it to market. The result, however, may be a product that won't work.

Pyruvate is a classic example of this phenomenon. Researchers found that this supplement promoted fat loss in subjects taking 16 to 25 grams a day, but selling it with that "standard serving" would have been prohibitively expensive. So it was sold with a recommended dose of $1/2$ to 2 grams a day—an amount for which there were no data showing effectiveness. At that dose, pyruvate probably does nothing except empty your wallet.

Yet another reason that it's hard to reach hard-and-fast conclusions about the efficacy of these supplements is that even studies that are conducted on mentally impaired subjects tend to occur outside the United States, usually in Europe. Regulation of dietary supplements isn't being implemented by the U.S. Food and Drug Administration—at least not for the time being—and herbal products aren't easily patented. If a company isn't going to be able to enjoy the windfall of having a product roped off from competition for several years via patent, little incentive

tion, some lousy stuff also gets published. You might see the first paper written on a previously unexplored topic, with the research having been done on a handful of subjects, using inadequate controls. Or maybe it's the 10th paper done on 400,000 subjects using state-of-the-art protocols. Either way, the public has no way to judge the evidence based on how it's reported. This phenomenon goes a long way toward explaining why scientists might claim that "vitamin XYZ" is good for you, bad for you, and doesn't make any difference, all at the same time.

Also, magazines devoted to health and fitness may be relying heavily on advertising dollars from supplement manufacturers, which can skew the magazine's objectivity. Editorial content that runs contrary to an important advertiser may be stricken from an article, or a product may be mentioned not based on an objective analysis of its usefulness but because an important advertiser markets it. These same sorts of conflicts of interest exist in television, radio—you name it.

Again, this doesn't mean that there isn't some very good information out there. Great books have been written, many of the magazines are reliable (although none that I know of are immune to pressure from advertisers), and there are some wonderful sites on the Internet. Just evaluate what you hear carefully, consider the source, and be aware of any potential conflicts of interest that might be coloring that information.

exists to pour a lot of research and development dollars into clinical trials on the front end. In contrast, herbal products that are proven safe and effective can be authorized for use in treating specific medical conditions in Germany and other European nations. This latter regulatory framework gives manufacturers a reason to research, develop, and market these products because they stand a legitimate chance of generating a return on their capital.

One final caveat as you begin evaluating these supplements: Most of them need to be taken for some time before having a noticeable effect, as the active ingredient takes time to accumulate in your system. The upside of having fewer negative side effects is balanced against a lower potency and longer time until effective dosages are reached.

The Truth about Supplements

Ginkgo biloba. Extracted from the dried leaves of the ancient ginkgo tree, this dean of brain-boosting supplements may clear your head. It seems to help widen constricted blood vessels, particularly the tiny microvessels that snake through the deep recesses of your brain, oxygenating the tissues in which many of your memories reside. Ginkgo may help inhibit the clotting of red blood cells, in turn reducing the buildup of plaque along arterial walls, which, left unchecked, can form clots and lead to a stroke. By preventing the buildup of plaque, blood flow is improved and more oxygen reaches all the brain cells. If you are young and healthy, however, ginkgo probably doesn't have much work to do inside your body. On the other hand, if you're in your mid- to late-30s and your primary sustenance for most of those years has been Ding Dongs, it might help slow an aging process that your unfit lifestyle has likely accelerated. Take 120 to 160 milligrams a day, divided among three servings.

Rhodiola rosea. Native to Siberia, *Rhodiola rosea* is purported to work by improving blood flow throughout the brain, and it also seems to raise the amount of basic b-endorphin in the blood plasma. That might help with stress management. One recent study took a group of college kids and plied them each with 100 milligrams of *Rhodiola rosea* for 20 days at exam time. Not only did the students have a better sense of well-being and more mental stamina, on average, but these improvements translated into better grades. Most *Rhodiola rosea* extract is standardized to contain 3 to 5 percent rosavins, the primary active ingredient. The majority of studies that showed positive effects used 2 to 10 milligrams of rosavins, or approximately 75 to 200 milligrams of rhodiola root.

Ginseng. Derived from the root of *Panax ginseng* in Asia, this supplement has a venerable history dating back centuries in Chinese medicine. There are numerous types of ginseng, and depending on whether the source is Asian or North American, the effects may vary. Ginseng contains many bioactive components, called ginsenosides, and depending on the preparation and plant source (i.e., root, leaf, flower, or stem and seed), their quantity, activity, and potency may vary widely. Because the purity and standardization of the preparations used in research studies are generally not available to the public, supplements on the market usually cannot replicate the results seen in scientific studies. A review of the literature suggests that the jury is still out on ginseng's efficacy. In one rat study, among subjects made to breathe a stingy 7.6 percent oxygen—remember, they are just rats, before you get all misty-eyed—the survival rate of those taking ginseng nearly doubled. Needless to say, this study has yet to be duplicated using humans. And there's the rub: It won't be. Take 100 milligrams two times a day, standardized for 4 percent ginsenosides.

L-tyrosine. When manufactured by the body, tyrosine becomes a precursor of the neurotransmitters dopamine, which modulates feelings of well-being, and norepinephrine and epinephrine, which provide a jolt of energy. Not surprisingly, people lacking ty-rosine tend to feel depressed, tired, and stressed out. Given that tyrosine stokes these neurotransmitters, the thinking goes, might not taking the supplement L-tyrosine make you happier, better able to handle stress, sharper mentally, and more energetic? The re-search, much of it conducted by the military, sug-gests that supplemental tyrosine can help delay the onset of fatigue. Tyrosine doesn't, however, seem to have an effect on the quantity and quality of sleep it-self. A study published in the journal *Nutritional Neuroscience* in 2003 found that taking tyrosine sup-plements had no discernible effect on sleep-deprived adult males. The supplement has also failed tests of its ability to enhance endurance. The recommended dosage is 1 to 3 grams daily.

Vitamin E. This fat-soluble vitamin is a pow-erful antioxidant that protects your cells against damage from free radicals. Perhaps by protecting the brain from radiation and various chemicals, vitamin E does appear to play a role in slowing memory loss due to aging or Alzheimer's disease. Also, by thin-ning your blood slightly, it may prevent plaque ac-cumulation and blockage in small blood vessels in the brain. Results of both the National Health and Nutrition Examination Survey and the Continuing Survey of Food Intakes of Individuals indicated that most Americans don't consume the adult RDA of 15 milligrams. Epidemiological studies also suggest that older people with high levels of vit-amin E in their bloodstream have better memory than those who don't, a finding supported in an-imal studies as well. Most studies investigating general prevention against oxidative damage have used 600 IU of d-alpha-tocopherol, the natural form of vitamin E, per day.

St. John's wort. Long before Paxil, Zoloft, and Prozac, there was this popular mood elevator, which works by inhibiting the reuptake of serotonin. Any number of well-controlled studies suggest that St. John's wort can help lift mood. In an analysis of 23 randomized trials involving over 1,700 patients, re-searchers found St. John's wort significantly superior to a placebo and as effective as standard antidepres-sants but with fewer side effects. The standard is 300 milligrams, standardized to 0.3 percent hyper-icum, taken three times a day. St. John's wort can in-terfere with other medications and may have side effects. Consult with your physician before begin-ning to supplement.

Kava (or Kava Kava). In Germany and France, this supplement is used as a drug for conditions in-cluding mild anxiety and sleep disorders. The pop-ular press has promoted it as a remedy for anxiety, and a booster of mental alertness and concentration. But while it has been found to be effective for mild anxiety and some sleep disorders, there are concerns over its safety. Kava has been associated with liver toxicity, and may interfere with medications. Con-sult with your physician prior to using Kava. The recommended dose is 1.7 to 3.4 grams daily (or, if you're measuring the active component Kava py-rones, take 60-120 milligrams.

Others to watch. The medical community hasn't come to any conclusions about the following sup-plements, but you may want to keep your eye on them-some very preliminary research shows they may affect mood and cognitive performance:

acetyl-L carnitine (ALC)
ashwagandha
creatine
huperzine A
vinpocetine

THE ALL-DAY-ENERGY MEAL PLAN

IF YOU'RE FALLING ASLEEP AT YOUR DESK IN THE MIDDLE OF THE AFTERNOON, you may be eating too much sugar, drinking too much coffee, skipping meals, or eating too infrequently. To turn things around, consume small meals frequently throughout the day. Eat a small lunch and rely on snacks to avoid the crash. Combine protein, carbs, and fat all day long for timed-release energy. Focus your sugar consumption around your workouts so that it becomes an effective tool in your diet. Drink plenty of fluids and sip from a sports drink and a water bottle during your workout to keep energy levels high.

Daily Assumptions*†

2,470 calories
309 grams carbohydrates
159 grams protein
66 grams fat

Daily Breakdown*†

8 bread
5 fruit
4 milk
9 teaspoons added sugar
6 vegetable
6 very lean protein
6 lean protein
1 medium-fat protein
5 fat

Note: Occasionally, a fat-free product, like mustard or cooking spray, is included on the menus. These do not count toward your daily breakdown but should not be overused.

*Use every day.

† Based on a 185-pound man.

THE MENU

DAY 1

Breakfast

2 bread	1 cup Shredded Wheat
1 milk	1 cup fat-free milk
2 fruit	1/2 cup grapefruit juice
	3/4 cup blueberries
1 medium-fat protein	1 egg, scrambled on a nonstick pan
1 very lean protein	2 egg whites, scrambled with whole egg
1 fat	1 1/2 tablespoons ground flaxseed
	Tea
	Water
	Oil-free cooking spray (for eggs)

Snack

1 bread	1/2 whole-wheat pita
1 vegetable	Salad with 1 cup lettuce, 1/4 cup tomato, 1/4 cup cucumber
1 lean protein	1 ounce part-skim mozzarella

Lunch

2 bread	2 slices whole-grain bread
2 vegetable	Salad with 2 cups romaine lettuce, 1/2 cup tomato, 1/2 cup cucumber
3 very lean protein	3 ounces sliced turkey
1 fat	1 tablespoon low-fat vinaigrette
	Dijon mustard

Dinner

3 bread	1 large baked sweet potato
1 milk	1 cup fat-free milk
3 vegetable	1½ cups steamed asparagus
4 lean protein	4 ounces salmon, grilled
2 fat	2 teaspoons each olive oil and lemon juice (for asparagus)

Pre-Workout Snack

1 milk	1 cup fat-free milk
1 fruit	1 apple, sliced
1 lean protein	1 tablespoon peanut butter
1 fat	Included (peanut butter)

Workout

| 6 teaspoons added sugar | 12-ounce sports drink |
| | Water |

Post-Workout

POWER SMOOTHIE

Blend until smooth. Drink 15 to 30 minutes after your workout.

2 fruit	⅓ cup frozen strawberries
	½ cup mango
	½ cup orange juice
1 milk	1 cup fat-free milk
3 teaspoons added sugar	1 tablespoon honey
2 very lean protein	14 grams whey protein powder

DAY 2

Breakfast

Combine yogurt, fruit, and honey. Combine muffin and egg for sandwich.

2 bread	1 whole-wheat English muffin
1 milk	1 cup fat-free unsweetened yogurt
2 fruit	1¼ cups fresh strawberries
1 medium-fat protein	1 whole egg, hard-cooked
1 very lean protein	2 eggs, hard-cooked (discard yolks)
1 fat	1½ tablespoons ground flaxseed (add to yogurt)
	Water

Snack

1 soy	1/2 cup soy nuts
1 vegetable	Vegetable sticks
1 lean protein	Included (soy nuts)

Lunch

2 bread	1 slice whole-grain bread
	1 ounce croutons
2 vegetable	Large salad with romaine lettuce, tomato, grilled eggplant, roasted red pepper
	Fat-free dressing
3 very lean protein	3 ounces skinless white-meat chicken, grilled with lime juice
1 fat	1 teaspoon olive oil for roasted vegetables

Dinner

3 bread	1 cup cooked pasta
	1 slice garlic bread
1 milk	1 ounce reduced-fat cheese
3 vegetable	2 cups ratatouille (over pasta)
	Salad with 1 cup lettuce, 1/4 cup tomato, 1/4 cup cucumber
	2 tablespoons fat-free dressing
4 lean protein	4 ounces lean ground beef
2 fat	2 teaspoons olive oil (in ratatouille)

Pre-Workout Snack

1 milk	1 cup fat-free milk
1 fruit	1 apple, sliced
1 lean protein	1 tablespoon peanut butter
1 fat	Included (peanut butter)

Workout

6 teaspoons added sugar	12-ounce sports drink
	Water

Post-Workout

POWER SMOOTHIE

Blend until smooth. Drink 15 to 30 minutes after your workout.

2 fruit	1/3 cup frozen strawberries
	1/2 large banana
	1/2 cup orange juice
1 milk	1 cup fat-free milk
3 teaspoons added sugar	1 tablespoon honey
2 very lean protein	14 grams whey protein powder

DAY 3

Breakfast

2 bread	2 slices whole-wheat bread
1 milk	1 cup fat-free cottage cheese
2 fruit	4 ounces freshly squeezed orange juice (with pulp)
	$1/2$ cup sliced pineapple
1 medium-fat protein	1 egg, sunny-side up, cooked in a nonstick pan
1 very lean protein	2 egg whites (add to sunny-side up egg)
1 fat	$1^1/2$ tablespoons ground flaxseed
	Water
	Oil-free cooking spray (for eggs)

Snack

1 bread	$1/2$ bagel
1 vegetable	Tomato, sprouts
1 lean protein	1 ounce low-fat Swiss cheese

Lunch

2 bread	$2/3$ cup rice
2 vegetable	1 cup Chinese vegetables, stir-fried with garlic, onion, fresh ginger
3 very lean protein	3 ounces scallops, stir-fried
1 fat	1 teaspoon oil (for stir-frying)

Dinner

3 bread	2-inch square of corn bread
	1 cup kidney beans (add to chili)
1 milk	1 ounce fat-free cheese, grated (for chili)
3 vegetable	1 cup chopped cooked tomatoes with chili seasoning
	$1/2$ onion, garlic (for seasoning)
	Salad with 1 cup lettuce, $1/4$ cup tomato, $1/4$ cup cucumber
4 lean protein	Included (in beans)
	2 ounces soy crumbles (add to chili)
2 fat	1 slice bacon, cooked very crisp (crumble into chili)
	Included (in corn bread)

Pre-Workout Snack

1 milk	1 cup fat-free milk
1 fruit	1 apple, sliced
1 lean protein	1 tablespoon peanut butter
1 fat	Included (in peanut butter)

Workout

6 teaspoons added sugar	12-ounce sports drink
	Water

Post-Workout

POWER SMOOTHIE

Blend until smooth. Drink 15 to 30 minutes after your workout.

2 fruit	⅓ cup frozen peaches
	½ cup mango
	½ cup orange juice
1 milk	1 cup fat-free milk
3 teaspoons added sugar	1 tablespoon honey
2 very lean protein	14 grams whey protein powder

DAY 4

Breakfast

2 fruit	1 cup raspberries
	½ cup orange juice
1 milk	1 cup fat-free milk (½ cup for French toast)

FRENCH TOAST

Combine milk, egg, egg whites, and flaxseed. Dip bread and fry until golden.

2 bread	2 slices whole-wheat bread
1 medium-fat protein	1 egg
1 very lean protein	2 egg whites
1 fat	1½ tablespoons ground flaxseed
	Water
	Oil-free cooking spray (for eggs)
	1 tablespoon no-sugar maple-flavored syrup

Snack

1 bread	12 Wheat Thins
1 vegetable	1 cup sliced bell pepper
1 lean protein	¼ cup cottage cheese
	No-calorie sweetener to taste (for cottage cheese)

Lunch

FAJITAS

Combine ingredients.

2 bread	1/3 cup Spanish rice
	1 tortilla
2 vegetable	1 cup sautéed onions and peppers
	2 tablespoons salsa
3 very lean protein	3 ounces skinless white-meat chicken, grilled with lime juice
1 fat	1 teaspoon olive oil (for cooking)

Dinner

3 bread	1 ounce croutons (for salad)
	1 cup chicken noodle soup
	4 reduced-fat crackers
1 milk	1 cup fat-free milk
3 vegetable	3 cups salad with lettuce, tomato, cucumber, pepper
4 lean protein	4 ounces swordfish, grilled with ginger and scallions
2 fat	8 black or 10 green large olives
	2 tablespoons reduced-fat dressing

Pre-Workout Snack

1 milk	1 cup fat-free milk
1 fruit	1 apple, sliced
1 lean protein	1 tablespoon peanut butter
1 fat	Included (in peanut butter)

Workout

6 teaspoons added sugar	12-ounce sports drink
	Water

Post-Workout

POWER SMOOTHIE

Blend until smooth. Drink 15 to 30 minutes after your workout.

2 fruit	1/3 cup frozen strawberries
	1/2 cup mango
	1/2 cup orange juice
1 milk	1 cup fat-free milk
3 teaspoons added sugar	1 tablespoon honey
2 very lean protein	14 grams whey protein powder

DAY 5

Breakfast

2 bread	1 cup quick oats (not instant)
1 milk	1 cup fat-free milk
2 fruit	1/2 cup diced apples
	1¼ cups strawberries, sliced
1 medium-fat protein	1 egg, hard-cooked
1 very lean protein	2 eggs, hard-cooked (discard yolks)
1 fat	1½ tablespoons ground flaxseed
	Water

Snack

1 bread	3/4 ounce baked tortillas
1 vegetable	Salsa
1 lean protein	1 ounce low-fat cheddar cheese

Lunch

2 bread	3/4 cup minestrone soup
	1/2 cup cooked linguini
2 vegetable	Salad with 1 cup lettuce, 1/4 cup tomato, 1/4 cup cucumber
	Fat-free dressing
	1/2 cup marinara sauce
3 very lean protein	3 ounces shrimp, grilled
1 fat	1 teaspoon olive oil (for cooking)

Dinner

3 bread	1 large pita
	1 ounce croutons
1 milk	1/2 cup fat-free yogurt
	1/2 cup fat-free milk
3 vegetable	Salad with 2 cups romaine lettuce, 1/2 cup tomato, 1/2 cup cucumber
	Garlic, onion (for sandwich)
4 lean protein	4 ounces lean lamb, grilled with lime juice
2 fat	2 tablespoons vinaigrette

Pre-Workout Snack

1 milk	1 cup fat-free milk
1 fruit	1 apple, sliced
1 lean protein	1 tablespoon peanut butter
1 fat	Included (in peanut butter)

Workout

6 teaspoons added sugar	12-ounce sports drink
	Water

Post-Workout

POWER SMOOTHIE

Blend until smooth. Drink 15 to 30 minutes after your workout.

2 fruit	$1/3$ cup frozen strawberries
	$1/2$ cup frozen raspberries
	$1/2$ cup orange juice
1 milk	1 cup fat-free milk
3 teaspoons added sugar	1 tablespoon honey
2 very lean protein	14 grams whey protein powder

DAY 6

Breakfast

2 bread	2 slices multigrain toast
1 medium-fat protein	1 egg, scrambled in a nonstick pan
1 very lean protein	2 egg whites (scrambled with whole egg)
	Oil-free cooking spray (for eggs)

SMOOTHIE

Blend until smooth.

1 milk	1 cup fat-free milk
2 fruit	$1/2$ cup orange juice
	1 fresh peach
1 fat	$1^{1}/2$ tablespoons ground flaxseed or 1 teaspoon flaxseed oil
	Water

Snack

1 bread	1 slice whole-wheat bread
1 vegetable	Tomato, lettuce, mustard (on sandwich)
1 lean protein	1 ounce lean ham

Lunch

2 bread	1 whole-wheat bagel
2 vegetable	$1/2$ cup carrot sticks, onions, tomatoes
3 very lean protein	3 ounces smoked salmon
1 fat	3 tablespoons reduced-fat cream cheese

Dinner

3 bread	2 slices rye bread
	$1/2$ cup pasta salad
1 milk	1 cup fat-free milk
3 vegetable	1 cup coleslaw
	$1/2$ cup chopped vegetables (cucumbers, carrots, onions; mix into tuna)
4 lean protein	4 ounces tuna in olive oil, drained
2 fat	3 teaspoons mayonnaise

Pre-Workout Snack

1 milk	1 cup fat-free milk
1 fruit	1 apple, sliced
1 lean protein	1 tablespoon peanut butter
1 fat	Included (in peanut butter)

Workout

6 teaspoons added sugar	12-ounce sports drink
	Water

Post-Workout

POWER SMOOTHIE

Blend until smooth. Drink 15 to 30 minutes after your workout.

2 fruit	$1/3$ cup frozen strawberries
	$1/2$ large banana
	$1/2$ cup orange juice
1 milk	1 cup fat-free milk
3 added sugar	1 tablespoon honey
2 very lean protein	14 grams whey protein powder

DAY 7

Breakfast

2 bread	1 cup Shredded Wheat
1 milk	1 cup fat-free milk
2 fruit	2 cups raspberries
1 medium-fat protein	1 egg, hard-cooked
1 very lean protein	2 eggs, hard-cooked (discard yolks)
1 fat	$1^1/2$ tablespoons ground flaxseed
	Water

Snack

1 bread	1 tortilla
1 vegetable	Sliced vegetables
	Salsa
1 lean protein	1 ounce low-fat Mexican cheese, shredded

Lunch

2 bread	1 small multigrain roll
	3 ounces baked yam
2 vegetable	Sliced tomato, lettuce (for sandwich)
	1/2 cup radishes, celery, carrots
3 very lean protein	3 ounces grilled chicken
2 fat	2 tablespoons low-fat ranch dressing (for dipping)
	1 teaspoon olive oil (for chicken)

Dinner

3 bread	3-inch square of corn bread
	1 ounce croutons
1 milk	1/2 cup fat-free milk
	1 ounce fat-free cheese, shredded
3 vegetable	3 cups salad with lettuce, tomato, cucumber, pepper
4 lean protein	4 ounces salmon, poached
2 fat	2 tablespoons low-fat Caesar dressing
	Included (in corn bread)

Pre-Workout Snack

1 milk	1 cup fat-free milk
1 fruit	1 apple, sliced
1 lean protein	1 tablespoon peanut butter
1 fat	Included (in peanut butter)

Workout

6 teaspoons added sugar	12-ounce sports drink
	Water

Post-Workout

POWER SMOOTHIE

Blend until smooth. Drink 15 to 30 minutes after your workout.

2 fruit	1/3 cup frozen melon
	1/2 cup mango
	1/2 cup orange juice
1 milk	1 cup fat-free milk
3 teaspoons added sugar	1 tablespoon honey
2 very lean protein	14 grams whey protein powder

THE ANTI-INSOMNIAC MEAL PLAN

YOU MAY TOSS AND TURN FROM TOO MUCH CAFFEINE, ALCOHOL, AND SUGAR, OR from food eaten too late at night. To get a better night's rest, work out in the morning, increase your consumption of tryptophan and carbs at dinner (to increase melatonin and serotonin), don't drink coffee after noon, reduce your sugar consumption, and favor low-GI carbohydrate sources.

Daily Assumptions*†

2,500 calories
314 grams carbohydrates
156 grams protein
69 grams fat

Daily Breakdown*†

8 bread
6 fruit
4 milk
10 teaspoons added sugar
6 vegetable
6 very lean protein
6 lean protein
1 medium-fat protein
5 fat

Note: Occasionally, a fat-free product, like mustard or cooking spray, is included on the menus. These do not count toward your daily breakdown but should not be overused.

*Use every day.

† Based on a 185-pound man.

DAY 1

Pre-Workout Snack

SMOOTHIE
Blend until smooth.

1 milk	1 cup fat-free milk
1 fruit	1/2 cup orange juice
2 very lean protein	14 grams whey protein powder
	Ice cubes

Workout

8 teaspoons added sugar	16-ounce sports drink
	Water

Breakfast

2 bread	1 cup Shredded Wheat
1 milk	1 cup fat-free milk
2 fruit	2 tablespoons raisins
	1/2 large banana
2 teaspoons added sugar	Tea with 2 teaspoons honey
2 very lean protein	4 egg whites, scrambled in a nonstick pan
1 fat	1 1/2 tablespoons ground flaxseed
	Water
	Oil-free cooking spray (for eggs)

Snack

1 milk	1 cup reduced-fat plain yogurt
1 fruit	1 1/4 cups strawberries
1 fat	Included (in yogurt)

Lunch

2 bread	1 whole-grain roll
	½ cup brown rice
2 vegetable	1 cup steamed asparagus
6 lean protein	6 ounces broiled salmon, with lemon

Snack

1 bread	½ ounce pretzels
1 vegetable	8 mini carrots
1 fat	10 peanuts

Dinner

3 bread	1 medium sweet potato, baked
	1 medium to small ear of corn
1 milk	1 cup fat-free milk
2 fruit	2 kiwis
3 vegetable	3 cups salad with lettuce, tomato, cucumber, pepper
2 very lean protein	2 ounces sliced turkey
1 medium-fat protein	1 egg, hard-cooked
2 fat	4 tablespoons reduced-fat dressing

DAY 2

Pre-Workout Snack

SMOOTHIE

Blend until smooth.

1 milk	1 cup fat-free milk
1 fruit	½ cup orange juice
2 very lean protein	14 grams whey protein powder
	Ice cubes

Workout

| 8 teaspoons added sugar | 16-ounce sports drink |
| | Water |

Breakfast

Combine yogurt, fruit, and honey. Combine muffin and egg for sandwich.

2 bread	1 whole-wheat English muffin
1 milk	1 cup fat-free unsweetened yogurt
2 fruit	1$\frac{1}{4}$ cups fresh strawberries
2 teaspoons added sugar	2 teaspoons honey for yogurt
2 very lean protein	4 eggs, hard-cooked (discard yolks)
1 fat	1$\frac{1}{2}$ tablespoons ground flaxseed
	Water

Snack

1 milk	1 cup reduced-fat plain yogurt
1 fruit	1 cup blueberries
1 fat	Included (in yogurt)

Lunch

2 bread	1 cup bowtie pasta
2 vegetable	1 cup grilled eggplant and roasted red peppers
6 lean protein	6 ounces shrimp, grilled
	Fat-free dressing
	Oil-free cooking spray for shrimp

Snack

1 bread	$\frac{1}{2}$ whole-wheat pita
1 vegetable	Romaine lettuce, mushrooms, other veggies
1 fat	1 tablespoon Thousand Island dressing

Dinner

3 bread	1 cup cooked pasta
	1 slice garlic bread
1 milk	1 ounce reduced-fat cheese
2 fruit	2 cups blueberries
3 vegetable	2 cups ratatouille (over pasta)
	Salad with 1 cup lettuce, $\frac{1}{4}$ cup tomato, $\frac{1}{4}$ cup cucumber
2 very lean protein	2 ounces lean ground turkey
1 medium-fat protein	1 egg (mix with turkey for meatballs)
2 fat	2 tablespoons fat-free dressing
	2 teaspoons olive oil (for cooking ratatouille)

DAY 3

Pre-Workout Snack

SMOOTHIE

Blend until smooth.

1 milk	1 cup fat-free milk
1 fruit	1/2 cup orange juice
2 very lean protein	14 grams whey protein powder
	Ice cubes

Workout

8 teaspoons added sugar	16-ounce sports drink
	Water

Breakfast

2 bread	2 slices whole-wheat bread
1 milk	1 cup fat-free cottage cheese (on bread; sprinkle with brown sugar and cinnamon)
2 fruit	4 ounces freshly squeezed orange juice (with pulp)
	1/2 cup sliced pineapple
2 teaspoons added sugar	2 teaspoons brown sugar
2 very lean protein	4 egg whites, fried in a nonstick skillet
1 fat	1 1/2 tablespoons ground flaxseed
	Water
	Oil-free cooking spray (for eggs)

Snack

1 milk	1 cup reduced-fat plain yogurt
1 fruit	1/2 large banana, sliced
1 fat	Included (in yogurt)

Lunch

2 bread	1 cup rice
2 vegetable	1 cup Chinese vegetables, stir-fried with garlic, onion, fresh ginger
6 lean protein	6 ounces scallops, stir-fried in heated nonstick wok
	Oil-free cooking spray (for scallops)

Snack

1 bread	1/2 bagel
1 vegetable	Tomato, sprouts
1 fat	3 tablespoons reduced-fat cream cheese

Dinner

3 bread	2-inch square of corn bread
	1 cup kidney beans (add to chili)
1 milk	1 cup fat-free grated cheese (for chili)
2 fruit	1 mango
3 vegetable	1 cup chopped cooked tomatoes with chili seasoning, ½ onion, garlic for seasoning
2 very lean protein	Included (in beans)
1 medium-fat protein	2 ounces soy crumbles (for chili)
2 fat	1 slice bacon, cooked very crisp (crumble into chili)

DAY 4

Pre-Workout Snack

SMOOTHIE

Blend until smooth.

1 milk	1 cup fat-free milk
1 fruit	½ cup orange juice
2 very lean protein	14 grams whey protein powder
	Ice cubes

Workout

8 teaspoons added sugar	16-ounce sports drink
	Water

Breakfast

2 fruit	1 cup raspberries
	½ cup orange juice
1 milk	1 cup fat-free milk (½ cup for French toast)

FRENCH TOAST *(See recipe directions on page 44.)*

2 bread	2 slices whole-wheat bread
2 very lean protein	4 egg whites
1 fat	1½ tablespoons ground flaxseed
	Water
	Oil-free cooking spray
	2 teaspoons no-calorie sweetener

Snack

1 milk	1 cup reduced-fat plain yogurt
1 fruit	1 peach, sliced
1 fat	Included (in yogurt)
	No-calorie sweetener to taste

Lunch

FAJITAS

Combine ingredients.

2 bread	1/3 cup Spanish rice
	1 tortilla
2 vegetable	1 cup sautéed onions and peppers
	2 tablespoons salsa
6 lean protein	6 ounces swordfish, grilled with lime juice
	Oil-free cooking spray for vegetables

Snack

1 bread	12 Wheat Thins
1 vegetable	1 cup sliced bell pepper
1 fat	1 ounce soft ripened cheese

Dinner

3 bread	1 ounce croutons for salad
	1 cup chicken noodle soup
	4 reduced-fat crackers
1 milk	1 fat-free milk
2 fruit	1 cup chunky applesauce
3 vegetable	3 cups salad with lettuce, tomato, cucumber, pepper
2 very lean protein	2 ounces skinless white-meat chicken, grilled with ginger and scallions
1 medium-fat protein	1 egg, hard-cooked, sliced
2 fat	8 black or 10 green olives, large
	2 tablespoons reduced-fat dressing

DAY 5

Pre-Workout Snack

SMOOTHIE

Blend until smooth.

1 milk	1 cup fat-free milk
1 fruit	1/2 cup orange juice
2 very lean protein	14 grams whey protein powder
	Ice cubes

Workout

8 teaspoons added sugar	16-ounce sports drink
	Water

Breakfast

2 bread	1 cup quick oats (not instant)
1 milk	1 cup fat-free milk
2 fruit	1/2 cup diced apples
	1 1/4 cups sliced strawberries
2 teaspoons added sugar	2 teaspoons brown sugar
2 very lean protein	4 eggs, hard-cooked (discard yolks)
1 fat	1 1/2 tablespoons ground flaxseed
	Water

Snack

1 milk	1 cup reduced-fat plain yogurt
1 fruit	1 cup raspberries
1 fat	Included (in yogurt)

Lunch

2 bread	3/4 cup minestrone soup
	1 small potato, baked
2 vegetable	Salad with 1 cup lettuce, 1/4 cup tomato, 1/4 cup cucumber
	Fat-free dressing
	1 cup broccoli
6 lean protein	6 ounces shrimp, grilled
	Oil-free cooking spray (for grilling shrimp)

Snack

1 bread	3/4 ounce baked tortillas
1 vegetable	Salsa
1 fat	2 tablespoons guacamole

Dinner

3 bread	1 large pita
	1 ounce croutons
1 milk	1/2 cup fat-free yogurt
	1/2 cup fat-free milk
2 fruit	4 figs
3 vegetable	Salad with 2 cups romaine lettuce, 1/2 cup tomato, 1/2 cup cucumber
	Garlic, onion for sandwich
2 very lean protein	2 ounces skinless white-meat chicken, grilled with lime juice
1 medium-fat protein	1 egg, hard-cooked, chopped
2 fat	2 tablespoons vinaigrette

DAY 6

Pre-Workout Snack

SMOOTHIE

Blend until smooth.

1 milk	1 cup fat-free milk
1 fruit	½ cup orange juice
2 very lean protein	14 grams whey protein powder
	Ice cubes

Workout

8 teaspoons added sugar	16-ounce sports drink
	Water

Breakfast

2 bread	2 slices multigrain bread, toasted
2 very lean protein	4 egg whites, scrambled
	Oil-free cooking spray (for eggs)

SMOOTHIE

Blend until smooth.

1 milk	1 cup fat-free milk
2 fruit	½ cup orange juice
	1 fresh peach
2 teaspoons added sugar	2 teaspoons honey
1 fat	1½ tablespoons ground flaxseed or 1 teaspoon flaxseed oil
	Water

Snack

1 milk	1 cup reduced-fat plain yogurt
1 fruit	½ cup unsweetened chunky applesauce with cinnamon
1 fat	Included (in yogurt)

Lunch

2 bread	1 whole-wheat bagel
2 vegetable	½ cup carrot sticks
	Onion, tomato
6 lean protein	6 ounces smoked salmon
	2 tablespoons fat-free cream cheese

Snack

1 bread	1 slice whole-wheat bread
1 vegetable	Tomato, lettuce, mustard
1 fat	$^1/_8$ avocado

Dinner

3 bread	2 slices rye bread
	$^1/_2$ cup pasta salad
1 milk	1 cup fat-free milk
2 fruit	$^1/_4$ honeydew
3 vegetable	1 cup coleslaw
	$^1/_2$ cup chopped vegetables (cucumbers, carrots, onions; mix into turkey)
2 very lean protein	2 ounces cubed turkey
1 medium-fat protein	1 ounce cubed hard-cooked egg (mix into turkey)
2 fat	1 tablespoon mayonnaise
	Included (in coleslaw and pasta salad)

DAY 7

Pre-Workout Snack

SMOOTHIE

Blend until smooth.

1 milk	1 cup fat-free milk
1 fruit	$^1/_2$ cup orange juice
2 very lean protein	14 grams whey protein powder
	Ice cubes

Workout

8 teaspoons added sugar	16-ounce sports drink
	Water

Breakfast

2 bread	1 cup Shredded Wheat
1 milk	1 cup fat-free milk
2 fruit	2 cups raspberries
2 teaspoons added sugar	2 teaspoons sugar
2 very lean protein	4 eggs, hard-cooked (discard yolks)
1 fat	$1^1/_2$ tablespoons ground flaxseed
	Water

Snack

1 milk	1 cup reduced-fat plain yogurt
1 fruit	1 cup blackberries
1 fat	Included (in yogurt)

Lunch

2 bread	1 small multigrain roll
	3 ounces baked yam
2 vegetable	1/2 cup green beans
	1/2 cup radishes, celery, carrots
6 lean protein	6 ounces fresh ham steak
	2 tablespoons fat-free ranch dressing (for dipping)

Snack

1 bread	1 tortilla
1 vegetable	1/2 cup sliced veggies
	1/2 cup salsa
1 fat	2 tablespoons reduced-fat sour cream

Dinner

3 bread	3-inch square of corn bread
	1 ounce croutons
1 milk	1/2 cup fat-free milk
	1/2 ounce fat-free shredded cheese
2 fruit	2 kiwis
3 vegetable	3 cups salad with lettuce, tomato, cucumber, pepper
2 very lean protein	2 ounces grilled chicken
1 medium-fat protein	1 egg, hard-cooked, chopped (for salad)
2 fat	2 tablespoons low-fat Caesar dressing
	Included (in corn bread)

THE MOOD-BOOST MEAL PLAN

IF YOU'RE FEELING MOODY, ODDS ARE YOU'RE not eating enough healthy fats, eating the right carbs at the wrong times, or underconsuming fruits and vegetables. You might also be drinking too much alcohol. To boost your mood, exercise in the morning to get the endorphins pumping, and have some caffeine beforehand to kick-start your workout. Eat carbs ranking low on the glycemic index; select turkey, whey, dairy, and other protein sources high in tryptophan; and increase healthy fats in your diet by eating fish five times a week. Add flaxseed to your diet: The alpha-linolenic acid and omega 3s it contains have antidepressant effects.

Daily Assumptions*†

2,500 calories
313 grams carbohydrates
131 grams protein
79 grams fat

Daily Breakdown*†

8 bread
5 fruit
4 milk
10 teaspoons added sugar
6 vegetable
4 very lean protein
4 lean protein
1 medium-fat protein
10 fat

Note: Occasionally, a fat-free product, like mustard or cooking spray, is included on the menus. These do not count toward your daily breakdown but should not be overused.

*Use every day.

† Based on a 185-pound man.

THE MENU

DAY 1

Pre-Workout Snack

SMOOTHIE
Blend until smooth.

1 milk	1 cup fat-free milk
1 fruit	½ cup orange juice
2 very lean protein	14 grams whey protein powder
	Ice cubes

Workout

8 teaspoons added sugar	16-ounce sports drink
	Water

Breakfast

2 bread	1 cup Shredded Wheat
1 milk	1 cup fat-free milk
2 fruit	½ large banana
	2 tablespoons raisins
2 teaspoons added sugar	Tea with 2 teaspoons honey
1 medium-fat protein	1 egg, scrambled on a nonstick pan
1 fat	1½ tablespoons ground flaxseed
	Water
	Oil-free cooking spray (for egg)

Snack

1 milk	1 cup fat-free milk
1 fruit	1 apple, sliced
2 fat	1 tablespoon peanut butter (for dipping apples)

Lunch

2 bread	1 small whole-grain roll
	⅓ cup brown rice
2 vegetable	1 cup steamed asparagus
4 lean protein	4 ounces salmon, broiled
3 fat	1 tablespoon olive oil (for dipping bread or drizzling on fish)

Snack

1 bread	¾ ounce pretzels
1 vegetable	8 mini carrots
1 fat	2 tablespoons reduced-fat ranch dressing

Dinner

3 bread	1 medium baked potato
	1 medium ear corn on the cob
1 milk	1 cup fat-free milk
1 fruit	½ papaya
3 vegetable	3 cups tossed salad with lettuce, tomato, cucumber, pepper
2 very lean protein	2 ounces sliced turkey
3 fat	8 black or 10 green olives, large
	4 tablespoons reduced-fat dressing

DAY 2

Pre-Workout Snack

SMOOTHIE

Blend until smooth.

1 milk	1 cup fat-free milk
1 fruit	½ cup orange juice
2 very lean protein	14 grams whey protein powder
	Ice cubes

Workout

8 teaspoons added sugar	16-ounce sports drink
	Water

Breakfast

Combine yogurt, fruit, and honey. Combine muffin and egg for sandwich.

2 bread	1 whole-wheat English muffin
1 milk	1 cup fat-free unsweetened yogurt
2 fruit	1½ cups fresh blueberries
2 teaspoons added sugar	2 teaspoons honey
1 medium-fat protein	1 egg, hard-cooked
1 fat	1½ tablespoons ground flaxseed
	Water

Snack

SMOOTHIE

Blend until smooth.

1 milk	1 cup fat-free milk
1 fruit	½ large banana
2 fat	1 tablespoon peanut butter
	Ice

Lunch

2 bread	1 slice whole-grain bread
	1 ounce croutons
2 vegetable	Salad with romaine lettuce, tomato, grilled eggplant, roasted red pepper
4 lean protein	3 ounces white-meat turkey
	1 ounce fresh mozzarella
3 fat	3 teaspoons olive oil and balsamic vinegar (on salad or as part of roasted vegetables)

Snack

1 bread	3 cups popped light popcorn
1 vegetable	½ cup V8 juice
1 fat	Included (in popcorn)

Dinner

3 bread	1 cup cooked pasta
	1 slice garlic bread
1 milk	1 ounce reduced-fat cheese
1 fruit	12 grapes
3 vegetable	2 cups ratatouille (over pasta)
	Tossed salad with 1 cup lettuce, ¼ cup tomato, ¼ cup cucumber
2 very lean protein	2 ounces lean soy ground meat crumbles (for ratatouille)
3 fat	2 tablespoons reduced-fat dressing
	1 teaspoon butter (for garlic bread)

DAY 3

Pre-Workout Snack

SMOOTHIE

Blend until smooth.

1 milk	1 cup fat-free milk
1 fruit	¹/₂ cup orange juice
2 very lean protein	14 grams whey protein powder
	Ice cubes

Workout

8 teaspoons added sugar	16-ounce sports drink
	Water

Breakfast

2 bread	2 slices whole-wheat bread
1 milk	1 cup fat-free cottage cheese (on bread; sprinkle with brown sugar and cinnamon)
2 fruit	4 ounces freshly squeezed orange juice (with pulp)
	¹/₂ cup sliced pineapple
2 teaspoons added sugar	2 teaspoons brown sugar
1 medium-fat protein	1 egg, cooked sunny-side up in a nonstick pan
1 fat	1¹/₂ tablespoons ground flaxseed
	Water
	Oil-free cooking spray (for egg)

Snack

TRAIL MIX

Chop apricots and almonds. Mix.

1 milk	1 cup fat-free milk
1 fruit	4 halves dried apricots
2 fat	18 almonds

Lunch

2 bread	1 cup rice
2 vegetable	1 cup Chinese vegetables, stir-fried with garlic, onion, fresh ginger
4 lean protein	4 ounces lean pork, stir-fried
3 fat	3 teaspoons oil (for stir-frying)

Snack

1 bread	3 cups fat-free or low-fat microwave popcorn
1 vegetable	1 cup celery
1 fat	½ tablespoon peanut butter (for celery)

Dinner

3 bread	2-inch square of corn bread
	1 cup kidney beans (add to chili)
1 milk	1 ounce fat-free grated cheese (for chili)
1 fruit	½ cup mixed citrus salad
3 vegetable	1 cup chopped cooked tomatoes with chili seasoning
	½ onion, garlic for seasoning
	Tossed salad with 1 cup lettuce, ¼ cup tomato, ¼ cup cucumber
2 very lean protein	Included (in beans)
3 fat	1 slice bacon, cooked very crisp and crumbled into chili
	2 tablespoons reduced-fat dressing for salad
	Included (in corn bread)

DAY 4

Pre-Workout Snack

SMOOTHIE

Blend until smooth.

1 milk	1 cup fat-free milk
1 fruit	½ cup orange juice
2 very lean protein	14 grams whey protein powder
	Ice cubes

Workout

8 teaspoons added sugar	16-ounce sports drink
	Water

Breakfast

2 fruit	2 cup raspberries
1 milk	1 cup fat-free milk (½ cup for French toast)

FRENCH TOAST (*See recipe directions on page 44.*)

2 bread	2 slices whole-wheat bread
2 teaspoons added sugar	2 teaspoons maple syrup
1 medium-fat protein	1 egg
1 fat	1½ tablespoons ground flaxseed
	Water
	Oil-free cooking spray

Snack

1 milk	1 cup fat-free cottage cheese
	No-calorie sweetener to taste (for cottage cheese)
1 fruit	10 pitted, halved cherries
2 fat	10 walnut halves, chopped (add to cottage cheese)

Lunch

FAJITAS

Combine ingredients.

2 bread	⅓ cup Spanish rice
	1 tortilla
2 vegetable	1 cup sautéed onions and peppers
	2 tablespoons salsa
4 lean protein	4 ounces skinless white-meat chicken, grilled with lime juice
3 fat	2 teaspoons olive oil (for cooking)
	2 tablespoons guacamole

Snack

1 bread	½ bagel
1 vegetable	1 cup tomato juice
1 fat	3 tablespoons reduced-fat cream cheese

Dinner

3 bread	1 ounce croutons for salad
	1 cup chicken noodle soup
	4 reduced-fat crackers
1 milk	1 cup fat-free milk
1 fruit	⅛ honeydew
3 vegetable	3 cups salad with lettuce, tomato, cucumber, pepper
2 very lean protein	2 ounces baby shrimp (for salad)
3 fat	8 black or 10 green olives, large
	4 tablespoons reduced-fat dressing

DAY 5

Pre-Workout Snack

SMOOTHIE

Blend until smooth.

1 milk	1 cup fat-free milk
1 fruit	1/2 cup orange juice
2 very lean protein	14 grams whey protein powder
	Ice cubes

Workout

8 teaspoons added sugar	16-ounce sports drink
	Water

Breakfast

2 bread	1 cup quick oats (not instant)
1 milk	1 cup fat-free milk
2 fruit	1 apple, diced
	1 1/4 cups strawberries, sliced
2 teaspoons added sugar	2 teaspoons brown sugar
1 medium-fat protein	1 egg, hard-cooked
1 fat	1 1/2 tablespoons ground flaxseed
	Water

Snack

1 milk	1 cup fat-free milk

TRAIL MIX

Combine ingredients.

1 fruit	3 dates, chopped
2 fat	8 pecan halves

Lunch

2 bread	3/4 cup minestrone soup
	1/2 cup cooked linguini
2 vegetable	Salad with 2 cups romaine lettuce, 1/2 cup tomato, 1/2 cup cucumber
	1/2 cup marinara sauce
4 lean protein	4 ounces shrimp, grilled
3 fat	2 teaspoons olive oil (for cooking)
	2 tablespoons reduced-fat dressing

Snack

NACHOS

Combine ingredients and heat.

1 bread	³/₄ ounce baked snack chips
1 vegetable	¹/₂ cup salsa
1 fat	¹/₂ ounce shredded cheddar cheese

Dinner

3 bread	1 cup chickpeas, ground, seasoned, and pan-fried for falafel
	1 pita
1 milk	¹/₂ cup fat-free yogurt (for falafel)
	¹/₂ cup fat-free milk
1 fruit	¹/₄ cantaloupe
3 vegetable	3 cups tossed salad with cucumber, tomato, sprouts, garlic, onion
2 very lean protein	Included (in chickpeas)
3 fat	Included (in falafel)

DAY 6

Pre-Workout Snack

SMOOTHIE

Blend until smooth.

1 milk	1 cup fat-free milk
1 fruit	¹/₂ cup orange juice
2 very lean protein	14 grams whey protein powder
	Ice cubes

Workout

8 teaspoons added sugar	16-ounce sports drink
	Water

Breakfast

2 bread	2 slices multigrain bread, toasted
1 medium-fat protein	1 egg, scrambled on a nonstick pan
	Oil-free cooking spray (for egg)

SMOOTHIE

Blend until smooth.

1 milk	1 cup fat-free milk
2 fruit	¹/₂ cup orange juice
	1 fresh peach
2 teaspoons added sugar	2 teaspoons honey
1 fat	1¹/₂ tablespoons ground flaxseed or 1 teaspoon flaxseed oil
	Water

Snack

1 milk	1 cup fat-free milk
1 fruit	1/4 cantaloupe
2 fat	40 pistachios

Lunch

2 bread	1 whole-wheat bagel
2 vegetable	1/2 cup carrot sticks
	Onion and tomato
4 lean protein	4 ounces smoked salmon
3 fat	3 tablespoons cream cheese

Snack

1 bread	12 Wheat Thins
1 vegetable	1 cup sliced bell pepper
1 fat	2 tablespoon reduced-fat dressing (for dipping)

Dinner

3 bread	1 ounce croutons
	2-inch square of corn bread
1 milk	1 cup fat-free milk
1 fruit	1/2 sliced mango (for salad)
3 vegetable	3 cups salad with lettuce, tomato, cucumber, pepper
2 very lean protein	2 ounces fresh crab (for salad)
3 fat	4 pecan halves, chopped (for salad)
	4 tablespoons reduced-fat dressing

DAY 7

Pre-Workout Snack

SMOOTHIE

Blend until smooth.

1 milk	1 cup fat-free milk
1 fruit	1/2 cup orange juice
2 very lean protein	14 grams whey protein powder
	Ice cubes

Workout

8 teaspoons added sugar	16-ounce sports drink
	Water

Breakfast

2 bread	1 cup Shredded Wheat
1 milk	1 cup fat-free milk
2 fruit	2 cups raspberries
2 teaspoons added sugar	2 teaspoons sugar
1 medium-fat protein	1 egg, hard-cooked
1 fat	1 1/2 tablespoons ground flaxseed
	Water

Snack

Combine ingredients.

1 milk	1 cup fat-free plain yogurt
1 fruit	1 apple, diced
2 fat	10 walnut halves, chopped
	Cinnamon and no-calorie sweetener to taste

Lunch

2 bread	1 small multigrain roll
	3 ounces baked yam
2 vegetable	Sliced tomato and lettuce (for sandwich)
	1/2 cup radishes, celery, carrots
4 lean protein	3 ounces dark-meat chicken, grilled with lime juice
	1 ounce Swiss cheese
3 fat	3 tablespoons regular ranch dressing (for dipping)
	1 teaspoon butter (for yam)

Snack

1 bread	1 tortilla
1 vegetable	1/2 cup salsa
1 fat	1/8 avocado

Dinner

3 bread	2 slices rye bread
	1/2 cup pasta salad
1 milk	1 cup fat-free milk
1 fruit	3/4 cup fresh pineapple
3 vegetable	1 cup coleslaw
	1/2 cup chopped vegetables (cucumbers, carrots, onions; mix into tuna)
2 very lean protein	2 ounces tuna in water, drained
3 fat	2 tablespoons reduced-fat mayonnaise

THE NO-STRESS MEAL PLAN

IF YOU'RE FEELING STRESSED OUT, YOU MAY BE DRINKING TOO MUCH CAFFEINE, eating too much sugar and refined foods, and not eating enough fruits and vegetables. To calm down, increase your consumption of whey protein and dairy, consume more carbs during the day to stimulate serotonin release, stick with carbs that have a low to moderate glycemic index, avoid caffeine, and increase your consumption of antioxidants (like blueberries, strawberries, and spinach), B vitamins, nuts, and nut butters.

Daily Assumptions*†

2,500 calories
281 grams carbohydrates
159 grams protein
84 grams fat

Daily Breakdown*†

8 bread
5 fruit
4 milk
3 teaspoons added sugar
6 vegetable
6 very lean protein
6 lean protein
1 medium-fat protein
8 fat

Note: Occasionally, a fat-free product, like mustard or cooking spray, is included on the menus. These do not count toward your daily breakdown but should not be overused.

*Use every day.

† Based on a 185-pound man.

THE MENU

DAY 1

Breakfast

2 bread	1 cup Shredded Wheat
1 milk	1 cup fat-free milk
2 fruit	1/2 large banana
	1 cup blueberries
1 medium-fat protein	1 egg, scrambled on a nonstick pan
1 very lean protein	2 egg whites, scrambled with whole egg
1 fat	1 1/2 tablespoons ground flaxseed
	Tea with no-calorie sweetener
	Water
	Oil-free cooking spray (for eggs)

Snack

1 bread	1/2 whole-wheat pita
1 vegetable	Romaine lettuce, mushrooms, other veggies
1 lean protein	1 ounce part-skim mozzarella
1 fat	10 peanuts

Lunch

2 bread	2 slices whole-grain bread
3 very lean protein	3 ounces sliced turkey
2 vegetable	Salad with 2 cups romaine lettuce, 1/2 cup tomato, 1/2 cup cucumber
2 fat	1 tablespoon vinaigrette (for salad)
	8 black olives
	Dijon mustard (for sandwich)

Dinner

3 bread	1 large sweet potato baked
1 milk	1 cup fat-free milk
3 vegetable	1½ cups steamed asparagus
4 lean protein	4 ounces salmon, grilled
3 fat	1 tablespoon each olive oil and lemon juice (for asparagus)

Pre-Workout Snack

1 milk	1 cup fat-free milk
1 fruit	1 apple, sliced
1 lean protein	1 tablespoon peanut butter
1 fat	Included (peanut butter)

Workout

Water

Post-Workout

SMOOTHIE

Blend until smooth. Drink 15 to 30 minutes after your workout.

2 fruit	⅓ cup frozen strawberries
	½ cup mango
	½ cup orange juice
1 milk	1 cup fat-free milk
3 teaspoons added sugar	1 tablespoon honey
2 very lean protein	14 grams whey protein powder

DAY 2

Breakfast

Combine yogurt, fruit, and honey. Combine muffin and egg for sandwich.

2 bread	1 whole-wheat English muffin
1 milk	1 cup fat-free unsweetened yogurt
	No-calorie sweetener (for yogurt)
2 fruit	2½ cups fresh strawberries
1 medium-fat protein	1 egg, hard-cooked
1 very lean protein	2 eggs, hard-cooked (discard yolks)
1 fat	1½ tablespoons ground flaxseed
	Water

Snack

1 bread	$\frac{1}{2}$ cup soy nuts
1 vegetable	1 cup celery sticks
1 lean protein	Included (in soy nuts)
1 fat	1 tablespoon salad dressing (for dipping)

Lunch

2 bread	1 slice whole-grain bread
	1 ounce croutons
2 vegetable	Large salad with romaine lettuce, tomato, grilled eggplant, roasted red pepper
3 very lean protein	3 ounces skinless white-meat chicken, grilled with lime juice
2 fat	2 tablespoons reduced-fat dressing
	1 teaspoon olive oil (for roasted vegetables)

Dinner

3 bread	1 cup cooked pasta
	1 slice garlic bread
1 milk	1 ounce reduced-fat cheese
3 vegetable	2 cups ratatouille (over pasta)
	Salad with 1 cup lettuce, $\frac{1}{4}$ cup tomato, $\frac{1}{4}$ cup cucumber
	2 tablespoons fat-free dressing
4 lean protein	4 ounces lean ground beef
3 fat	1 teaspoon butter (for garlic bread)
	2 teaspoons olive oil (for cooking ratatouille)

Pre-Workout Snack

1 milk	1 cup fat-free milk
1 fruit	1 apple, sliced
1 lean protein	1 tablespoon peanut butter
1 fat	Included (in peanut butter)

Workout

Water

Post-Workout

SMOOTHIE

Blend until smooth. Drink 15 to 30 minutes after your workout.

2 fruit	$\frac{1}{3}$ cup frozen strawberries
	$\frac{1}{2}$ large banana
	$\frac{1}{2}$ cup orange juice
1 milk	1 cup fat-free milk
3 teaspoons added sugar	1 tablespoon honey
2 very lean protein	14 grams whey protein powder

DAY 3

Breakfast

2 bread	2 slices whole-wheat bread
1 milk	1 cup fat-free cottage cheese (on bread; sprinkle with no-calorie sweetener and cinnamon)
	No-calorie sweetener
2 fruit	4 ounces freshly squeezed orange juice (with pulp)
	$^1/_2$ cup sliced pineapple
1 medium-fat protein	1 egg, cooked sunny-side up in a nonstick pan
1 very lean protein	2 egg whites, added to sunny-side up egg
1 fat	$1^1/_2$ tablespoons ground flaxseed
	Water
	Oil-free cooking spray (for eggs)

Snack

1 bread	$^1/_2$ bagel
1 vegetable	Tomato, sprouts
1 lean protein	1 ounce Swiss cheese
1 fat	1 tablespoon sunflower seeds

Lunch

2 bread	1 cup rice
2 vegetable	1 cup Chinese vegetables, stir-fried with garlic, onion, fresh ginger
3 very lean protein	3 ounces scallops, stir-fried
2 fat	2 teaspoons oil (for stir-frying)

Dinner

3 bread	2-inch square of corn bread
	1 cup kidney beans (add to chili)
1 milk	1 ounce fat-free grated cheese (for chili)
3 vegetable	1 cup chopped cooked tomatoes with chili seasoning, $^1/_2$ onion, garlic for seasoning
	Salad with 2 cups romaine lettuce, $^1/_2$ cup tomato, $^1/_2$ cup cucumber
4 lean protein	2 ounces soy crumbles (add to chili)
	Included (in beans)
3 fat	2 slices bacon, cooked very crisp and crumbled into chili
	Included (in corn bread)

Pre-Workout Snack

1 milk	1 cup fat-free milk
1 fruit	1 apple, sliced
1 lean protein	1 tablespoon peanut butter
1 fat	Included (in peanut butter)

Workout

Water

Post-Workout

SMOOTHIE

Blend until smooth. Drink 15 to 30 minutes after your workout.

2 fruit	$^{1}/_{3}$ cup frozen peaches
	$^{1}/_{2}$ cup mango
	$^{1}/_{2}$ cup orange juice
1 milk	1 cup fat-free milk
3 teaspoons added sugar	1 tablespoon honey
2 very lean protein	14 grams whey protein powder

DAY 4

Breakfast

2 fruit	2 cups raspberries
1 milk	1 cup fat-free milk ($^{1}/_{2}$ cup for French toast)

FRENCH TOAST (*See recipe directions on page 44.*)

2 bread	2 slices whole-wheat bread
1 medium-fat protein	1 egg
1 very lean protein	2 egg whites
1 fat	$1^{1}/_{2}$ tablespoons ground flaxseed
	1 tablespoon no-calorie maple-flavored syrup
	Water
	Oil-free cooking spray

Snack

1 bread	12 Wheat Thins
1 vegetable	1 cup sliced bell pepper
1 lean protein	$^{1}/_{4}$ cup cottage cheese
1 fat	8 black olives
	No-calorie sweetener to taste

Lunch

FAJITAS

Combine ingredients.

2 bread	$^1/_3$ cup Spanish rice
	1 tortilla
2 vegetable	1 cup sautéed onions and peppers
	2 tablespoons salsa
3 very lean protein	3 ounces skinless white-meat chicken, grilled with lime juice
2 fat	1 teaspoon olive oil (for cooking)
	$^1/_8$ avocado

Dinner

3 bread	1 ounce croutons (for salad)
	1 cup chicken noodle soup
	4 crackers
1 milk	1 cup fat-free milk
3 vegetable	3 cups salad with lettuce, tomato, cucumber, pepper
4 lean protein	4 ounces swordfish, grilled with ginger and scallions
3 fat	8 black or 10 green olives, large
	2 tablespoons dressing

Pre-Workout Snack

1 milk	1 cup fat-free milk
1 fruit	1 sliced apple
1 lean protein	1 tablespoon peanut butter
1 fat	Included (in peanut butter)

Workout

Water

Post-Workout

SMOOTHIE

Blend until smooth. Drink 15 to 30 minutes after your workout.

2 fruit	$^1/_3$ cup frozen strawberries
	$^1/_2$ cup mango
	$^1/_2$ cup orange juice
1 milk	1 cup fat-free milk
3 teaspoons added sugar	1 tablespoon honey
2 very lean protein	14 grams whey protein powder

DAY 5

Breakfast

2 bread	1 cup quick oats (not instant)
1 milk	1 cup fat-free milk
2 fruit	1 apple, diced
	1¼ cups sliced strawberries
	No-calorie sweetener
1 medium-fat protein	1 egg, hard-cooked
1 very lean protein	2 eggs, hard-cooked (discard yolks)
1 fat	1½ tablespoons ground flaxseed
	Water

Snack

1 bread	¾ ounce baked tortillas
1 vegetable	½ cup salsa
1 lean protein	1 ounce cheddar cheese
1 fat	Included (in cheese)

Lunch

2 bread	¾ cup minestrone soup
	½ cup cooked linguini
2 vegetable	Salad with 1 cup lettuce, ¼ cup tomato, ¼ cup cucumber, fat-free dressing
	½ cup marinara sauce
3 very lean protein	3 ounces shrimp, grilled
2 fat	2 teaspoons olive oil (for cooking shrimp)

Dinner

3 bread	1 large pita
	1 ounce croutons
1 milk	½ cup fat-free yogurt (with dill, for lamb)
	½ cup fat-free milk
3 vegetable	Salad with 2 cups romaine lettuce, ½ cup tomato, ½ cup cucumber
	Garlic, onion (for sandwich)
4 lean protein	4 ounces lean lamb, grilled with lime juice
3 fat	3 tablespoons vinaigrette

Pre-Workout Snack

1 milk	1 cup fat-free milk
1 fruit	1 apple, sliced
1 lean protein	1 tablespoon peanut butter
1 fat	Included (in peanut butter)

Workout

Water

Post-Workout

SMOOTHIE

Blend until smooth. Drink 15 to 30 minutes after your workout.

2 fruit	$^1/_3$ cup frozen strawberries
	$^1/_2$ cup frozen raspberries
	$^1/_2$ cup orange juice
1 milk	1 cup fat-free milk
3 teaspoons added sugar	1 tablespoon honey
2 very lean protein	14 grams whey protein powder

DAY 6

Breakfast

2 bread	2 slices multigrain toast
1 medium-fat protein	1 egg, scrambled on a nonstick pan
1 very lean protein	2 egg whites, scrambled with whole egg
	Oil-free cooking spray (for eggs)

SMOOTHIE

Blend until smooth.

1 milk	1 cup fat-free milk
2 fruit	$^1/_2$ cup orange juice
	1 fresh peach
	No-calorie sweetener
1 fat	$1^1/_2$ tablespoons ground flaxseed or 1 teaspoon flaxseed oil

Snack

1 bread	1 slice whole-wheat bread
1 vegetable	Tomato, lettuce, mustard
1 lean protein	1 ounce lean ham
1 fat	1 ounce Swiss cheese

Lunch

2 bread	1 whole-wheat bagel	
2 vegetable	1/2 cup carrot sticks	
	Onion, tomato	
3 very lean protein	3 ounces smoked salmon	
2 fat	2 tablespoons cream cheese	

Dinner

3 bread	2 slices rye bread
	1/2 cup pasta salad
1 milk	1 cup fat-free milk
3 vegetable	1 cup coleslaw
	1/2 cup chopped vegetables (cucumbers, carrots, onions; mix into tuna)
4 lean protein	4 ounces tuna in olive oil, drained
3 fat	2 tablespoons mayonnaise (for tuna)
	Included (in coleslaw, pasta salad)

Pre-Workout Snack

1 milk	1 cup fat-free milk
1 fruit	1 apple, sliced
1 lean protein	1 tablespoon peanut butter
1 fat	Included (in peanut butter)

Workout

Water

Post-Workout

SMOOTHIE

Blend until smooth. Drink 15 to 30 minutes after your workout.

2 fruit	1/3 cup frozen strawberries
	1/2 large banana
	1/2 cup orange juice
1 milk	1 cup fat-free milk
3 teaspoons added sugar	1 tablespoon honey
2 very lean protein	14 grams whey protein powder

DAY 7

Breakfast

2 bread	1 cup Shredded Wheat
1 milk	1 cup fat-free milk
2 fruit	2 cups raspberries
	No-calorie sweetener
1 medium-fat protein	1 egg, hard-cooked
1 very lean protein	2 eggs, hard-cooked (discard yolks)
1 fat	1½ tablespoons ground flaxseed
	Water

Snack

1 bread	1 tortilla
1 vegetable	Sliced veggies
	½ cup salsa
1 lean protein	1 ounce shredded Mexican cheese
1 fat	Included (in cheese)

Lunch

2 bread	1 small multigrain roll
	3 ounces baked yam
2 vegetable	Sliced tomato, lettuce (for sandwich)
	½ cup radishes, celery, carrots
3 very lean protein	3 ounces grilled chicken
2 fat	2 tablespoons low-fat ranch dressing (for dipping)
	1 teaspoon olive oil (for grilling chicken)

Dinner

3 bread	3-inch square of corn bread
	1 ounce croutons
1 milk	½ cup fat-free milk
	1 ounce fat-free shredded cheese
3 vegetable	3 cups salad with lettuce, tomato, cucumber, pepper
4 lean protein	4 ounces salmon, poached
3 fat	2 tablespoons low-fat Caesar dressing
	Included (in cheese, corn bread)

Pre-Workout Snack

1 milk	1 cup fat-free milk
1 fruit	1 apple, sliced
1 lean protein	1 tablespoon peanut butter
1 fat	Included (in peanut butter)

Workout

Water

Post-Workout

SMOOTHIE

Blend until smooth. Drink 15 to 30 minutes after your workout.

2 fruit	$^{1}/_{3}$ cup frozen melon
	$^{1}/_{2}$ cup mango
	$^{1}/_{2}$ cup orange juice
1 milk	1 cup fat-free milk
3 teaspoons added sugar	1 tablespoon honey
2 very lean protein	14 grams whey protein powder

CHAPTER THREE

Food and Weight Loss

FOLLOW OUR SIMPLE RULES TO SUCCESS
AND YOU'LL SHED FAT FAST

The 1990s have been dubbed the "The Bubble Decade," a reference to the once-inflated share prices of technology stocks. Alas, it applies equally to America's expanding waistline. Now the bubble has burst, and companies across the nation are shrinking to survive. Perhaps it's time to jettison the excess baggage you've been carrying around your waistline as well?

As many of those corporations have learned, getting lean and mean again usually requires going back to basics. Whether you're obese, somewhat overweight, or searching for traces of the six-pack abs that faded a few Coronas back, shaping up means rediscovering exercise and better eating. This chapter is your map back.

So how did we get lost in the first place? To paraphrase President Clinton, it's the calories, stupid. Thanks largely to modern food-processing technology, way too many calories are way too accessible to way too many people. The percentage of U.S. men categorized as obese nearly doubled—to 20 percent—between 1991 and 2000, according to the

National Center for Chronic Disease Prevention and Health Promotion. A recent National Health and Nutrition survey says that 31 percent of all Americans can now be classified as obese. (Expand that cohort to include the merely overweight, and the percentage balloons to more than 60.) Grimmer still is this number: More than 90 percent of the people who diet away excess pounds gain them back later.

The problem isn't lack of information—there's certainly no shortage of that. Rather, it's that the smorgasbord of diets and advice inundating the market has had little impact on the gut of America. Many of those books are marketing driven—they use hooks and extreme programs, creating diets that are simplistic and one-dimensional. This hook-driven approach may sell books, but it doesn't give you the information that you need to really lose the weight and keep it off. My approach may not be sexy, and it certainly isn't a simple, quick fix. Yet I can promise you something that other diets cannot: The advice you are about to read is based on real science conducted in real labs on real people who lost weight and kept it off. It's the stuff that works.

Before you learn how to lose weight, however, you first must know how your body works from the inside out and how you can use that information to your advantage. Keep reading.

Metabolism 101

Here's the simplest part. To lose weight, you must create an *energy imbalance* by consuming fewer calories than you burn. Of course, things are a bit more complex than that. Eat too few calories and you risk slowing your metabolism, for one. Eat the right types of calories and you can speed up your metabolism, coaxing your body to waste calories. Eat the wrong types of calories and you'll feel hungrier on more food.

So, as you can see, weight loss is not as simple as cutting all of your meal sizes in half and calling it a day. To understand why, you must understand how your metabolism works; and to understand that, you must understand some basic terms.

■ **Metabolism.** This often-used but seldom-understood term refers to the chemical processes occurring within a living cell or organism that are necessary for the maintenance of life. In humans, much of that activity involves the breakdown of materials (i.e., calories) to provide the energy needed to keep that organism's systems functioning; the remainder involves the synthesis of materials necessary for life.

■ **Metabolic rate.** The rate at which energy is produced in your body. It's how much energy you burn per unit of work.

■ **Basal metabolic rate.** This is the amount of energy it takes to power your body's involuntary processes, such as your heartbeat and kidney function. In other words, your basal metabolic rate equals the number of calories your body burns when you are lying on your back in a near-catatonic state. By providing you with enough energy to keep the nerves in your brain firing, it gives you enough to keep your lungs pumping, your heart beating, your organs functioning, and your immune system up and running.

■ **Resting metabolic rate.** People move, of course, so they burn more calories than their basal metabolic rate. Your basal metabolic rate plus the extra few calories you burn by getting up in the morning, going to the bathroom, and lying down again equals your resting metabolic rate. Resting metabolic rate only slightly exceeds your basal metabolic rate. Added to your resting metabolic rate are the calories that you expend for activity. The more you move, the more energy you burn. Sitting at a computer burns little; running a marathon burns a lot.

■ **Thermic effect of food.** Your body burns calories as it digests, absorbs, and processes food. Collectively, this is called the thermic effect of food. This expenditure is considerable, accounting for as much as 10 percent of the energy you burn in a day. Some foods take more energy for your body to break down than others, so gravitating toward foods with a high thermic effect can help boost your overall metabolism.

■ **Leptin.** This protein circulates in your bloodstream and, like the hormone insulin, is a key hormone in the weight-management equation. Leptin regulates your food intake as well as your body's energy expenditure. When cells in your brain sense a rise in leptin, they signal other parts of your nervous system to turn down your appetite and turn up your metabolism. When researchers inject animal subjects with leptin, the critters lose weight through a suppression of their food intake and an increase in their metabolic rate and energy expenditure.

What's happening in the animals—and perhaps in humans, as well—is that as the body senses it's getting fatter, it cranks up the fat-burning process in response. Normally, leptin helps keep the body in a blissful state of homeostasis. If you eat a few too many calories, leptin rises, causing your metabolic rate to heat up and burn those calories off. Trouble is, in some people, the brain can become less responsive to increasing levels of leptin. So even though fat cells are filling up, the brain doesn't react.

■ **Body composition.** A number of experts say that body composition (your ratio of lean tissue, such as muscle and bones, to fat) is in fact the most important predictor of metabolic rate. Particularly important is muscle, where energy is produced. Even when your muscles are not actively moving, they are burning calories as they break down and rebuild proteins. That's why the more muscle you have, the easier it is to lose fat. Whether you're sleeping, watching the Tour de France on TV, or pedaling in the race next to Lance Armstrong, the more muscle you have, the more calories you burn.

Your body composition has a huge impact on metabolic rate, and you can dictate your body composition to a large extent—that's what a lot of this book is about.

Many other factors determine your rate of energy expenditure. Your gender has an influence; so do age, height, weight, and genetics. Yes, at least some of your metabolism is hardwired inside your DNA. I often see evidence of this in my private practice: I meet one guy who's eating 3,500 calories a day, and then I meet another guy eating 2,500—and they look exactly the same. When it comes to metabolism, some guys are naturally faster and some guys are naturally slower, for reasons having to do with pituitary production and other primitive controls located in the brain stem.

Why Diets Almost Always Fail

Nutritionists agree that most diets aren't worth the paper they're printed on. They realize that the key to losing weight is adopting a sound, sustainable eating plan and then sticking with it, rather than opting for some wacko quick fix.

Diets don't last. The problem with virtually all diets is the short-term mindset into which they feed. Most guys approach diets as an all-or-nothing proposition. Rather than making small, even incremental changes in lifestyle that can last a lifetime, diets encourage you to turn your life inside out for two weeks or so. Yet once those two weeks are over and you return to your old habits, guess what? Your body returns to its former state as well. If there's a rule of thumb to be had in this regard, it's that small changes last and big ones don't. Saying that you'll change everything you're doing wrong starting on Monday morning and straight-line it from there might sound impressive—and earn you some pats on the back—but it doesn't change your underlying behavior patterns. It's the slow, steady route that ultimately leads to success.

Diets make you hungry. Diets also typically treat fat loss as a function of nutrition only, when training is equally important. The diet world is all about tearing down, and sports nutrition is all about building up. In the *Power Food* program, you'll lose weight by creating a calorie deficit—your body will burn more calories than you eat. You'll create that deficit, however, mostly through training and not through drastic dieting. The calories you burn in the weight room added to the metabolism boost you get from muscle growth will kick your body into fat-burning mode—without making you hungry.

Diets make you tired. A chronic problem with diets is that so many of them are simply too low in calories. Because they don't provide enough energy for you to do your workouts and accomplish everything else you need to do in a day, they're a short-term solution at best. Even when weight-loss programs incorporate exercise—and, astonishingly, many don't—they typically ask you to eat like a gerbil and then train like a hamster by running or cycling endlessly in place. You may shed a few pounds in the short run, but you'll also forsake muscle, and the resulting metabolic downshift will soon take you back to square one. Whether it's being done on a treadmill, a stationary bike, or a squeaky metal cylinder, endless cardio performed on restricted calories is a road to nowhere, literally and figuratively.

This is especially true if you're following one of the ultra-low-carb diets that are so popular now. Carbohydrates are the primary energy source for physical activity, and decades of research has shown that low-carb diets don't adequately support strenuous physical activity or athletic performance for extended periods of time. In contrast, a diet moderate in carbs will supply enough energy for the average Joe to stay active and still burn fat. Endurance exercise requires more carbohydrates than strength training does, but in neither case will training be optimized without sufficient carbs.

Diets cannibalize your muscle. Diets also tend to pay too little attention to supporting muscle mass during periods of caloric restriction. This is important for more than just aesthetic reasons. As I've already discussed, when you lose muscle, your basal metabolic rate drops, and you don't burn as many calories.

Most guys try to burn off the fat first and then build the muscle. To do that, you have to lower your calories so far that you don't have the energy to train hard in the gym. You burn more muscle than fat, lowering your metabolic rate and setting the stage for weight gain. On the other hand, if you follow the *Power Food* plan, you'll train hard, build muscle, burn fat, and keep the fat off forever because you have raised your metabolic rate.

The *Power Food* Fat-Loss Rules

Now that you know what doesn't work, here are the 20 *Power Food* keys to successful fat loss. Drum roll, please.

1. **Fat is less important than calories.** You may have heard that your body lays down fat whenever it has more calories than it needs to satisfy its energy requirements, and that it deposits fat calories more easily than it deposits calories from protein or carbs. Fat also has twice as many calories as protein and carbs do per unit volume—9 versus 4 per gram. So if you're going to cut out an ounce of something from your diet, fat gives you the best bang for your buck.

   That said, you could double your fat consumption, or halve it, and still lose weight. Calories offer no such latitude—they constitute the

---

Stealthy Eating

If you're a reasonably health-conscious guy and you eat out now and then, you know full well that, nutritionally speaking, ordering at a restaurant is basically a crapshoot. The key, then, is to make sound ordering decisions. Following these six recommendations would be a good starting point.

- When ordering pasta, choose the red sauce over a white alternative.
- When ordering a steak, choose a lean cut such as sirloin.
- Make your appetizer a large salad. Request low-fat dressing on the side.
- Split your dessert with your dinner companion. Doing so can save you in the neighborhood of 300 calories and 20 grams of fat.
- Keep your plate balanced with a steak, chicken breast, or other protein source; a steamed veggie; a salad; and a sweet potato or rice.
- Go easy on the bread basket, or you'll be sporting one yourself.

bottom-line number that will determine how much weight you gain or, in this case, lose. At the end of the day, to burn fat and shift the energy balance away from fat accumulation, you need to consume fewer calories than you expend. One pound of body fat equals 3,500 calories, so if your goal is to lose 20 pounds, you need to create a deficit of 70,000 calories over time.

Also, all fats aren't created equal when it comes to fat storage. Remember fish oils and omega-3 fats, those healthy fats I wrote about at length in chapter 2? Well, they may play a role in downshifting the machinery of fat building. So don't throw the baby out with the bathwater. Focus on eating healthy fats such as nuts, seeds, nut butters, olives, olive oil, avocados, and fatty fish, and lay off the Snickers bars and Cinnabons. With a little calorie control, your abs and your arteries will both benefit.

2. **Limit your intake of processed foods.** The over-processing of food may be the most insidious contributor to America's bulging waistline. Not only does it remove vitamins, minerals, phytochemicals, fiber, and other stuff that's good for you, it also replaces them with fat and carbs like sugars. As a result, they'll be absorbed into your bloodstream rapid-fire. As I've already discussed, high-glycemic-index carbs trigger a heavy release of the anabolic hormone insulin, which quickly lowers blood sugar, making you feel hungry and tired. And if you're not a serious athlete needing to store those sugar calories for muscle fuel, you'll put them into fat storage faster than you can say "spare tire."

I recommend you consume your carbs in the form of whole grains, vegetables, fruits, beans, nuts, and seeds, which allow for timed release into the bloodstream without the overbearing insulin response. If you're not sure whether a food falls into the highly processed category, here are some hints.

- Just about all highly processed foods come in either a box or a bag and are often shrink-wrapped as well.
- The ingredients label will probably read more like your high school chemistry homework assignments than something edible.
- Processed foods don't exist in nature; there's no tree that grows Cheetos or Oreo cookies, for example. These foods had to be processed to assume their current form, and to manufacture them, companies need to add things that otherwise wouldn't be there.

3. **Eat smaller, more-frequent meals.** "Wait a minute! Here I am trying to lose fat—and you're telling me I can eat more?" Slow down, hot shot. Not more—more *often*. Take what you currently ingest, and along with making the other dietary adjustments recommended here, divide that consumption among five to seven meals a day.

The goal here is twofold: to keep your metabolism humming along, and to prevent the sort of intense hunger pangs that bring willpower to its knees. Once you get really, really hungry, you probably won't be very selective. You'll feel like you need to eat quickly because you're starving, causing you to outrace the "fullness" signal that would normally get transmitted to your stomach. So not only will you eat pork rinds that have been sitting in the back of your cupboard since 1976, you'll eat the whole bag. (Note: See "Calories In, Calories Out" on page 15 for more info on this.)

Excluding sleep, you should almost never go longer than 4 hours without eating. However, an even better interval is to eat every 2½ to 3 hours—literally like clockwork. If you're eating three times a day, a good way to start changing your frequency is to take roughly the same amount of food and spread it over four or five meals.

When you eat consistently throughout the day, your muscles will have plenty of fuel for exercise, wherever it falls in your schedule. Eating at shorter intervals will also help flatten out excessive rises and dips in your blood sugar. As an added bonus, you burn calories every time you eat and digest food, so grazing, as it's called, helps you chisel off a few extra calories versus consuming the same amount of food in larger, less frequent chunks.

4. **Pump up your protein consumption.** Diet fads are often like old girlfriends: They can be hard to shake, but sometimes the one that you thought was nutty turns out to be a princess instead.

Although I don't promote super-low-carb/high-protein diets, this eating approach has taught us all a few important facts about protein and its importance in weight loss.

For instance, you need protein to build the muscles that boost your metabolism. When you restrict calories, your body will seek out protein to meet those energy demands unmet by carbs and fat. This siphoning-off process reduces the amount of protein available for muscle building. The effect will be magnified if your calorie restriction targets carbs especially (which is why super-low-carbohydrate diets aren't the way to go). To provide an adequate amount of protein for all of the body's important functions, you need to consume more protein. How much more? That

depends on the source of the calorie deficit and the diet plan that you're following. If you don't exercise but you're cutting calories in an attempt to lose weight, you need to eat about 60 percent more protein than someone who's not trying to lose weight. A study conducted in Japan in 1987 estimated that on an energy-restricted diet, sedentary guys need to eat 0.6 grams per pound of body weight per day to achieve protein balance.

If you're a vegetarian, you'll need to eat even more. By the way, vegetarians also need more protein when they're dieting. The plant proteins on which they rely are considered lower-quality proteins because they're less-complete than animal proteins. Except for soy, all plant proteins lack adequate levels of at least one amino acid, and as a result, they must be combined with complementary plant proteins. All else being equal, vegetarians should consume up to 10 percent more protein than meat eaters should. They'll need about 0.66 grams of protein per pound of body weight. (Remember, this research is on sedentary guys. If you're exercising, expect to eat more.)

5. **Trade fatty protein for lean.** If you've got more body fat than you'd like, I'll bet the farm that the culprit isn't lean protein sources such as egg

A DAY'S WORTH OF PROTEIN

A TYPICAL GUY (185 POUNDS) NEEDS TO EAT ABOUT 181 GRAMS OF PROTEIN in a day to build and maintain muscle mass and lose fat. Here's one way to get it.

Food	Protein (grams)	Food	Protein (grams)
3 cups fat-free milk	24	6-ounce chicken breast	42
1 whole egg	7	6 ounces salmon	42
3 egg whites	14	30 grams whey protein powder	30
½ cup cottage cheese	14	**Total**	**181**
2 tablespoons peanut butter	8		

whites, chicken, turkey, and lean red meat. Most guys simply don't sit in front of *Monday Night Football* and gorge themselves silly with skinless turkey breast meat.

In addition to helping build muscle, lean protein helps stoke the fat-burning fires—its thermogenic effect is 20 to 30 percent, compared with an anemic 3 to 12 percent for carbs. If you don't have a blender and some protein powder already, buy them. When you crave a cheeseburger, fried chicken, or something else loaded with saturated fat, reach for a protein shake instead.

6. **Try to spread your protein consumption throughout the day.** To capitalize on the thermogenic effect of high-protein foods, consume them frequently throughout the day. This allows for the most efficient absorption of protein and helps maintain high levels of internal energy production to promote weight loss.

7. **Control your portions by emphasizing low-energy-density foods.** The National Weight Control Registry is a database that looks retrospectively at people who have successfully achieved and then maintained weight loss. When you sift through the data, two prerequisites for successful weight loss recur: on the expenditure side, exercise; and on the consumption side, portion control.

To control your portion sizes, favor foods that are low in something called energy density. The term refers to calories per gram, and the higher the energy density, the easier it is to overeat—more calories are packed into a smaller portion. Lower-energy-density foods include things like fruits and vegetables; higher-energy-density foods tend to be high in fat and sugar. (Energy density is different from nutrient density; vegetables, for example, have a low energy density but a high nutrient density.)

8. **Don't be an extremist concerning fats and carbs.** On the one hand, you have the extreme diet advocated by the late Dr. Robert Atkins, which is very, very low in carbohydrates. On the other, you have the Dean Ornish extreme, where fewer than 10 percent of calories come from fat. Who's right? The data suggest that the ideal probably lies somewhere between the two.

Carbs provide the lion's share of the fuel for your workouts. If you cut carbs to the point where you can no longer sustain the desired intensity of your workouts—which is exactly what would happen if you followed some of these ultra-low-carb diets that are all the rage now—you'll be shooting yourself in the foot.

Eat mixed meals, such as the ones outlined in the meal plans throughout this book, and at the end of the day, your diet will be balanced, which is what you're after. Eating protein, fat, or both with carbs slows the latter's absorption, preventing your blood sugar and insulin from going on roller coaster rides. If you have a bagel for breakfast, for example, find one with some whole grain in it or some seeds on top, and spread some all-natural peanut butter on it.

9. **Reduce your liquid calories.** I often hear from clients who complain, "I hardly eat anything, yet I'm still fat." Often, once I do a little detective work, I realize they are telling the truth. They truly are not eating much, but they are drinking a lot. The calories in sodas and fruit juices—not to mention beer—add up quickly, often more quickly than most people realize. Liquid calories reach well beyond beverages, however. Salad dressings, sauces, and spreads account for more unconscious calorie consumption.

Your goal, then, should be to replace soft drinks with water, limit your intake of fruit juices, replace dressings with low-fat versions or something else entirely, and forego sweeteners altogether. Just switching from a regular 12-ounce Coke to the diet version can make a huge difference calorie-wise. A guy who drinks 10 Cokes a week can save 1,000 calories during that period just by switching to 5 regulars and 5 diets. That's one-third of a pound right there. Just drinking water with your popcorn instead of having a belly-buster-size soda can save you an additional 500 calories.

Don't booze it up, either. Drinking alcohol is a surefire way to add inches to your waist (they don't call it a beer belly for nothing). Study after study has correlated increasing alcohol consumption with increasing waist measurements in men and women. Or you can just look at your Uncle Elmer, who kills a six-pack every weekend and hasn't seen his shoes since LBJ was president.

10. **Water yourself.** Water is another key component of weight management. In a phrase, drink up. In fact, most guys who have managed to lose weight successfully—meaning once off, the fat stayed off—will tell you that they used water as an appetite suppressant. In fact, the well-known psychologist Kelly Brownell, Ph.D., who has been studying weight loss for years, developed a behavioral-modification program for weight loss that lists drinking water among its 10 best strategies.

Water does more than just make you feel full, however. As a healthy, noncaloric beverage, it provides a great alternative to the two or three cans of soda a day that many guys drink. That's a great way to excise a couple hundred empty calories out of your diet.

Water also flushes out your internal systems. Most environmental contaminants are fat soluble, so, the reasoning goes, even when they enter the human body, they're benign. They just go into fat cells and sit there. On a weight-loss diet, however, you're mobilizing those fat stores and marching them into your bloodstream, where they need to go before being passed out of the body. The toxins reentering your bloodstream may have been sitting in storage, dormant, for a decade or more. Some of them—DDT and PCBs, for example—may actually slow your metabolism. You want to flush these out ASAP, and water is the key to doing just that.

When your body is well hydrated, it also helps your kidneys and liver go full tilt in processing fat and other toxins. In contrast, when you're dehydrated, your liver has to work overtime to help the kidneys with detoxification, diminishing its ability to remove fat. Finally, when you drink plenty of water, your cells stay well hydrated, and cells that are well hydrated—or volumized, as the process is often called—promote more-efficient and more-effective protein metabolism. Because you're trying to build muscle while you lose fat, the last thing you want to do is slow down protein metabolism. If you're dehydrated, it will.

11. **Eat more fiber.** Eating 30 to 40 grams daily will keep you feeling fuller longer than you would otherwise. Not only does fiber occupy a lot of room in your stomach, but water-soluble fiber, the type found in oatmeal, apples, and beans, also absorbs some fat from your digestive tract, moving it through your system quickly enough to diminish your body's ability to digest fat. Even if we're talking about only an extra gram or two of fat every day, that's another 9 to 18 calories that get eliminated along with the fiber you're eating.

Fiber does more than escort excess calories out of your gut and help you to eat less. It also gives food a crisp, crunchy texture and a great mouth feel. When you're hankering for something crunchy and you think you want potato chips or Fritos, try sprinkling some salt on a carrot or a piece of celery instead. Nowadays people treat saltshakers like they're radioactive—

Soy Wonders

You've probably heard mixed reviews on soy and its place in a man's diet. Two things are important where weight loss and soy are concerned:

1. Because soybeans are high in fiber, they slow digestion and help control your insulin response. What's more, they enhance fat oxidation by stimulating the release of the hormone glucagon in a way that animal sources don't.

2. Nonvegetarians, who are trying to lose fat while holding onto muscle, should not rely heavily on soy to satisfy their protein needs. Even though soy has a complete distribution of essential amino acids to support health and growth in general, research is beginning to show that, when eaten as the sole source of complete protein, soy doesn't support muscle building and repair as well as animal protein does. Some soy is great, but animal protein will help boost your results.

it's almost taboo to see one on a table—and that's unnecessary. Unless you are a guy with hypertension (high blood pressure), don't be scared of it. I'm not saying you should eat a salt-shaker, but when you're looking for that crispy, salty taste, lightly salted vegetables might do the trick.

Along with fibrous vegetables, good fiber sources include whole-grain breads, Shredded Wheat and Kashi cereals (there are others, too), fruits, and vegetables such as soybeans. Try something as simple as eating an orange rather than drinking a glass of orange juice. There's a big difference in the way they're metabolized. Because of the fiber in the orange, it takes a lot longer to digest it than a glass of juice.

12. **Consume starchy carbs earlier in the day, and water-rich carbs later.** Your insulin sensitivity is highest in the morning. There appears to be a circadian rhythm to the way your body secretes insulin, and rates of insulin secretion fall around 6:00 P.M. At this point, your body becomes less capable of handling carbohydrates as efficiently. So frontload the breads, rice, oatmeal, potatoes, and other starchy complex carbs in your diet. Later in the day, begin to favor low-calorie vegetables, such as tomatoes, cucumbers, onions, broccoli, peppers, mushrooms, spinach, lettuce, and other so-called wet-carb sources. You can probably save a few calories from fat storage every day simply by giving your body different types of carbs at the times it can handle them most efficiently. Although that may not sound like much, every little bit helps.

13. **Pull yourself together.** Your lifestyle has to be compatible with fat loss. For example, if you don't exercise, your dietary changes will produce limited results at best. In particular, getting enough sleep is a huge success factor in weight loss. Shortchanging it will slow your metabolism. Elevated stress is a problem, too, as it will stoke the release of the catabolic hormone cortisol. Marijuana and cocaine will depress your testosterone levels. All of the above will conspire to make your body lose muscle and store nutrients as fat. Not only do you need to watch what you eat, but you also must complement your food plan with a weight-loss-friendly life plan.

14. **Reduce the amount of fast food you eat.** Although it's admittedly an extreme example, a Carl's Jr. Double Western Bacon Cheeseburger saddles you with 900 calories and 49 grams of fat along with its 49 grams of protein. The average powder shake will give you the same amount of protein with 300 calories and a stingy 2.5 fat grams.

Insert Fork in Mouth, Chew, Then Swallow

We've all seen them: Grown men who eat as if they were participating in one of those hot-dog-eating contests at the county fair—you know, the ones where some guy ends up shoving 19 wieners into his pie hole in under 2 minutes. Those displays involve an undeniable element of showmanship, but when a guy takes the same approach during a formal dinner party, he's sealing his fate as a social pariah.

It makes you wonder where this impulse to speed-eat comes from. For many guys, it probably dates back to childhood. Maybe your parents ate like that, and you copied them. Maybe you shared the table with a pack of hungry siblings, whom you needed to outrace in order to get your fair share at mealtime. An overweight friend of mine knows exactly why he eats so fast: As a child, he had to sit around the table with a horribly dysfunctional family, so he ate as fast as he could to get away from them as quickly as possible. Old habits die hard, and as you age, the time pressures on your dining only grow. Eating on the run is the norm these days, which is one reason that fast food has become so ubiquitous.

Regardless of where the habit developed, eating too fast is a major contributor to being overweight. The faster you eat, the more calories you can shove in before your brain registers that you're eating. During the same time that one guy is eating 300 or 400 calories, another guy might be shoving in 800. If you're the 800 dude, you need to slow down, start chewing your food well, and pay more attention to what you've eaten. When you eat really fast, you get a feeling at the end that you don't even know what you've eaten. You don't even feel like you've had a meal, so you continue to look for food.

If you rely heavily on this prefab cuisine and want to lose body fat, you don't necessarily have to go cold turkey, but you *do* have to cut back—way back. To that end, consider two complementary strategies. One is to say, "Look, when I go to McDonald's, a Quarter Pounder with Cheese and fries is my thing, and I'm not messing with that." If so, consider dropping the frequency of your drive-thrus from four times a week to two. Or you could say, "Instead of a Double Whopper with Cheese, I could have a Whopper with Cheese, and regular fries instead of supersize fries." Switching from a bacon-cheeseburger to a grilled chicken sandwich sans mayo saves about 500 calories.

The dining-out dilemma isn't limited to fast food. Restaurant meals often come in proportions that range from above average to obscene. Try brown-bagging your lunch for a few days instead of eating out. You'll be amazed at how easy it is to go from a 1,000-calorie lunch to one containing 400 calories.

15. **Eat slower.** People who are overweight almost always eat so fast that they outrace their body's fullness signals. They shove in a whole bunch of calories before their brain registers that they've eaten. If that sounds familiar, you need to train yourself to slow down. To do so, concentrate on what you are doing: *eating.* That means, at least until you get the hang of chewing and tasting your food, do nothing else while you eat—no television watching, no newspaper reading, no Internet surfing, and no report writing.

16. **Eat fish often.** When you study the experiences of most guys who have dieted successfully, one of the common denominators that jumps out, usually ranking among the top-five factors, is eating more fish. For many years, nutritionists assumed you lost weight when you ate fish because it has fewer calories, pound for pound, than red meat does. Now, however, it appears that reasons go above and beyond calories.

Most important, the type of fat found in fish appears to enhance the efficiency of the hormone leptin. That's one more reason that incorporating a daily meal of fatty fish like salmon, halibut, or shellfish may help decrease the size of fat cells and assist with fat loss.

17. **Stick to the low end of the glycemic index.** Carbs are all categorized according to a sliding scale, the glycemic index (GI). This index ranks each carbohydrate according to how quickly the body converts it to glucose and shuttles it into your bloodstream. The higher the number, the faster your body converts that food to glucose. You can find a good, user-friendly list of the glycemic index of foods on the Internet at www.glycemicindex.com.

    Keep in mind that these numbers aren't etched in stone, partly because human digestion varies by individual. Also, the digestion speed of any carbohydrate is affected by what it's being digested with. Fiber, protein, and fat all tend to slow digestion. And you can forget gaining many benefits if you stuff yourself with any carb, even low-GI ones.

    Regardless, diets containing largely low-GI foods promote fat loss better than those loaded with high-GI foods. This was demonstrated in a recent study published in the journal *Diabetes Care.* For five weeks, one group of guys ate carbs that were predominantly low GI, and another group ate high-GI carbs. The low-GI diet produced greater losses in abdominal fat and overall fat, and spared more muscle.

18. **Switch from saturated and hydrogenated fats to monounsaturated fats.** The kinds of fat you eat can influence your energy expenditure and body weight. Energy is released through heat production in a process called *nonshivering thermogenesis,* which is controlled by uncoupling proteins (UCP) in the cells of brown fat, white fat, and muscle. Researchers interested in finding out if diet can influence this process investigated possible dietary enhancements of thermogenesis in rats. They found that olive oil, which is high in monounsaturated fats, increased the activity of the UCPs, and hence of metabolic rates. Because of the short duration of the study, published in the *American Journal of Clinical Nutrition,* no differences in body weight were recorded between the rats fed olive oil and those fed other fats. The authors speculate that because UCPs are found in the muscle of humans, this may pose a promising new area in obesity research.

19. **Exercise.** No surprise here, given what you've learned so far. Fat loss comes down to 50 percent training, 50 percent nutrition. It doesn't work otherwise. In fact, the meal plans throughout this book are for physically active men. To be blunt, if you're sedentary, none of this will work as well as it should. You're not going to achieve the results that you want *unless you exercise.*

    Why not? If you're sedentary and you cut calories, you'll start to lose more muscle than

Exercise and Protein

Here's yet another benefit of moderate exercise: It makes your body use protein more efficiently. In fact, you get more work out of each protein gram when you exercise at 40 to 50 percent of your max, even while dieting. If you want to lose weight by burning more calories through exercise rather than by cutting calories, you might not need much more protein.

When exercising at higher intensities, though, the same protein-efficiency effect doesn't apply. In fact, exercising at 65 percent or more of your max while dieting may decrease protein efficiency, which would require even more consumption to compensate.

you want, your metabolic rate will dip, and you'll be burning fewer calories, which will force you to cut calories even more. As you get thinner, you'll actually be getting less toned and flabbier. The minute you add back calories, you're going to get fat again—make that fat*ter.*

20. **Avoid the fat-free and carb-free trap.** Many guys read a label that says "fat-free ice cream," and they think not only that it's okay for them to eat it, but that they can have a double- or triple-size portion to boot. The snack foods and packaged cookies and cakes that are promoted as fat-free and carb-free and that come in strange colors and strange shapes are highly engineered foods. They may be fat-free thanks to Olestra and other fat replacements, but they're chock-full of chemicals. The low-carb and carb-free products are just as high in calories, due to added fat and carb replacements. They've been taken apart and reassembled by some dude in a lab coat, not Mother Nature. The finished products are often so unnatural that I hesitate to call many of them food. They certainly don't look like it.

In addition to all the added chemicals, these fat-free and reduced-fat products are often still quite high in carbohydrates because companies replace some of the fat with sugar. Worst of all, perhaps, are fat-free cakes and cookies. They taste nightmarishly bad, and after you've eaten them, you still won't feel satisfied. You won't have achieved the pleasure sensation you're looking for. You will have consumed a bunch of calories and a lot of carbohydrates, but you'll still want to go eat something else.

What you end up with are chemical-laden products with virtually the same number of calories as the products they're replacing. However, they're probably even higher in carbohydrates, which likely affects your fat-loss diet more negatively than the fat would have in the first place. How could that be? Because your insulin levels spike, and the calories con-

The Fat–Heart Disease Connection

One caveat to this anti-fat-free-food diatribe concerns people who have heart disease already, or who are at high risk of getting it. Those individuals, whose goal isn't necessarily to lose body fat but to decrease the amount of fat in their diet, can benefit from these kinds of foods. The research has borne this out. For people sticking with a low-fat, low-cholesterol diet, fat-reduced foods can give them some variety that they otherwise couldn't have. They're happy just to have something that resembles whatever this food originally was, and they're disciplined enough to not overeat it.

But for the general population, there are no data showing that most reduced-fat foods can help you lose weight. In no way should these products be considered health foods, no matter how manufacturers spin them. Just because they're a little less unhealthy than they were before doesn't mean they're healthy.

vert to fat, rather than being used as energy or stored as glycogen in your muscles. When you eat fat and protein, your insulin levels barely change. So take a single-portion serving of the food that you really want rather than settle for its reduced-fat cousin.

There are a few exceptions to this rule. Examples include selected reduced-fat nonprocessed foods such as low-fat or fat-free yogurt, cream cheese, and milk, where the manufacturer has skimmed off some or all of that fat but left the underlying product essentially intact. They've siphoned off mostly saturated fats and left all the good parts. Baked chips rather than fried chips are also good: They really hit the spot for most guys, who often prefer the baked stuff to oily fried chips. The baked ones aren't fat-free—there is a certain amount of natural fat in the corn—and they aren't promoted as such. They're very crunchy and tasty, and once you're sticking them in salsa, it doesn't make any difference taste-wise. Just remember: Don't eat the whole bag.

The Last Rule

I've saved possibly the most important weight-loss tactic until last. To shed fat, you must wean yourself off foods that contain an additive called high-fructose corn syrup (HFCS).

Far more insidious than reduced-fat foods is the rise of HFCS, a sweetener manufactured from cornstarch. Although corn syrups contain varying proportions of glucose and other simple sugars, HFCS starts out with a high proportion of glucose, which is then treated with an enzyme that converts part of that glucose to fructose, which is much sweeter. The

WHY I DON'T BELIEVE IN LOW-CARB DIETS

ALTHOUGH DEVOTEES OF LOW-CARB DIETS CLAIM that theirs is the ideal ratio of carbs to protein in order to maintain the most muscle mass during weight loss, several studies suggest that a better approach combines moderate carbs with high protein. One study put one group on a high-carb, low-protein diet, and another on a moderate-carb, high-protein diet. On average, subjects in the moderate-carb group lost 8.1 more pounds of body weight overall (and 7.3 more pounds of body fat) than those in the high-carb group. So there was pretty good weight and fat loss on the moderate-carb diet.

One of the knocks against high-protein, low-carb eating is its potential for inducing an abnormal physiological state called *ketosis*. In this condition, blood-sugar levels drop so low and insulin secretion is reduced so dramatically that fat stores are broken down and converted by the liver to ketone bodies for energy. The body can't use all the ketone bodies without carbs, so they accumulate in the bloodstream and spill out in urine. Symptoms of ketosis include acetone-smelling breath and body odor, and loss of appetite. Fat loss and diminished appetite are desirable for dieters, but if carbohydrate levels remain too low, ketosis may turn into *ketoacidosis*, a potentially life-threatening condition. Such diets also result in lower levels of serotonin, the neurotransmitter in the brain responsible for mood elevation. If you think your girlfriend is crabby when she first wakes up, you ain't seen nothin' until she tries a low-carb diet. Does this sound like a diet to follow for a lifetime?

Although ketosis results in high fat metabolism and appetite loss, you can achieve the same results without it. Moderate-carb, high-protein diets promote successful fat loss, but they're healthy, too. By following a moderate-carb, high-protein diet, you'll feel more satisfied and have greater control over what and how much you eat. You'll be easier to get along with, smell better, and feel more like going for a workout. In the long run, you'll have kept the important disease-fighting phytochemicals and fibers in your diet that come only from carb-containing plant foods like fruits, vegetables, grains, beans, nuts, and seeds. Who wants to be skinny and die from colon cancer?

result of this process is a very inexpensive replacement for traditional cane sugar. The HFCS found in beverages contains about 55 percent fructose, and the HFCS in some food products may contain up to 90 percent fructose.

The commercial use of HFCS began in the 1970s, and I first heard about it in 1980, while attending grad school. I was taking a course called Food Science, which involved the study of how food ingredients work during cooking and processing. During a lecture on sweetening agents in food, my professor said something to this effect: "High-fructose corn syrup has recently been introduced into the food supply. Compared with sucrose, it is a very inexpensive sweetener and will likely replace sugar in most processed foods. Our understanding of how fructose works in the body is very limited, and we have no idea how this will affect the population once it is found almost everywhere in large amounts in the processed food supply." How prophetic. By 1985, HFCS accounted for approximately 35 percent of the total amount (measured by dry weight) of all sweeteners in the U.S. food supply. In 1970, per capita use of HFCS was $\frac{1}{2}$ pound; by 1997, the last year for which such data were collected, the number was $62\frac{1}{2}$ pounds. By that time, the average American was consuming 97 grams of HFCS, or 388 calories' worth, per day.

Yikes.

Eight years later, those figures are without a doubt significantly higher. After all, the major source of HFCS is soft drinks, and they're more popular than ever. In a 1998 study on soft-drink consumption titled "Liquid Candy," the nonprofit Center for Science in the Public Interest reported that Americans are drinking twice as much soda as they did a quarter-century ago. The average American teenage male today drinks between 1.6 and 2 cans of soda per day, depending on the study you use. Two cans daily is equal to 40 grams, or 160 calories, of fructose every day (because HFCS is 55 percent fructose), good for just under 10 percent of a guy's energy need. Remember, that's just from soda—it doesn't take into account other sources of fructose in your diet.

Might there be a connection between this rise in fructose consumption and the remarkable increase in obesity over the past two decades? Researchers from the Department of Nutrition at the University of California, Davis; the U.S. Department of Agriculture Western Human Nutrition Research Center at Davis; the Monell Chemical Sense Institute; and the University of Pennsylvania, Philadelphia, have recently published a landmark review of the scientific literature on fructose, weight gain, and the insulin resistance syndrome, known as Syndrome X. They theorize that fructose in the form of the ingredient HFCS may be primarily responsible for the epidemic of obesity and abnormalities seen as part of Syndrome X, including insulin resistance, impaired glucose tolerance, hyperinsulinemia, hypertriacylglycerolemia, and hypertension.

How could one substitute ingredient be wreaking such havoc with America's waistline? The problem is the way the human body metabolizes it. The body prefers to turn glucose into energy or store it as glycogen, the fuel in muscle cells. Not so with fructose, which the body metabolizes in the liver and prefers turning into fat. Studies have shown that although ingesting fructose increases the rate of fat production, ingesting the same number of calories of glucose does not cause the same response.

Not only does fructose turn preferentially into fat, it also shuts down the mechanisms your body has for preventing fat accumulation. Numerous studies on animals—and a handful on some human guinea pigs—have shown that fructose doesn't stimulate the production of two key hormones that are intimately involved in the regulation of energy balance—the dietary dynamic duo, insulin and leptin. Unlike glucose, fructose doesn't stimulate the secretion of insulin from the pancreas. If you want to lose body fat, this is a bad deal. Here's why: Insulin helps control the accumulation of body fat, inhibiting food intake and increasing energy expenditure. That's why your body secretes insulin after you eat carbohydrates. Along with ushering glucose into cells, insulin signals how much food you've eaten and tells you when it's time to stop. Flick off that insulin switch altogether and there's nothing to turn off your appetite. This increases the likelihood of gaining weight or even becoming obese.

Because HFCS flies under insulin's radar screen, leptin also gets left in the lurch. After all, leptin is waiting to receive its cue from insulin, after which leptin abates hunger and increases energy production. When HFCS is consumed, this cascade of events is bypassed, crippling the body's in-house mechanisms for calorie control and energy balance.

Though animal studies consistently show that high-fructose diets have an alarming connection to weight gain, a smattering of studies have begun to study the same effect in humans. What these researchers have done is add 300 calories a day from soft drinks to their subjects' diets. Usually, when that sort of energy is added to a person's diet, the body figures out a way to balance it out over time, reaching a steady state. However, when those calories come in the form of fructose-laden soft drinks, the body doesn't balance it out. The net result is weight gain, likely for the reasons I've just discussed.

One study used overweight subjects to gauge what effect a sucrose-sweetened beverage might have on their food consumption and weight, compared with the effect on the same parameters of beverages sweetened with noncaloric sweeteners.

THE FOOD CONSPIRACY

How food manufacturers make you fat

AS SOON AS THERE'S A BIG HUE AND CRY ABOUT something like HFCS or trans fats, companies like snack food manufacturers typically evaluate it as a marketing opportunity rather than a public health issue. By removing the dubious ingredient, they can come up with new products and start selling all over again.

The question, though, is what they're replacing that ingredient with. For example, we ended up with trans fats in foods when the public demanded that saturated fat–laden lard be removed from packaged snacks and baked goods. The food industry had to come up with something that would replace the lard but still give consumers the same taste, texture, mouth-feel, and shelf life that they had come to expect from those foods. Thus, hydrogenated fats were born—and now we want them eliminated from our food supply as well. So now we've got fractionated fats: fats made up of the extracted saturated fat fraction of otherwise healthy fats like sunflower, safflower, and canola oils. Do you see a trend?

Sucrose, a.k.a. table sugar, is a disaccharide—half glucose, half fructose—so you can figure that the sucrose drinks were about half fructose. Ten weeks into the study, members of the sucrose group had higher energy intakes (up 28 percent), body weight, fat mass, and blood pressure than they did when they started. In contrast, the group drinking the artificially sweetened beverages measured lower in all four categories than they had at the start of the study.

Another study looked at the effect of liquid and solid carbs on consumption and body weight. Subjects added extra carbs to their diet by eating jelly beans or drinking soda before eating on their own. During the four-week period when they were eating jelly beans, the subjects' energy intake remained balanced; they were compensating for the extra calories. However, during the four-week "liquid" period, the extra calories weren't compensated for, and total daily calorie intake increased by 17 percent. Body weight and BMI both increased significantly, indicating that the liquid-carb calories went unrecognized by the physiological systems that control energy balance.

In spite of the fact that fructose is commonly known as "fruit sugar," these warnings about the perils of HFCS shouldn't be extended to the fructose occurring naturally in fruits and vegetables. Fruits contain only a small amount of fructose, and they house it inside a nutritious package of fiber and other healthful nutrients, which counteract the effect of fructose in the body. In the form of big slugs of HFCS, however, mounting evidence strongly suggests that fructose is an undesirable ingredient in the diet. Although small amounts are probably not

SUGAR SHOTS

CONSIDER THESE STATISTICS BEFORE YOU DOWN THAT CAN OF SODA.

■ Per capita consumption of added sugars has risen by 28 percent since 1983. The average American consumes at least 64 pounds of sugar per year, and the average teenage boy at least 109 pounds.

■ The typical American gets 16 percent of his or her calories from added sugars. Children (age 6 to 11) get 18 percent of their calories from added sugars. Teenagers (age 12 to 19) get 20 percent of their calories from added sugars.

■ The USDA projects that if consumption trends continue, added-sugar intake will increase almost 20 percent by 2005.

■ People who consume diets high in added sugars consume lower levels of fiber; vitamins A, C, E, and folate; magnesium; calcium; and other nutrients. By displacing protective nutrients and foods in the diet, added sugars may increase the risk of osteoporosis, cancer, high blood pressure, heart disease, and other health problems. For instance, drinking soft drinks instead of milk may increase the risk of osteoporosis.

■ Calorie-dense foods, which are typically high in sugar and/or fat, contribute to obesity. Between 1976 to 1980 and 1988 to 1994, overweight rates in teenage boys rose from 5 to 12 percent, in teenage girls from 7 to 11 percent, and in adults from 25 to 35 percent.

harmful and wouldn't interfere with energy metabolism, the large amounts found in soft drinks and many processed foods may be at the root of the body's inability to maintain energy balance and control body weight.

The soft drink and corn industry are combating these claims by saying that HFCS has no more fructose than sugar. Yet the HFCS commonly used in foods probably has about 5 percent more fructose than sugar. Second, HFCS is found in a much wider variety of foods than table sugar ever was. According to a study in the *Journal of Obesity Research,* worldwide consumption of total sugar, including HFCS increased by 74 calories per day from 1962 to 2000. Sugar consumption in the United States increased by even more, rising by 83 calories per day from 1977 to 1996. In the end, we're getting much more fructose than ever before.

What to Expect

If you're serious about eating better and willing to lift weights and do cardio consistently, you can probably lose that lard hanging over your belt faster than you think. The guy whose physique is shot to hell to begin with will almost always achieve the most dramatic improvements at first, if only because he has the most room for improvement. It's sort of like the bounce you get after a market crash—not a cause for celebration, per se, but a reflection of how bad things had gotten. It's not unheard of for guys in really bad shape to lose 2 to 4 pounds a week right off the bat, although such a rapid rate of loss will undoubtedly be short-lived.

With the exception of the "beginner's effect," you can expect to lose 1½ pounds in a week. That's a good thing. Lose any more than that and you'll likely rob your body of muscle cells, the calorie-burning

IF NOT FRUCTOSE, THEN WHAT?

HERE'S SOME ADVICE FOR CUTTING BACK ON HIGH FRUCTOSE CORN SYRUP (HFCS).

Can the soda. I've already talked about drinking more water instead of soda, and that's certainly the first alternative that comes to mind. The second is skim milk, and the third is 100 percent fruit juice. If you can't imagine a day without a soda, have a diet one instead. If you can stomach the taste, it's a decent alternative. Another is mixing 1 part grape juice with 3 parts sparkling water. You get your antioxidants in a great-tasting spritzer.

Bring back the sugar bowl and the honey pot. Avoid presweetened foods, which most likely were sweetened with HFCS, and sweeten them at home. For example, buy plain, unflavored yogurt and mix in some honey to sweeten it. Buy unsweetened cereals such as Kashi and add a few teaspoons of sugar at home. Use seltzer water and add some flavored syrup to make your own Italian soda. You will never add as much sugar as the food manufacturers do, and your food will taste better as well.

Read every label. Watch out for foods laced with HFCS. Candy, ice cream, frozen yogurt, Popsicles, fruit bars, ketchup, pasta sauce, soups, and even hamburger buns use HFCS in varying amounts. When you add these foods to a couple of cans of soda every day, you've got a heavy load of fructose. Read ingredient labels to educate yourself and to make informed choices.

machines within the machine. Losing too much too soon can also throw your hormones out of whack.

Before you start losing that weight, however, you need to pinpoint your destination and figure out how much fat you need to lose. Sounds simple enough, but this can be a surprisingly tough question to answer. For the average person, the readings you get from the scale are nearly meaningless. The scale measures body weight, when what really matters is body composition. At the extreme, it's pretty obvious that someone who is 100 pounds overweight has a body-weight problem, but the more common and more subtle problem concerns someone who has too much fat relative to the amount of muscle he's carrying on his frame.

Another tool that people use that's not entirely reliable is the Ideal Body Weight Chart, which gives ideal weights for specific heights. (You might have seen one of these taped to the inside of the exam room door the last time you sat and waited—and waited—for your physician.) The Ideal Body Weight charts are flawed because their supporting data was not collected in a scientific fashion. Ultimately, the recommendations aren't meaningful.

A more useful tool is the Body Mass Index, commonly known as the BMI, which is your weight in kilograms divided by your height in meters squared. The BMI is useful because it represents a relationship between body mass and risk of chronic disease. If you're an average guy, the greater your BMI, the higher your health risk. For guys who aren't average—who fall outside the usual norms of body type—the BMI is problematic at best. If you are thin, but poorly muscled and overly fat (after you've been ill, for example), your BMI might actually register as normal even though you're probably not very healthy. Conversely, an athlete who is very muscular with a low percent of body fat would likely register as overweight with a high BMI.

To make the BMI a more accurate tool, it has been combined with the measurement of waist circumference to give you some notion of how much fat you're carrying. If your BMI is normal but your waist measurement is high, then you probably have a beer belly and need to lose some fat. If you're a bodybuilder, your BMI will probably be in the overweight range, but you're lean and your waist will be well within the range of normal. If your BMI is high and so is your waist circumference, you've got some work to do.

Step 1. Calculate your body mass index using the chart on page 000.

Step 2. Measure your waist circumference by wrapping a flexible measuring tape around your abdomen just above your belly button.

Step 3. Look at your results. If your BMI is greater than 25 and your waist circumference is more than 40 inches, you're too fat. As you lose weight, continue to calculate your BMI and waist measurement. Once one or both is in the normal range, you may have reached your goal.

Even more accurate than the BMI is to know your body composition, the percentage of lean muscle and body fat on your frame. That's really the ideal way to figure out how much fat you need to lose. Do you know what this is, offhand? Didn't think so. Most guys don't. I have a research-quality tool (called a bioelectrical impedance meter) that I use to measure body composition; and, even with that, guys need to follow a fairly elaborate protocol over the 12 hours before measurement to ensure accuracy. The absolute best way to measure body composition is through a very expensive medical scanning device called DEXA (Dual Energy X-ray Absorptiometry)› But that level of accuracy is usually not necessary for the average guy. Though there are bathroom versions of bioelectrical impedance scales on the market, the readings they give can be fairly unreliable, especially if you get on the scale just after you've worked out or stepped out of the shower.

For the sake of practicality and reliability, use the

BMI and the measurement of your waist circumference to give you some notion of how much fat you're carrying. Once you put those numbers together, you should have some idea of where you fall along the body-fat continuum.

Getting Started

If your fat-loss diet isn't built on what you realistically can do, it's doomed to failure. If it isn't formulated in the context of your lifestyle and personal preferences, the most sophisticated plan in the world is useless. It's got to be something that you really can do, that you're really going to follow. Whether you're speaking with a nutritionist, watching a nutrition show on TV, or reading a book like *Power Food,* evaluate the different suggestions being made and say, "This I like, this I can do, this I'm already doing, so I can continue. . . ." Build from there. Don't try to turn yourself into something you're not. Only the most-intense Type-A personalities can do that. Everybody else who follows the route reaches a dead end soon enough.

Right off the bat, you need to evaluate your own diet the way I evaluated Matt's. Keep a food journal to figure out how many calories you're taking in now, and in what form. Log everything you eat and drink for a week, and then use either a book or an online program to translate this consumption into total calories. This will give you a baseline from which you can make adjustments. It will also establish a pattern of what you like to eat, which might not be obvious even to you until you see it in print. Without question, jotting down what, when, and how much you eat and drink is the best way to understand where you are nutrition-wise.

That's the information I use to plan a guy's diet, and you can do the same. If you eat a specific cereal at the same time every day, and it's a good choice, use that. In that situation, I wouldn't ask the client to ditch that cereal in favor of oatmeal. I use what

---

Trading Places

Losing fat is as much about making good decisions as it is about anything else. Along those lines, here are five items you should include in your diet and four others that you should give the heave-ho. Items are ranked in no particular order.

Five items you should eat:
- Soy nuts
- Grapefruit
- Fat-free yogurt
- 100 percent protein-enriched (low-GI) pasta with a tomato-base sauce
- Fresh spinach for salads

Four items you should avoid:
- Hot dogs
- Bologna
- Onion rings
- Beer

---

they're already doing. Like I said, though, it has to be a good cereal. If it were Crunchy Marshmallow Surprise, I would definitely find something better.

Starting from that foundation, you can begin systematically adding in all the things you need to add in while subtracting what needs to go. But even the things you want to keep must be adapted to your new diet if you're trying to control calories. Through time, the not-so-healthy stuff will go, because as you look back over your day's consumption, the focus will always be, "What haven't I eaten that I really need to eat?" That's the mindset I try to foster in clients, and it's the correct mindset for you. When 7:00 P.M. arrives and you're hungry, think, "What do I still need to eat?" Don't look back and obsess over what you ate that you shouldn't have eaten. That doesn't matter anymore—it's over. It's all about what you still need to eat. And 95 percent

CALCULATE YOUR BODY-MASS INDEX

THIS CHART WORKS FOR MEN'S BODIES. Find your height in the left column. Then find your weight in that row. The number at the top of that column is your BMI.

BODY MASS INDEX

HEIGHT (IN.)	19	20	21	22	23	24	25	26	27	28	29	30	31	32	33	34	35
58	91	96	100	105	110	115	119	124	129	134	138	143	148	153	158	162	167
59	94	99	104	109	114	119	124	128	133	138	143	148	153	158	163	168	173
60	97	102	107	112	118	123	128	133	138	143	148	153	158	163	168	174	179
61	100	106	111	116	122	127	132	137	143	148	153	158	164	169	174	180	185
62	104	109	115	120	126	131	136	142	147	153	158	164	169	175	180	186	191
63	107	113	118	124	130	135	141	146	152	158	163	169	175	180	186	191	197
64	110	116	122	128	134	140	145	151	157	163	169	174	180	186	192	197	204
65	114	120	126	132	138	144	150	156	162	168	174	180	186	192	198	204	210
66	118	124	130	136	142	148	155	161	167	173	179	186	192	198	204	210	216
67	121	127	134	140	146	153	159	166	172	178	185	191	198	204	211	217	223
68	125	131	138	144	151	158	164	171	177	184	190	197	203	210	216	223	230
69	128	135	142	149	155	162	169	176	182	189	196	203	209	216	223	230	236
70	132	139	146	153	160	167	174	181	188	195	202	209	216	222	229	236	243
71	136	143	150	157	165	172	179	186	193	200	208	215	222	229	236	243	250
72	140	147	154	162	169	177	184	191	199	206	213	221	228	235	242	250	258
73	144	151	159	166	174	182	189	197	204	212	219	227	235	242	250	257	265
74	148	155	163	171	179	189	194	202	210	218	225	233	241	249	256	264	272
75	152	160	168	176	184	192	200	208	216	224	232	240	248	256	264	272	279
76	156	164	172	180	189	197	205	213	221	230	238	246	254	263	271	279	287

Source: National Heart, Lung, and Blood Institute

of the time, that will be fruits and vegetables, so that's what you should eat. Day by day, you'll realize earlier and earlier that you haven't eaten your fruits and vegetables, and you'll respond accordingly. It won't take long until you've dropped a whole bunch of stuff from your diet that you thought you could never give up.

The meal plans in this chapter will give you a rough rule of thumb for daily nutrition. You can either follow them to a T, or you can use the amounts of suggested food groups and vary them as needed. The main point is that you should eat the foods on your list first and the ones not on your list second. At the end of the day, when you are rummaging through the fridge and not sure what to eat, it may help to ask yourself the following:

CLASSIFICATION OF OVERWEIGHT AND OBESITY BY BMI, WAIST CIRCUMFERENCE, AND ASSOCIATED DISEASE RISKS

| | BMI (kg/m²) | Obesity Class | DISEASE RISK* RELATIVE TO NORMAL WEIGHT AND WAIST CIRCUMFERENCE | |
			Men 102 cm (40 in) or less Women 88 cm (35 in) or less	Men › 102 cm (40 in) Women › 88 cm (35 in)
Underweight	‹18.5		—	—
Normal	18.5–24.9		—	—
Overweight	25.0–29.9		Increased	High
Obesity	30.0–34.9	I	High	Very High
	35.0–39.9	II	Very High	Very High
Extreme Obesity	40.0†	III	Extremely High	Extremely High

*Disease risk for type 2 diabetes, hypertension, and CVD.

† Increased waist circumference can also be a marker for increased risk even in persons of normal weight.

Source: National Heart, Lung, and Blood Institute

Have I consumed enough water and fluids?

Did I have all of my milk today?

Have I eaten all of my fruits in a variety of colors?

Did I have enough vegetables?

Have I eaten any nuts or nut butter?

What about healthy oils, olives, or avocado?

Do I need some more protein?

For Guys Who Want a Six-Pack

When summer rolls around, you might decide that you want to go from being in better, leaner shape to being in no-woman-on-the-beach-will-be-able-to-resist-my-Michelangelo-worthy-body shape. Alas, the most potent symbol of that process, the six-pack, has always been obscured as much by myth as by stubborn layers of fat. Years ago, the sit-up was lauded as the premier ab exercise, when in fact the crunch was a more stomach-specific movement. Hundreds of reps done every day became the common prescription, but that almost always represented overtraining.

In reality, whether or not your stomach is flat has more to do with diet and genetics than anything else, including training. And staying in bed for two or three years eating Ding Dongs is most assuredly not the answer. It's almost a cliché at this point, but next to finding parents with better genes, in order to expose those ab muscles lurking under your belly fat, you're going to have to pay even more attention to what you put into it than you have so far in this chapter.

Because you've already burned some of your body fat with our 20 rules for fat burning, what you need to do now is walk a fine line. You really need to know what you're doing to achieve the results you're after. You're going to have to do some fairly intense cardiovascular work in order to burn fat and achieve your goal, but at the same time you need to fuel that effort. Here are some tips.

Putting an End to Nighttime Eating

One of the most intractable challenges facing a guy who wants to eat better is the nighttime craving. If you get these a lot, you probably need to eat more during the day. Also, make sure you're really hungry and not just thirsty. Guys often misconstrue hunger for thirst, and thirst for hunger. When clients say to me, "I wake up in the middle of the night hungry," aside from revamping their diet so that they're getting more calories and fluids during the day, I suggest that before they eat anything, they drink something. If nothing else, it makes them wait a minute before reaching for some sort of instant gratification. If you give it maybe 5 or 10 minutes, by the time you've prepared, say, a cup of decaffeinated tea, you may realize that you're not really hungry but that you were bored, or worried. Or maybe you're really tired and you should just go to sleep.

Late-night cravings can also be masking emotional issues. Is there a reason you're avoiding going to bed? I've encountered clients who feel like they're in okay relationships, but they consistently avoid going to bed, and they stay up and eat instead. Often they aren't aware of what they're doing, and they certainly don't verbalize it. Maybe it's because of a partner, or maybe it's because there is no partner, but they avoid going to bed because it's depressing. When you've got the TV on or you're sitting at the computer, food keeps you company and you don't have that sense of being alone. It's much more common than people realize.

Eat 250 fewer calories. To shed body fat without sacrificing much, if any, of your hard-earned muscle, try dropping your calories by 250 or so a day, although that figure will vary by individual. If you're a 5-foot, 11-inch, 270-pound bodybuilder like two-time Mr. Olympia Ronnie Coleman, you'll have to cut significantly more calories than that to achieve your desired result. If your build falls closer to Gary Coleman's, however, a smallish calorie cut will pack a punch worthy of the diminutive former sitcom star with an appropriately short fuse. Most of you should fall somewhere between those two living legends— probably 250 to 300 calories.

Cut out the empty calories. Start making the calories you consume really count. In particular, avoid simple sugars, particularly those found in junk foods and sweets. You need to watch out for anything that might provide excess calories. It's easy to grab a bag of M&Ms and think you're not doing much damage by eating a handful, but those extra hundred or so calories might put you over the top and not allow your body to burn extra fat.

Eat only the best fats. Emphasize monounsaturated fats (like olive oil), polyunsaturated fats (such as corn and soybeans), and essential fatty acids (like oily fish), and limit your intake of saturated fats (such as fatty meats and cheese) and trans fatty acids (like French fries and packaged cookies). Where fat normally might account for roughly 25 percent of your calories, it should account for only 20 percent or so if you want killer abs. Don't go much lower than that, though. Fat plays important roles in providing energy, enhancing the absorption of fat-soluble vitamins, making testosterone, and supporting the immune system, so don't shortchange yourself there.

Make every carb count. Focus on consuming complex, low-GI carbohydrates like those found in oatmeal, vegetables, and whole-grain breads and cereals. Be careful about reducing your carbs excessively—such reductions often trick people into thinking they're burning fat. When you're training hard to get lean but want to maintain the gains you just worked so hard to achieve, you need to consume energy in the form of carbohydrates, not just protein. Although your calorie needs decrease, they decrease only slightly. Muscle requires more calories than body fat does, so you've got to feed them to keep them.

Keep in mind that for every gram of carbohydrate you store in muscle, you store anywhere from 3 to 4 grams of water. So if you don't eat many carbs, you lose water along with the carbs and, yes, you start to see better-defined muscles. But if your goal is to lose fat weight, you need to put in carbs to fuel those high-intensity workouts. Then, by creating just a small calorie deficit, fat supplies a little more of the energy and you start to see it coming off, leading to more-visible definition.

Good carb sources include sweet (not white) potatoes, brown rice, oatmeal, butternut squash, peas, and whole grains such as millet, quinoa, and wild rice. Because they have a low to moderate GI, these carbs cause smaller fluctuations in blood glucose and insulin than more rapidly digested sugars. That's important because insulin spikes will promote fat storage when you're trying to get lean, so remember to keep portion sizes under control.

Keep protein consumption high. Continue consuming roughly 1 gram of protein per pound of body weight per day. Protein sources often contain quite a bit of fat, though, so emphasize lean sources more than usual. If you've already switched from 2-percent-fat milk to 1-percent, try drinking skim milk during this phase. Emphasize lean meats like chicken and turkey, and remove visible fat from any type or cut of meat. Protein powders, which contain extremely limited amounts of fat, can be used very effectively here.

That's about as fancy as you need to get, though.

Be disciplined and use common sense, and there's no need to go overboard with fat-burning pills and potions. If you can hold true to that for four to six weeks, you'll see some serious results.

Little Herbal Helpers

Regarding pills and potions, they're often treated as the first line of defense against fat, when they should be the last. You're not going to lose weight just by taking a pill in the absence of dieting and exercise. But if you do those things, a few of the fat-loss supplements on the market might give you a slight edge with appetite control and fat burning. How slight is slight? Add a thermogenic to a good plan, and you might bump up your burn another 20 to 50 calories a day. Depending on your goals, that could be a significant windfall.

For other guys, the cost and the risks, such as they are, might outweigh the benefits. It's up to you.

EPHEDRA AND MA HUANG. These compounds have been virtually removed from the marketplace due to liabilities faced by the supplement manufacturers. However, similar ephedra-free products are discussed below.

SYNEPHRINE. This is one of a family of thermogenic compounds known as synephrine alkaloids, which are extracted from certain types of ripe citrus fruit. To know if the product you're considering contains it, check the fine print, not the front of the label. It'll probably be listed as *Citrus aurantium*—caffeine will probably be on there as well—and it's included in products with names such as Xenadrine, Ephedra-free and Phen-free.

To the extent that it works—studies suggest it may elevate metabolic rate, but no studies prove that it can help you successfully shed weight—it appears to do so by stimulating the central nervous system.

Dose: The doses used in research for synephrine have ranged from 40 to 58.5 milligrams.

Warnings: This and products like it aren't for the faint of heart, literally and figuratively. Synephrine's possible side effects resemble those of ephedrine: dizziness, headache, tremor, euphoria, insomnia, dry mouth, increased blood pressure, heart palpitations, and constipation. Also, check the label for health conditions that contraindicate its use. Regardless, check with your physician before using products containing synephrine.

7-KETO DEHYDROEPIANDROSTERONE. In the one major study using this thyroid supplement, 7-Keto showed promise. All subjects exercised and reduced their calories moderately for eight weeks, but only a portion took the supplement. They lost three times as much weight—6.4 pounds versus 2.1—and experienced a 2.2 percent decline in body fat that the others didn't.

Dose: For research, 200 milligrams a day. The typical product on the market contains 25 to 50 milligrams.

Warnings: The "sterone" in this might make you wonder if 7-Keto will turn you into a baritone, but a subset of subjects in the aforementioned study showed no change in testosterone levels. Measurements of more than 20 blood markers also showed no problems. But this was a short-term study; no long-term studies have been conducted.

PYRUVATE. This naturally occurring substance helps kick-start something called the Krebs cycle, which ultimately leads to adenosine triphosphate (ATP) being produced (see page 196). It may also stimulate cellular respiration and inhibit fat production.

Whether it does much as a supplement is debatable. Much of the research on pyruvate was done using very, very fat women as subjects, so it's tough to extrapolate the fat loss shown there to men looking to shed a few pounds.

Dose: 2 grams a day—much less than what's been used in studies, which is one reason a lot of skepticism surrounds pyruvate. There's no evidence to show it will do much of anything in those amounts.

Warnings: Read label instructions.

VITAMIN/MINERAL SUPPLEMENTS. You should be taking one of these daily anyway, but because deficiencies in minerals such as chromium can slow fat loss, there's a specific connection here.

Dose: 100 percent of daily value.

Warnings: Read label instructions.

CARNITINE. Made in the body from two amino acids, this serves various protective purposes, particularly relating to the heart. It also increases fat metabolism, raising some hope that it might be an effective fat-loss supplement.

The research results have been equivocal. So far, there isn't much here to get excited about.

Dose: 500 milligrams taken twice daily.

Warnings: Follow label instructions.

Foods That Promote Weight Loss

Eat these foods to turn up your metabolism:

Chili peppers	Olive oil
Fatty fish: salmon, herring, mackerel, black cod	Olives
	Soy
	Tomatoes
Flaxseed	Water
Green tea	Whole fruits
Milk	Whole grains
Nuts	Yogurt

GREEN TEA. The data here look good, but the research is still young. In 1999, scientists in Switzerland studied whether a green tea extract in capsular form could increase energy expenditure and fat utilization in 10 men over 24 hours. The green tea extract increased energy expenditure by 4 percent relative to a placebo treatment, which shakes out to about 82 calories in 24 hours. Fat utilization also increased. When compared with caffeine alone, energy expenditure increased by 3 percent.

Dose: Depends on the form in which you're taking it. Overall, the studies showing benefits have used extracts rather than the beverage.

Warnings: The researchers in Switzerland also examined the heart rates of the subjects because of the possible negative cardiovascular effects of caffeine. None of the subjects reported any side effects, including no significant differences in heart rate.

Foods That Undermine Weight Loss

Eat these foods with caution:

Fried foods	Sugar
High-fructose corn syrup	Sugar-sweetened soft drinks and beverages
Refined carbohydrates: cookies, cakes, candies, snack foods, chips	White breads and refined grains and cereals

MEAL PLAN FOR THE ACTIVE OVERWEIGHT GUY

THIS PLAN IS FOR THE GUY WHO WORKS OUT but just doesn't know how to eat. Armed with a diet plan that gives him enough fuel for exercise, he should shed the pounds fast. The key here is cutting out some carbs by reducing consumption of refined foods and keeping consumption of alcohol to a minimum, while including plenty of high-quality proteins, vegetables, and fruit.

Daily Assumptions*†

2,239 calories
265 grams carbohydrates
153 grams protein
63 grams fat

Daily Breakdown*†

7 bread
5 fruit
3 milk
6 teaspoons added sugar
5 vegetable
8 very lean protein
5 lean protein
1 medium-fat protein
5 fat

Note: Occasionally, a fat-free product, like mustard or cooking spray, is included on the menus. These do not count toward your daily breakdown but should not be overused.

*Use every day.

† Based on a 185-pound man.

THE MENU

DAY 1

Breakfast

2 bread	1 cup Shredded Wheat
1 milk	1 cup fat-free milk
1 fruit	1 cup fresh raspberries
1 medium-fat protein	1 egg, scrambled on a nonstick pan
1 very lean protein	2 egg whites, scrambled with whole egg
1 fat	1$\frac{1}{2}$ tablespoons ground flaxseed
	Water
	Oil-free cooking spray (for eggs)

Lunch

2 bread	2 slices whole-wheat bread
2 vegetable	Salad with 2 cups romaine lettuce, $\frac{1}{2}$ cup tomato, $\frac{1}{2}$ cup cucumber
1 fruit	1 nectarine
4 very lean protein	4 ounces turkey
1 fat	2 tablespoons low-fat dressing

Dinner

3 bread	1 sweet potato, baked
	1 small multigrain roll
1 fruit	1 slice watermelon
2 vegetable	1 cup cooked broccoli and/or cauliflower
5 lean protein	5 ounces salmon, grilled
2 fat	8 Kalamata olives
	1 teaspoon butter

Pre-Workout Snack

1 fat	10 peanuts
1 milk	1 cup fat-free unsweetened yogurt
1 vegetable	1 cup veggie sticks
	Water

Workout

Water

Post-Workout

SMOOTHIE

Blend until smooth.

1 milk	1 cup fat-free milk
2 fruit	1/2 cup orange juice
	1/2 cup frozen pineapple
	1/2 cup frozen strawberries
6 teaspoons added sugar	2 tablespoons honey
3 very lean protein	21 grams whey protein powder

DAY 2

Breakfast

Combine yogurt, fruit, and honey. Combine muffin and egg for sandwich.

2 bread	1 whole-wheat English muffin
1 milk	1 cup fat-free unsweetened yogurt
1 fruit	1 1/4 cups fresh strawberries
1 medium-fat protein	1 egg, hard-cooked
1 very lean protein	2 eggs, hard-cooked (discard yolks)
1 fat	1 1/2 tablespoons ground flaxseed
	Water

Lunch

2 bread	2 slices whole-grain bread
2 vegetable	Large salad with romaine lettuce, tomato, grilled eggplant, roasted red pepper
	Fat-free dressing
1 fruit	1 kiwi, sliced
4 very lean protein	4 ounces skinless white-meat chicken, grilled with lime juice
1 fat	1 teaspoon olive oil (for grilling)

Dinner

3 bread	1 cup cooked pasta
	1 slice garlic bread
1 fruit	1 cup strawberries
2 vegetable	1 cup ratatouille (over pasta)
	Salad with 1 cup lettuce, 1/4 cup tomato, 1/4 cup cucumber
5 lean protein	5 ounces lean ground beef (added to ratatouille)
2 fat	2 tablespoons low-fat dressing
	1 teaspoon butter (for garlic bread)

Pre-Workout Snack

1 fat	1 tablespoon almond butter
1 milk	1 cup fat-free milk
1 vegetable	1 cup veggie sticks
	Water

Workout

	Water

Post-Workout

SMOOTHIE

Blend until smooth.

1 milk	1 cup fat-free milk
2 fruit	1/2 cup orange juice
	1/2 cup frozen pineapple
	1/2 cup frozen strawberries
6 teaspoons added sugar	2 tablespoons honey
3 very lean protein	21 grams whey protein powder

DAY 3

Breakfast

2 bread	2 slices whole-wheat bread
1 milk	1 cup fat-free cottage cheese (on bread; sprinkle with no-calorie sweetener and cinnamon)
1 fruit	4 ounces freshly squeezed orange juice (with pulp)
1 medium-fat protein	1 egg, cooked sunny-side up on a nonstick pan
1 very lean protein	2 egg whites, cooked with sunny-side up egg
1 fat	1 1/2 tablespoons ground flaxseed
	Water
	Oil-free cooking spray (for eggs)

Lunch

2 bread	1 cup rice
2 vegetable	1 cup Chinese vegetables, stir-fried with garlic, onion, fresh ginger
1 fruit	1/2 cup citrus sections
4 very lean protein	4 ounces scallops, stir-fried
1 fat	1 teaspoon oil (for stir-frying)

Dinner

3 bread	2-inch square of corn bread
	1 cup kidney beans (add to chili)
1 fruit	1 pear
2 vegetable	1 cup chopped cooked tomatoes, with chili seasoning
	1/2 onion, garlic for seasoning
	Salad with 1 cup lettuce, 1/4 cup tomato, 1/4 cup cucumber
5 lean protein	Included (in beans)
	3 ounces soy crumbles (for chili)
2 fat	2 slices bacon, cooked very crisp and crumbled into chili
	Included (in corn bread)

Pre-Workout Snack

1 fat	1 tablespoon ranch dressing (for dipping)
1 milk	1 cup fat-free milk
1 vegetable	1 cup veggie sticks
	Water

Workout

Water

Post-Workout

SMOOTHIE

Blend until smooth.

1 milk	1 cup fat-free milk
2 fruit	1/2 cup orange juice
	1/2 cup frozen pineapple
	1/2 cup frozen strawberries
6 teaspoons added sugar	2 tablespoons honey
3 very lean protein	21 grams whey protein powder

DAY 4

Breakfast

1 fruit	1 cup raspberries
1 milk	1 cup fat-free milk (1/2 cup for French toast)

FRENCH TOAST *(See recipe directions on page 44.)*

2 bread	2 slices whole-wheat bread
1 medium-fat protein	1 egg
1 very lean protein	2 egg whites
1 fat	1 1/2 tablespoons ground flaxseed
	Water
	Oil-free cooking spray
	1 tablespoon no-sugar maple-flavored syrup

Lunch

1 fruit	3/4 cup blueberries

FAJITAS

Combine ingredients.

2 bread	2 tortillas
2 vegetable	1 cup sautéed onions and peppers
	2 tablespoons salsa
4 very lean protein	4 ounces skinless white-meat chicken, grilled with lime juice
1 fat	1 teaspoon olive oil (for cooking)

Dinner

3 bread	1 ounce croutons (for salad)
	1 cup chicken noodle soup
	4 crackers
1 fruit	1 nectarine
2 vegetable	Salad with 2 cups romaine lettuce, 1/2 cup tomato, 1/2 cup cucumber
5 lean protein	5 ounces swordfish, grilled with ginger and scallions
2 fat	2 tablespoons dressing

Pre-Workout Snack

1 fat	10 mixed nuts
1 milk	1 cup fat-free unsweetened yogurt
1 vegetable	1 cup V8 juice
	Water

Workout

Water

Post-Workout

SMOOTHIE

Blend until smooth.

1 milk	1 cup fat-free milk
2 fruit	½ cup orange juice
	½ cup frozen pineapple
	½ cup frozen strawberries
6 teaspoons added sugar	2 tablespoons honey
3 very lean protein	21 grams whey protein powder

DAY 5

Breakfast

2 bread	1 cup quick oats (not instant)
1 milk	1 cup fat-free milk
1 fruit	1 cup apples, diced
1 medium-fat protein	1 egg, scrambled on a nonstick pan
1 very lean protein	2 egg whites, scramble with whole egg
1 fat	1½ tablespoons ground flaxseed
	Water
	Oil-free cooking spray (for eggs)

Lunch

2 bread	1 cup cooked linguini
2 vegetable	Salad with 1 cup lettuce, ¼ cup tomato, ¼ cup cucumber
	Fat-free dressing
	½ cup marinara sauce
1 fruit	½ grapefruit, sectioned
4 very lean protein	4 ounces shrimp, grilled
1 fat	1 teaspoon olive oil (for cooking)

Dinner

3 bread	1 large pita
	1 ounce croutons
1 fruit	2 large figs
2 vegetable	Salad with 2 cups romaine lettuce, $1/2$ cup tomato, $1/2$ cup cucumber
5 lean protein	5 ounces lean lamb, grilled with lime juice
2 fat	2 tablespoons vinaigrette

Pre-Workout Snack

1 fat	1 tablespoon peanut butter
1 milk	1 cup fat-free milk
1 vegetable	1 cup celery sticks
	Water

Workout

Water

Post-Workout

SMOOTHIE

Blend until smooth.

1 milk	1 cup fat-free milk
2 fruit	$1/2$ cup orange juice
	$1/2$ cup frozen pineapple
	$1/2$ cup frozen strawberries
6 teaspoons added sugar	2 tablespoons honey
3 very lean protein	21 grams whey protein powder

DAY 6

Breakfast

2 bread	2 slices multigrain toast
1 medium-fat protein	1 egg, scrambled on a nonstick pan
1 very lean protein	2 egg whites, scrambled with whole egg
	Oil-free cooking spray (for eggs)

SMOOTHIE

Blend until smooth.

1 milk	1 cup fat-free milk
1 fruit	$1/4$ cup orange juice
	$1/4$ cup fresh peaches
1 fat	$1 1/2$ tablespoons ground flaxseed
	No-calorie sweetener to taste
	Water

Lunch

2 bread	1 whole-wheat bagel
2 vegetable	$1/2$ cup carrot sticks
	Onion, tomato
1 fruit	$1/8$ honeydew
4 very lean protein	4 ounces smoked salmon
1 fat	$1^1/2$ tablespoons reduced-fat cream cheese

Dinner

3 bread	2 slices rye bread
	$1/2$ cup pasta salad
1 fruit	12 grapes
2 vegetable	1 cup coleslaw
	$1/2$ cup chopped vegetables (cucumbers, carrots, onions); mix into tuna
5 lean protein	5 ounces tuna in olive oil, drained
2 fat	2 tablespoons reduced-fat mayonnaise (for tuna)
	Included (in coleslaw, pasta salad)

Pre-Workout Snack

1 fat	1 tablespoon sunflower seeds
1 milk	1 cup fat-free cottage cheese
1 vegetable	1 cup sliced bell pepper
	Water

Workout

	Water

Post-Workout

SMOOTHIE

Blend until smooth.

1 milk	1 cup fat-free milk
2 fruit	$1/2$ cup orange juice
	$1/2$ cup frozen pineapple
	$1/2$ cup frozen strawberries
6 teaspoons added sugar	2 tablespoons honey
3 very lean protein	21 grams whey protein powder

DAY 7

Breakfast

2 bread	1 cup Shredded Wheat
1 milk	1 cup fat-free milk
1 fruit	3/4 cup blueberries
1 medium-fat protein	1 egg, hard-cooked, for egg salad
1 very lean protein	2 eggs, hard-cooked, for egg salad (discard yolks)
1 fat	1 1/2 tablespoons ground flaxseed
	1 tablespoon fat-free mayonnaise (for egg salad)
	Mustard (for egg salad)
	Water

Lunch

2 bread	1 large multigrain roll
2 vegetable	Sliced tomato, lettuce (for sandwich)
	1/2 cup radishes, celery, carrots
1 fruit	1 nectarine
4 very lean protein	4 ounces skinless white-meat chicken, grilled with lime juice
1 fat	2 tablespoons low-fat ranch dressing (for dipping)

Dinner

3 bread	3-inch square of corn bread
	1 ounce croutons
1 fruit	1 large tangerine
2 vegetable	Salad with 2 cups romaine lettuce, 1/2 cup tomato, 1/2 cup cucumber
5 lean protein	5 ounces salmon, poached
2 fat	2 tablespoons low-fat Caesar dressing
	Included (in corn bread)

Pre-Workout Snack

1 fat	2 tablespoons reduced-fat ranch dressing
1 milk	1 cup fat-free milk
1 vegetable	Cucumber

Workout

       Water

Post-Workout

SMOOTHIE

Blend until smooth.

1 milk	1 cup fat-free milk
2 fruit	$^{1}/_{2}$ cup orange juice
	$^{1}/_{2}$ cup frozen pineapple
	$^{1}/_{2}$ cup frozen strawberries
6 teaspoons added sugar	2 tablespoons honey
3 very lean protein	21 grams whey protein powder

THE SYNDROME-X MEAL PLAN

THIS IS FOR THE OVERWEIGHT GUY WHO ALREADY HAS SOME HEALTH ISSUES, such as diabetes or high blood pressure. The body of an old man is just around the corner. But if he changes his lifestyle, he can still salvage himself. He needs to put the brakes on refined foods, especially high-fructose corn syrup. He'll have to start reading labels in the grocery store before the food goes into the cart. And he's got to add healthy oils into his diet to replace all that refined sugar. Doing so will help him lose weight and improve his blood-sugar and -cholesterol profiles. (Make sure you read chapter 7 before continuing.)

Daily Assumptions*†

2,003 calories
196 grams carbohydrates
154 grams protein
67 grams fat

Daily Breakdown*†

5 bread
4 fruit
3 milk
5 vegetable
9 very lean protein
5 lean protein
1 medium-fat protein
6 fat
0 teaspoons added sugar

Note: Occasionally, a fat-free product, like mustard or cooking spray, is included on the menus. These do not count toward your daily breakdown but should not be overused.

*Use every day.

† Based on a 185-pound man.

THE MENU

DAY 1

Breakfast

1 bread	½ cup Shredded Wheat
1 milk	1 cup fat-free milk
1 fruit	1 cup fresh blueberries
1 medium-fat protein	1 egg, scrambled on a nonstick pan
1 very lean protein	2 egg whites, scrambled with whole egg
1 fat	1½ tablespoons ground flaxseed
	Water
	Oil-free cooking spray (for eggs)

Snack

1 bread	½ cup edamame
1 vegetable	1 cup vegetable sticks
1 very lean protein	Included (in edamame)

Lunch

1 bread	2 very small boiled potatoes (for salad Niçoise)
2 vegetable	Lettuce, tomato
	Green beans
4 very lean protein	4 ounces albacore tuna in water, drained
2 fat	2 tablespoons low-fat dressing
	8 black olives

Snack

1 fruit	½ cup unsweetened applesauce
1 lean protein	½ cup cottage cheese

Post-Workout

SMOOTHIE

Blend until smooth.

1 milk	1 cup fat-free milk
1 fruit	$1/2$ cup orange juice with calcium
3 very lean protein	21 grams whey protein powder

Dinner

2 bread	1 small ear corn on the cob
	1 slice crusty French bread
1 fruit	12 cherries
1 milk	1 cup fat-free milk
2 vegetable	1 cup grilled vegetables (peppers, zucchini, mushrooms, tomatoes)
4 lean protein	4 ounces dark-meat chicken, barbecued
3 fat	1 tablespoon garlic-infused olive oil (for dipping)

DAY 2

Breakfast

Combine yogurt, fruit, and honey. Combine muffin and egg for sandwich.

1 bread	$1/2$ whole-wheat English muffin
1 milk	1 cup fat-free unsweetened yogurt
1 fruit	$11/4$ cups fresh strawberries
1 medium-fat protein	1 egg, hard-cooked
1 very lean protein	2 eggs, hard-cooked (discard yolks)
1 fat	$11/2$ tablespoons ground flaxseed
	Water

Snack

1 bread	$1/2$ bagel
1 vegetable	Sliced tomato, onion
1 very lean protein	1 ounce lox or smoked salmon
	1 tablespoon fat-free cream cheese

Lunch

1 bread	1 slice whole-grain bread
2 vegetable	Large salad with romaine lettuce, tomato, grilled eggplant, roasted red pepper
4 very lean protein	4 ounces skinless white-meat chicken, grilled with lime juice
2 fat	Low-fat dressing
	2 teaspoons olive oil (for roasted vegetables)

Snack

| 1 fruit | 1/2 mango |
| 1 lean protein | 1 ounce reduced-fat ricotta cheese |

Post-Workout

SMOOTHIE

Blend until smooth.

1 milk	1 cup fat-free milk
1 fruit	1/2 cup orange juice with calcium
3 very lean protein	21 grams whey protein powder

Dinner

2 bread	1 cup cooked pasta
1 fruit	1 1/4 cups strawberries
1 milk	1 cup fat-free milk
2 vegetable	1 cup ratatouille (over pasta)
	Salad with 1 cup lettuce, 1/4 cup tomato, 1/4 cup cucumber
4 lean protein	4 ounces lean ground beef (add to ratatouille)
3 fat	1 tablespoon dressing

DAY 3

Breakfast

1 bread	1 slice whole-wheat bread
1 milk	1 cup fat-free cottage cheese (on bread; sprinkle with no-calorie sweetener and cinnamon)
1 fruit	4 ounces freshly squeezed orange juice (with pulp)
1 medium-fat protein	1 egg, cooked sunny-side up in a nonstick pan
1 very lean protein	2 egg whites, cooked with sunny-side up egg
1 fat	1 1/2 tablespoons ground flaxseed
	Water
	Oil-free cooking spray (for eggs)

Snack

1 bread	4 Wheat Thins
1 vegetable	1 cup diced bell pepper
1 very lean protein	3/4 cup fat-free cottage cheese

Lunch

1 bread	1/3 cup rice
2 vegetable	1 cup Chinese vegetables, stir-fried with garlic, onion, fresh ginger
4 very lean protein	4 ounces scallops, stir-fried
2 fat	2 teaspoons oil (for stir-frying)

Snack

1 fruit	1 cup sliced melon
1 lean protein	1 ounce reduced-fat cheddar cheese

Post-Workout

SMOOTHIE

Blend until smooth.

1 milk	1 cup fat-free milk
1 fruit	1/2 cup orange juice with calcium
3 very lean protein	21 grams whey protein powder

Dinner

2 bread	1 cup kidney beans (add to chili)
1 fruit	1 pear
1 milk	1 cup fat-free milk
2 vegetable	1 cup chopped cooked tomatoes with chili seasoning
	1/2 onion, garlic for seasoning
	Salad with 1 cup lettuce, 1/4 cup tomato, 1/4 cup cucumber
4 lean protein	Included (in beans)
	2 ounces soy crumbles (for chili)
3 fat	2 slices bacon, cooked very crisp, crumbled into chili
	1/8 avocado, diced

DAY 4

Breakfast

1 fruit	1 cup raspberries
1 milk	1 cup fat-free milk (1/2 cup for French toast)

FRENCH TOAST (*See recipe directions on page 44.*)

1 bread	1 slice whole-wheat bread
1 medium-fat protein	1 egg
1 very lean protein	2 egg whites
1 fat	1 1/2 tablespoons ground flaxseed
	Water
	Oil-free cooking spray

Snack

1 bread	1 slice multigrain bread
1 vegetable	Sliced tomato
1 very lean protein	1 ounce fat-free cheese

Lunch

FAJITAS

Combine ingredients.

1 bread	1 tortilla
2 vegetable	1 cup sautéed onions, peppers
	2 tablespoons salsa
4 very lean protein	4 ounces skinless white-meat chicken, grilled with lime juice
2 fat	2 teaspoons olive oil (for cooking)

Snack

1 fruit	1¼ cups strawberries
1 lean protein	1 ounce reduced-fat ricotta cheese

Post-Workout

SMOOTHIE

Blend until smooth.

1 milk	1 cup fat-free milk
1 fruit	½ cup orange juice with calcium
3 very lean protein	21 grams whey protein powder

Dinner

2 bread	1 ounce croutons for salad
	1 cup chicken noodle soup
1 fruit	1 nectarine
1 milk	1 cup fat-free milk
2 vegetable	Salad with 2 cups romaine lettuce, ½ cup tomato, ½ cup cucumber
4 lean protein	4 ounces swordfish, grilled with ginger and scallions
3 fat	2 tablespoons dressing
	1 teaspoon olive oil (for fish)

DAY 5

Breakfast

1 bread	½ cup quick oats (not instant)
1 milk	1 cup fat-free milk
1 fruit	1 apple, diced
1 medium-fat protein	1 egg, scrambled in a nonstick pan
1 very lean protein	2 egg whites, scrambled with whole egg
1 fat	1½ tablespoons ground flaxseed
	Water
	Oil-free cooking spray (for eggs)

Snack

1 bread	³/₄ ounce baked tortilla chips
1 vegetable	¹/₂ cup salsa
1 very lean protein	1 ounce shredded fat-free cheese

Lunch

1 bread	¹/₂ cup cooked linguini
2 vegetable	Salad with 1 cup lettuce, ¹/₄ cup tomato, ¹/₄ cup cucumber
	Fat-free dressing
	¹/₂ cup marinara sauce
4 very lean protein	4 ounces shrimp, grilled
2 fat	2 teaspoons olive oil (for cooking)

Snack

1 fruit	1 medium peach
1 lean protein	¹/₄ cup cottage cheese

Post-Workout

SMOOTHIE

Blend until smooth.

1 milk	1 cup fat-free milk
1 fruit	¹/₂ cup orange juice with calcium
3 very lean protein	21 grams whey protein powder

Dinner

2 bread	1 large pita
1 fruit	2 large figs
1 milk	1 cup fat-free milk
2 vegetable	Salad with 2 cups romaine lettuce, ¹/₂ cup tomato, ¹/₂ cup cucumber
4 lean protein	4 ounces lean lamb, grilled with lime juice
3 fat	2 tablespoons vinaigrette
	1 tablespoon cucumber-yogurt dressing (for lamb)

DAY 6

Breakfast

1 bread	1 slice multigrain toast
1 medium-fat protein	1 egg, scrambled
1 very lean protein	2 egg whites, scrambled with whole egg
	Oil-free cooking spray (for eggs)

SMOOTHIE

Blend until smooth.

1 milk	1 cup fat-free milk
1 fruit	$1/4$ cup orange juice
	1 fresh peach, small
1 fat	$1^1/_2$ tablespoons ground flaxseed
	Water

Snack

Place vegetables on pita, top with cheese, heat.

1 bread	1 small pita
1 vegetable	1 cup diced tomato, mushrooms
1 very lean protein	1 ounce fat-free mozzarella

Lunch

1 bread	$1/2$ whole-wheat bagel
2 vegetable	$1/2$ cup carrot sticks
	Onion, tomato
4 very lean protein	4 ounces smoked salmon
2 fat	2 tablespoons cream cheese

Snack

1 fruit	1 orange, small
1 lean protein	1 ounce turkey

Post-Workout

SMOOTHIE

Blend until smooth.

1 milk	1 cup fat-free milk
1 fruit	$1/2$ cup orange juice with calcium
3 very lean protein	21 grams whey protein powder

Dinner

2 bread	2 slices rye bread
1 fruit	12 grapes
1 milk	1 cup fat-free milk
2 vegetable	1 cup coleslaw
	$1/2$ cup chopped vegetables (cucumber, carrots, onion; mix into tuna)
4 lean protein	4 ounces tuna in olive oil, drained
3 fat	2 tablespoons mayonnaise
	Included (in coleslaw)

DAY 7

Breakfast

1 bread	½ cup Shredded Wheat
1 milk	1 cup fat-free milk
1 fruit	1 cup raspberries
1 medium-fat protein	1 egg, hard-cooked (for egg salad)
1 very lean protein	1 egg, hard-cooked (for egg salad; discard yolks)
1 fat	1½ tablespoons ground flaxseed
	1 tablespoon fat-free mayonnaise (for egg salad)
	Mustard (for egg salad)
	Water

Snack

1 bread	5 slices melba toast
1 vegetable	Celery sticks
1 very lean protein	¾ cup fat-free ricotta
	(Put dry onion soup mix into ricotta to make dip.)

Lunch

1 bread	1 small multigrain roll
2 vegetable	Sliced tomato, lettuce (for sandwich)
	½ cup radishes, celery, carrots
4 very lean protein	4 ounces skinless white-meat chicken, grilled with lime juice
2 fat	2 tablespoons ranch dressing (for dipping)

Snack

1 fruit	1 kiwi
1 lean protein	1 ounce low-fat ham

Post-Workout

SMOOTHIE

Blend until smooth.

1 milk	1 cup fat-free milk
1 fruit	½ cup orange juice with calcium
3 very lean protein	21 grams whey protein powder

Dinner

2 bread	3-inch square of corn bread
1 fruit	1 large tangerine
1 milk	1 cup fat-free milk
2 vegetable	Salad with 2 cups romaine lettuce, ½ cup tomato, ½ cup cucumber
4 lean protein	4 ounces salmon, poached
3 fat	4 tablespoons low-fat Caesar dressing
	Included (in corn bread)

THE LIGHT-SPEED WEIGHT-LOSS MEAL PLAN

I DESIGNED THIS MENU FOR THE GUY WHO WANTS TO LOSE **10** POUNDS FAST— by any means necessary. Don't forget that exercise is required to make this work without losing lots of muscle. You'll probably want to work out in the morning while your energy levels are high to gain the metabolic boost of exercise for an extra calorie burn all day long. But no matter what, if you follow this diet for much longer than 2 to 4 weeks, your tank will hit empty. This diet definitely cries out for supplementation. Take a multivitamin/mineral with antioxidants, plus 400 milligrams of calcium and 400 international units (IU) of vitamin D daily.

Daily Assumptions*†

1,800 calories
104 grams carbohydrates
184 grams protein
72 grams fat

Daily Breakdown*†

2 bread
2 fruit
2 milk
4 vegetable
15 very lean protein
6 lean protein
1 medium-fat protein
6 fat
0 teaspoons added sugar

Note: Occasionally, a fat-free product, like mustard or cooking spray, is included on the menus. These do not count toward your daily breakdown but should not be overused.

*Use every day.

† Based on a 185-pound man.

THE MENU

DAY 1

Pre-Workout Drink

4 very lean protein	28 grams whey protein powder
	Water, ice cubes

Breakfast

1 bread	½ cup Shredded Wheat
1 milk	1 cup fat-free milk
1 fruit	1 cup fresh blueberries
1 medium-fat protein	1 egg, scrambled on a nonstick pan
3 very lean protein	6 egg whites, scrambled with whole egg
1 fat	1½ tablespoons ground flaxseed
	Water
	Oil-free cooking spray (for eggs)

Snack

1 vegetable	1 cup vegetable sticks
2 fat	1 tablespoon peanut butter

Lunch

1 vegetable	Salad with 1 cup lettuce, ¼ cup tomato
	½ cup green beans
6 very lean protein	6 ounces albacore tuna in water, drained
2 fat	2 tablespoons low-fat dressing
	8 black olives

Snack

1 vegetable	1 cup vegetable sticks
2 very lean protein	½ cup low-fat cottage cheese

Dinner

1 bread	1 small ear corn on the cob
1 fruit	12 cherries
1 milk	1 cup fat-free milk
1 vegetable	½ cup grilled vegetables: peppers, zucchini, mushrooms, tomatoes
6 lean protein	6 ounces skinless dark-meat chicken, grilled with lime juice
1 fat	8 Kalamata olives

DAY 2

Pre-Workout Drink

4 very lean protein	28 grams whey protein powder
	Water, ice cubes

Breakfast

Combine yogurt, fruit, and honey. Combine muffin and egg for sandwich.

1 bread	½ whole-wheat English muffin
1 milk	1 cup fat-free unsweetened yogurt
1 fruit	1¼ cups fresh strawberries
1 medium-fat protein	1 egg, hard-cooked
3 very lean protein	6 eggs, hard-cooked (discard yolks)
1 fat	1½ tablespoons ground flaxseed
	Water

Snack

1 vegetable	Sliced tomato, onion
2 fat	2 ounces cream cheese

Lunch

1 vegetable	Large salad with romaine lettuce, tomato, grilled eggplant, roasted red pepper
6 very lean protein	6 ounces skinless white-meat chicken, grilled with lime juice
2 fat	Fat-free dressing
	2 teaspoons olive oil for roasted vegetables

Snack

1 vegetable	8 ounces V8 juice
2 very lean protein	2 ounces fat-free cheese

Dinner

1 bread	$^1/_2$ cup cooked pasta
1 fruit	$1^1/_4$ cups strawberries
1 milk	1 cup fat-free milk
1 vegetable	$^1/_2$ cup ratatouille (over pasta)
	Salad with 1 cup lettuce, $^1/_4$ cup tomato, $^1/_4$ cup cucumber
6 lean protein	6 ounces lean ground beef (add to ratatouille)
1 fat	2 tablespoons low-fat dressing

DAY 3

Pre-Workout Drink

4 very lean protein	28 grams whey protein powder
	Water, ice cubes

Breakfast

1 bread	1 slice whole-wheat bread
1 milk	1 cup fat-free cottage cheese (on bread; sprinkle with no-calorie sweetener and cinnamon)
1 fruit	4 ounces freshly squeezed orange juice (with pulp)
1 medium-fat protein	1 egg, cooked sunny-side up in a nonstick pan
3 very lean protein	6 egg whites, cooked with sunny-side up egg
1 fat	$1^1/_2$ tablespoons ground flaxseed
	Water
	Oil-free cooking spray (for eggs)

Snack

1 vegetable	Sliced radishes
2 fat	4 tablespoons low-fat ranch dressing

Lunch

1 vegetable	1 cup Chinese vegetables, stir-fried with garlic, onion, fresh ginger
6 very lean protein	6 ounces scallops, stir-fried
2 fat	2 teaspoons oil (for stir-frying)

Snack

1 vegetable	1 cup diced bell pepper
2 very lean protein	$^1/_2$ cup low-fat cottage cheese

Dinner

1 bread	½ cup kidney beans (add to chili)
1 fruit	1 pear
1 milk	1 cup fat-free milk
1 vegetable	½ cup chopped cooked tomatoes with chili seasoning
	½ onion, garlic for seasoning
6 lean protein	Included (in beans)
	5 ounces soy crumbles (for chili)
1 fat	⅛ avocado, diced

DAY 4

Pre-Workout Drink

4 very lean protein	28 grams whey protein powder
	Water, ice cubes

Breakfast

1 fruit	1 cup raspberries
1 milk	1 cup fat-free milk (½ cup for French toast)

FRENCH TOAST *(See recipe directions on page 44.)*

1 bread	1 slice whole-wheat bread
1 medium-fat protein	1 egg
3 very lean protein	6 egg whites
1 fat	1½ tablespoons ground flaxseed
	Water
	Oil-free cooking spray

Snack

1 vegetable	1 cup celery sticks
2 fat	1 tablespoon almond butter

Lunch

FAJITAS

Combine ingredients.

1 vegetable	½ cup sautéed onions, peppers
	2 tablespoons salsa
6 very lean protein	6 ounces skinless white-meat chicken, grilled with lime juice
2 fat	2 teaspoons olive oil (for cooking)

Snack

1 vegetable	Sliced tomato
2 very lean protein	2 ounces fat-free cheese

Dinner

1 bread	1 cup chicken noodle soup
1 fruit	1 nectarine
1 milk	1 cup fat-free milk
1 vegetable	Salad with 1 cup lettuce, $1/4$ cup tomato, $1/4$ cup cucumbers
6 lean protein	6 ounces swordfish, grilled with ginger and scallions
1 fat	2 tablespoons low-fat dressing
	1 teaspoon olive oil (for fish)

DAY 5

Pre-Workout Drink

4 very lean protein	28 grams whey protein powder
	Water, ice cubes

Breakfast

1 bread	$1/2$ cup quick oats (not instant)
1 milk	1 cup fat-free milk
1 fruit	1 apple, diced
1 medium-fat protein	1 egg, scrambled in a nonstick pan
3 very lean protein	6 egg whites, scrambled with whole egg
1 fat	$1^{1}/_{2}$ tablespoons ground flaxseed
	Water
	Oil-free cooking spray (for eggs)

Snack

1 vegetable	1 cup raw broccoli and/or cauliflower
2 fat	2 tablespoons Thousand Island dressing

Lunch

1 vegetable	Salad with 1 cup lettuce, $1/4$ cup tomato, $1/4$ cup cucumber
	Fat-free dressing
6 very lean protein	6 ounces shrimp, grilled
2 fat	2 teaspoons olive oil (for cooking)

Snack

1 vegetable	¼ cup salsa
	1 cup celery sticks
2 very lean protein	2 ounces shredded fat-free cheese

Dinner

1 bread	1 small pita
1 fruit	2 large figs
1 milk	1 cup fat-free milk
1 vegetable	Cucumber, tomato, sprouts
6 lean protein	6 ounces lean lamb, grilled with lime juice
1 fat	2 tablespoons low-fat cucumber-yogurt dressing (for lamb)

DAY 6

Pre-Workout Drink

4 very lean protein	28 grams whey protein powder
	Water, ice cubes

Breakfast

1 bread	1 slice multigrain bread, toasted
1 medium-fat protein	1 egg, scrambled in a nonstick pan
3 very lean protein	6 egg whites, scrambled with whole egg
	Oil-free cooking spray (for eggs)

SMOOTHIE
Blend until smooth.

1 milk	1 cup fat-free milk
1 fruit	¼ cup orange juice
	½ fresh peach
1 fat	1½ tablespoons ground flaxseed
	Water

Snack

1 vegetable	1 cup fresh raw green beans
2 fat	2 tablespoons sliced almonds

Lunch

Roll lox, cream cheese, veggies inside lettuce.

1 vegetable	Lettuce leaves, onion, tomato
6 very lean protein	6 ounces lox or smoked salmon
2 fat	2 tablespoons cream cheese

Snack

1 vegetable	1/2 cup diced tomatoes, mushrooms
2 very lean protein	2 ounces fat-free mozzarella

Dinner

1 bread	1 slice rye bread
1 fruit	12 grapes
1 milk	1 cup fat-free milk
1 vegetable	1/2 cup chopped vegetables (cucumbers, carrots, onions; mix into tuna)
6 lean protein	6 ounces tuna in olive oil, drained
1 fat	2 tablespoons reduced-fat mayonnaise

DAY 7

Pre-Workout Drink

4 very lean protein	28 grams whey protein powder
	Water, ice cubes

Breakfast

1 bread	1/2 cup Shredded Wheat
1 milk	1 cup fat-free milk
1 fruit	1 cup raspberries
1 medium-fat protein	1 egg, hard-cooked (for egg salad)
3 very lean protein	6 eggs, hard-cooked (for egg salad; discard yolks)
1 fat	1 1/2 tablespoons ground flaxseed
	1 tablespoon fat-free mayonnaise (for egg salad)
	Mustard (for egg salad)
	Water

Snack

1 vegetable	8 ounces V8 juice
2 fat	20 peanuts

Lunch

1 vegetable	Sliced tomato, lettuce (for sandwich)
	$1/2$ cup radishes, celery, carrots
6 very lean protein	6 ounces skinless white-meat chicken, grilled with lime juice
2 fat	2 tablespoons ranch dressing (for dipping)

Snack

1 vegetable	1 cup celery sticks
2 very lean protein	$3/4$ cup fat-free ricotta
	(Put dry onion soup mix into ricotta to make dip.)

Dinner

1 bread	1 small dinner whole wheat roll
1 fruit	1 large tangerine
1 milk	1 cup fat-free milk
1 vegetable	Salad with 1 cup lettuce, $1/4$ cup tomato, $1/4$ cup cucumber
6 lean protein	6 ounces salmon, poached
1 fat	2 tablespoons reduced-fat Caesar dressing

THE "NO MORE YO-YO DIETS" MEAL PLAN

THIS GUY HAS GONE ON AND OFF SO MANY DIETS, gained and lost pounds so many times, that his metabolic rate is in the cellar. When he diets, he basically fasts, eating as little as possible. He doesn't work out while he's dieting because he's too tired. He needs to get active, eat at regular intervals, and increase his caloric intake if he's ever going to have a chance of losing fat and gaining some muscle. That's the only way he can bump his metabolic rate back up to its starting point.

Daily Assumptions*†

2,003 calories
196 grams carbohydrates
154 grams protein
67 grams fat

Daily Breakdown*†

5 bread
4 fruit
3 milk
5 vegetable
9 very lean protein
5 lean protein
1 medium-fat protein
6 fat
0 teaspoons added sugar

Note: Occasionally, a fat-free product, like mustard or cooking spray, is included on the menus. These do not count toward your daily breakdown but should not be overused.

*Use every day.

† Based on a 185-pound man.

THE MENU

DAY 1

Pre-Workout Drink

1 milk	1 cup fat-free milk
1 fruit	½ cup orange juice with calcium
2 very lean protein	14 grams whey protein powder

Breakfast

1 bread	½ cup Shredded Wheat
1 milk	1 cup fat-free milk
1 fruit	¾ cup fresh blueberries
1 medium-fat protein	1 egg, scrambled on a nonstick pan
2 very lean protein	4 egg whites, scrambled with whole egg
1 fat	1½ tablespoons ground flaxseed
	Water
	Oil-free cooking spray (for eggs)

Snack

1 bread	½ cup edamame
1 vegetable	1 cup vegetable sticks
1 very lean protein	Included (in edamame)

Lunch

1 bread	2 very small boiled potatoes (for salad Niçoise)
2 vegetable	Lettuce, tomato
	Green beans
4 very lean protein	4 ounces albacore tuna in water, drained
2 fat	2 tablespoons low-fat dressing
	8 black olives

Snack

1 fruit	$^1/_2$ cup unsweetened applesauce
1 lean protein	$^1/_4$ cup cottage cheese

Dinner

2 bread	1 small ear corn on the cob
	1 slice crusty French bread
1 fruit	12 cherries
1 milk	1 cup fat-free milk
2 vegetable	1 cup grilled vegetables (peppers, zucchini, mushrooms, tomatoes)
4 lean protein	4 ounces barbecued chicken
3 fat	1 tablespoon garlic-infused olive oil (for dipping)

DAY 2

Pre-Workout Drink

1 milk	1 cup fat-free milk
1 fruit	$^1/_2$ cup orange juice with calcium
2 very lean protein	14 grams whey protein powder

Breakfast

Combine yogurt, fruit, and honey. Combine muffin and egg for sandwich.

1 bread	$^1/_2$ whole-wheat English muffin
1 milk	1 cup fat-free unsweetened yogurt
1 fruit	$1^1/_4$ cups fresh strawberries
1 medium-fat protein	1 egg, hard-cooked
2 very lean protein	4 eggs, hard-cooked (discard yolks)
1 fat	$1^1/_2$ tablespoons ground flaxseed
	Water

Snack

1 bread	$^1/_2$ bagel
1 vegetable	Sliced tomato, onion
1 very lean protein	1 ounce lox or smoked salmon
	1 tablespoon fat-free cream cheese

Lunch

1 bread	1 slice whole-grain bread
2 vegetable	Large salad with romaine lettuce, tomato, grilled eggplant, roasted red pepper
	Fat-free dressing
4 very lean protein	4 ounces skinless white-meat chicken, grilled with lime juice
2 fat	2 teaspoons olive oil (for roasted vegetables)

Snack

1 fruit	$^1/_2$ mango
1 lean protein	1 ounce reduced-fat ricotta cheese

Dinner

2 bread	1 cup cooked pasta
1 fruit	$1^1/_4$ cups strawberries
1 milk	1 cup fat-free milk
2 vegetable	1 cup ratatouille (over pasta)
	Salad with 1 cup lettuce, $^1/_4$ cup tomato, $^1/_4$ cup cucumber
4 lean protein	4 ounces lean ground beef (add to ratatouille)
3 fat	1 tablespoon dressing

DAY 3

Pre-Workout Drink

1 milk	1 cup fat-free milk
1 fruit	$^1/_2$ cup orange juice with calcium
2 very lean protein	14 grams whey protein powder

Breakfast

1 bread	1 slice whole-wheat bread
1 milk	1 cup fat-free cottage cheese (on bread; sprinkle with no-calorie sweetener and cinnamon)
1 fruit	4 ounces freshly squeezed orange juice (with pulp)
1 medium-fat protein	1 egg, cooked sunny-side up in a nonstick pan
2 very lean protein	4 egg whites, cooked with sunny-side up egg
1 fat	$1^1/_2$ tablespoons ground flaxseed
	Water
	Oil-free cooking spray (for eggs)

Snack

1 bread	4 Wheat Thins
1 vegetable	1 cup diced bell pepper
1 very lean protein	$^1/_4$ cup low-fat cottage cheese

Lunch

1 bread	$^1/_3$ cup rice
2 vegetable	1 cup Chinese vegetables, stir-fried with garlic, onion, fresh ginger
4 very lean protein	4 ounces scallops, stir-fried
2 fat	2 teaspoons oil (for stir-frying)

Snack

1 fruit	1 cup sliced melon
1 lean protein	1 ounce reduced-fat cheddar cheese

Dinner

2 bread	1 cup kidney beans (add to chili)
1 fruit	1 pear
1 milk	1 cup fat-free milk
2 vegetable	1 cup chopped cooked tomatoes with chili seasoning
	$^1/_2$ onion, garlic for seasoning
	Salad with 1 cup lettuce, $^1/_4$ cup tomato, $^1/_4$ cup cucumber
4 lean protein	Included (in beans)
	2 ounces soy crumbles (add to chili)
3 fat	2 slices bacon, cooked very crisp, crumbled into chili
	$^1/_8$ avocado, diced

DAY 4

Pre-Workout Drink

1 milk	1 cup fat-free milk
1 fruit	$^1/_2$ cup orange juice with calcium
2 very lean protein	14 grams whey protein powder

Breakfast

1 fruit	1 cup raspberries
1 milk	1 cup fat-free milk ($^1/_2$ cup for French toast)

FRENCH TOAST (*See recipe directions on page 44.*)

1 bread	1 slice whole-wheat bread
1 medium-fat protein	1 egg
2 very lean protein	4 egg whites
1 fat	$1^1/_2$ tablespoons ground flaxseed
	Water

Snack

1 bread	1 slice multigrain bread
1 vegetable	Sliced tomato
1 very lean protein	1 ounce fat-free cheese

Lunch

FAJITAS

Combine ingredients.

1 bread	1 tortilla
2 vegetable	1 cup sautéed onions, peppers
	2 tablespoons salsa
4 very lean protein	4 ounces skinless white-meat chicken, grilled with lime juice
2 fat	2 teaspoons olive oil (for cooking)

Snack

1 fruit	1¼ cups strawberries
1 lean protein	³⁄₄ cup reduced-fat ricotta cheese

Dinner

2 bread	1 ounce croutons (for salad)
	1 cup chicken noodle soup
1 fruit	1 nectarine
1 milk	1 cup fat-free milk
2 vegetable	Salad with 2 cups romaine lettuce, ¹⁄₂ cup tomato, ¹⁄₂ cup cucumber
4 lean protein	4 ounces swordfish, grilled with ginger and scallions
3 fat	2 tablespoons dressing
	1 teaspoon olive oil (for fish)

DAY 5

Pre-Workout Drink

1 milk	1 cup fat-free milk
1 fruit	¹⁄₂ cup orange juice with calcium
2 very lean protein	14 grams whey protein powder

Breakfast

1 bread	¹⁄₂ cup quick oats (not instant)
1 milk	1 cup fat-free milk
1 fruit	1 apple, diced
1 medium-fat protein	1 egg, scrambled in a nonstick pan
2 very lean protein	4 egg whites, scrambled with whole egg
1 fat	1¹⁄₂ tablespoons ground flaxseed
	Water
	Oil-free cooking spray (for eggs)

Snack

1 bread	$^3/_4$ ounce baked tortilla chips
1 vegetable	$^1/_2$ cup salsa
1 very lean protein	1 ounce shredded fat-free cheese

Lunch

1 bread	$^1/_2$ cup cooked linguini
2 vegetable	Salad with 1 cup lettuce, $^1/_4$ cup tomato, $^1/_4$ cup cucumber
	Fat-free dressing
	$^1/_2$ cup marinara sauce
4 very lean protein	4 ounces shrimp, grilled
2 fat	2 teaspoons olive oil (for cooking)

Snack

1 fruit	1 medium peach
1 lean protein	$^1/_4$ cup cottage cheese

Dinner

2 bread	1 large pita
1 fruit	2 large figs
1 milk	1 cup fat-free milk
2 vegetable	Salad with 2 cups romaine lettuce, $^1/_2$ cup tomato, $^1/_2$ cup cucumber
4 lean protein	4 ounces lean lamb, grilled with lime juice
3 fat	2 tablespoons vinaigrette
	1 tablespoon cucumber-yogurt dressing (for lamb)

DAY 6

Pre-Workout Drink

1 milk	1 cup fat-free milk
1 fruit	$^1/_2$ cup orange juice with calcium
2 very lean protein	14 grams whey protein powder

Breakfast

1 bread	1 slice multigrain bread, toasted
1 medium-fat protein	1 egg, scrambled in a nonstick pan
2 very lean protein	4 egg whites, scrambled with whole egg
	Oil-free cooking spray (for eggs)

SMOOTHIE

Blend until smooth.

1 milk	1 cup fat-free milk
1 fruit	1/4 cup orange juice
	1/2 fresh peach
1 fat	1 1/2 tablespoons ground flaxseed
	Water

Snack

Place vegetables on pita, top with cheese, heat.

1 bread	1 small pita
1 vegetable	1 cup diced tomato, mushrooms
1 very lean protein	1 ounce fat-free mozzarella

Lunch

1 bread	1/2 whole-wheat bagel
2 vegetable	1/2 cup carrot sticks
	Onion, tomato
4 very lean protein	4 ounces smoked salmon
2 fat	2 tablespoons cream cheese

Snack

1 fruit	1 small orange
1 lean protein	1 ounce turkey

Dinner

2 bread	2 slices rye bread
1 fruit	12 grapes
1 milk	1 cup fat-free milk
2 vegetable	1 cup coleslaw
	1/2 cup chopped vegetables (cucumbers, carrots, onions; mix into tuna)
4 lean protein	4 ounces tuna in olive oil, drained
3 fat	2 tablespoons mayonnaise
	Included (in coleslaw)

DAY 7

Pre-Workout Drink

1 milk	1 cup fat-free milk
1 fruit	1/2 cup orange juice with calcium
2 very lean protein	14 grams whey protein powder

Breakfast

1 bread	$\frac{1}{2}$ cup Shredded Wheat
1 milk	1 cup fat-free milk
1 fruit	1 cup raspberries
1 medium-fat protein	1 egg, hard-cooked (for egg salad)
2 very lean protein	4 eggs, hard-cooked (for egg salad; discard yolks)
1 fat	$1\frac{1}{2}$ tablespoons ground flaxseed
	1 tablespoon fat-free mayonnaise (for egg salad)
	Mustard (for egg salad)
	Water

Snack

1 bread	5 slices melba toast
1 vegetable	Celery sticks
1 very lean protein	$\frac{3}{4}$ cup fat-free ricotta
	(Stir dry onion soup mix into ricotta to make dip.)

Lunch

1 bread	1 small multigrain roll
2 vegetable	Sliced tomato, lettuce (for sandwich)
	$\frac{1}{2}$ cup radishes, celery, carrots
4 very lean protein	4 ounces skinless white-meat chicken, grilled with lime juice
2 fat	2 tablespoons ranch dressing (for dipping)

Snack

1 fruit	1 kiwi
1 lean protein	1 ounce low-fat ham

Dinner

2 bread	3-inch square of corn bread
1 fruit	1 large tangerine
1 milk	1 cup fat-free milk
2 vegetable	Salad with 1 cup romaine lettuce, $\frac{1}{2}$ cup tomato, $\frac{1}{2}$ cup cucumber
4 lean protein	4 ounces salmon, poached
3 fat	4 tablespoons low-fat Caesar dressing
	Included (in corn bread)

CHAPTER FOUR

Food and Muscle Gain

THESE PLANS FOR PACKING ON MUSCLE HELP EVEN THE WORST HARDGAINERS SEE RESULTS

You'd be hard-pressed to find a single establishment devoted to helping people gain weight. Weight-loss centers, of course. But weight-gain centers? Not a one.

Perhaps it's time to open shop. After all, there are millions of guys—commonly known as "hardgainers" or "ectomorphs"—who will never, ever pack on size without a specially tailored plan. Trying to outsmart your genes into creating a bigger, more impressive body than nature intended is one of the great fitness tricks.

But it can be done, and never is nutrition more important than when you're trying to coax your body into growth. Theoretically, you could keep your diet constant and train more intensely or more frequently, but trying to build muscle in the gym without sufficient fuel is an exercise in futility. You're going to need extra calories, and you don't have to get them from weight-gain shakes that taste like liquid cement. There's a better way. (*Note:* If your goal is to get stronger or have better muscle definition without adding too much mass, see the next chapter.)

The Science of Muscle Building

You probably know that lifting weights and eating lots of protein prompts your muscles to grow, but what's actually going on beneath your skin?

Your muscles are made up of fibers, and those fibers need to be damaged, or at least broken down, before their satellite cells can rebuild them bigger than before. Generally, your muscles can contract over and over again without a hitch, as they do during everyday tasks such as walking and brushing your teeth. When you apply a load that is greater than usual, however, your muscle fibers tear and proteins are damaged. If you were to look at your muscles under a microscope after you train, you'd actually see the torn fibers. With proper nutritional support and sufficient downtime, your body rebuilds them, only they don't just return to their original form—they get bigger and stronger, a process called *hypertrophy*. It's similar to how you learn a new software program on your computer. The first time you try to use it, you're forced to think really hard; and after a while, your brain hurts and you get a headache. Over time, the knowledge in your brain expands, and you can operate that same program headache-free.

To fuel hypertrophy, you need plenty of protein and its building blocks, amino acids. With protein on your side, you can push your body into an *anabolic* state—a state during which your body creates more muscle protein than it breaks down. (When the reverse occurs, you're in a *catabolic* state, not to be confused with a *catatonic* state, although that would make you quite catabolic, too. By the way, your body can't be anabolic and catabolic at the same time.)

This is not a workout book, and I'm not going to prescribe the muscle-building programs that will work in conjunction with your diet (although if you are looking for a good one, I suggest the *Men's Health Home Workout Bible.* It has almost every exercise imaginable and includes plans for guys with free weights, gym equipment, or no weights at all). What I can tell you is how to eat to maximize your workouts and keep you anabolic more often. The following nutritional strategies will help ensure that this rebuilding process works smoothly, allowing you to stay anabolic and not catabolic—or catatonic.

Eat, Eat, and Eat Some More

By now, you know that the muscle-building process doesn't work without food to fuel it. For people trying to lose weight, the key is to eat a lot and exercise even more. For you hardgainers, the key is exercising a little less and eating even more. Your question here is, of course: How do I know I'm eating enough?

It takes about 2,500 calories to add 1 pound of muscle, with "about" being the operative word—2,500 is an approximation for something that in reality is highly individualized and variable.

To begin with, as soon as you start eating more, your energy expenditure increases due to the thermic effect of food. Also, you'll probably amp up your weight training when eating for mass, so that, too,

---

Ten 100-Calorie Foods

When you're looking to add 100 or so calories to a meal, reach for one of these healthy alternatives, each of which gets you in the ballpark.

1 banana

1/2 plain bagel with low-fat cream cheese

8 ounces milk (2 percent fat)

1 bowl oatmeal

1/2 energy bar

Small handful raisins or dried fruit

Small handful nuts

1/2 medium cantaloupe

4 ounces low-fat vanilla yogurt

1 cup Cream of Wheat cereal

---

will cost you more calories. It takes still more energy to rebuild the muscle you're tearing down in the gym, and once it's been rebuilt, that tissue needs to be maintained. Here's another approximation: Every 10 pounds of muscle you add will require an additional 200 to 300 calories and 10 grams of protein a day.

If you're an average-size active male who wants to gain muscle, eat an additional 300 to 500 calories per day. Spread these extra calories over five or six meals a day. If you're eating fewer than five or six meals a day, you need to add meals until you reach that range. If you're already eating that frequently, start adding calories incrementally to existing meals. You'll be surprised at how easy it is to tack an extra 100 calories onto a meal. Adding an apple to your lunch gives you an extra 60 calories; topping it with a slice of mozzarella cheese or a tablespoon of peanut butter gets you over the century mark. So does a single banana or a glass of milk.

Here's some advice for fitting in the extra calories.

Drink your meals. Ready-to-mix powders allow you to drink those extra calories, which can come in handy when your time gets stretched tight. Note that these are not the weight-gain shakes of yesteryear (the ones that go down like melted tar). Many of the products on the market today are far more palatable. Rather than relying on protein powders—which, as their name suggests, are largely devoid of carbs—choose meal-replacement shakes. These combine carbohydrates with protein and even small amounts of fat. They're just what the doctor ordered after you've completed your workout, which, if you're not eating or drinking something then already, is the best starting place for tacking on those extra calories. By giving yourself protein and carbs immediately after exercise, you'll slow down the process of protein breakdown and boost protein manufacturing. As a colleague of mine says, "Put down your last weight and pick up your recovery drink."

Eat before your workouts. Another good way to shoehorn calories into your diet is to eat a meal 30 to 90 minutes before you work out, when your stomach should be able to handle 200 to 300 calories pretty easily. As a bonus, your pre-workout meal might decrease the catabolic effects of exercise, particularly if those calories contain an equal amount of carbs and protein along with some essential fatty acids.

Don't go overboard on calories. You don't have to eat everything in sight to put on size. Realistically, a daily increase of 20 percent or so is about the biggest jump in daily calories an average person can make without risk of adding significant additional fat. (You'll almost always add some fat when gaining muscle. It's rarely one or the other entirely, just as you're never losing only fat on a weight-loss regimen.) Trying to make a fast, radical shift in your lifestyle will raise the odds that you throw in the towel.

Rely on energy-dense foods. Certain otherwise-healthy foods can impede your progress en route to a bigger body. If you eat a humongous bran muffin for breakfast, chances are you won't be hungry for another 3 or 4 hours, and you'll miss an opportunity to consume more calories later.

In *The Volumetrics Weight Control Plan,* authors Barbara Rolls, Ph.D., and Robert Barnett point out

ANABOLIC POWER SHAKE

THIS IS AN IDEAL POST-EXERCISE RECOVERY SHAKE. Make it the night before, freeze it in a disposable plastic drink container, and throw it into your gym bag in the morning. It will thaw by the time you set down the last weight from your last rep. Leave some room under the lid so it won't burst open the container when it freezes.

1 cup frozen strawberries
1 cup low-fat or fat-free strawberry yogurt
25 grams whey protein powder
1 tablespoon honey
1 cup fat-free milk
1 cup orange juice fortified with vitamins C and E

2 to 5 grams creatine monohydrate
4 to 10 grams glutamine

Blend all ingredients until smooth. Best drunk immediately after exercise.

Contains 589 calories, 100 grams carbohydrates, 46 grams protein, 1 gram fat, 4 grams dietary fiber

that over the course of a day, most people tend to eat the same weight of food. The thrust of their suggestion for losing weight, then, is making sure that this usual quantity of food has fewer calories. One example they use is $1/4$ cup of raisins versus $1^2/3$ cups of grapes, both of which equal 100 calories. Although the calories are the same, eating the latter is more likely to make you feel full, Dr. Rolls' studies show, even if you eat less of it, thus consuming fewer calories.

That's great when you're trying to lose weight, but when you're trying to pack on size, you want to do the opposite. Although you want to pass on the chips, cookies, chocolate candy, and other types of high-calorie junk food, gravitate toward healthful, energy-dense foods such as nuts.

Don't eliminate low-energy-density foods, such as celery and lettuce, because many of them are in-credibly good for you. Just don't go overboard on them when you're shooting for size. They impart a feeling of fullness relatively quickly without adding a large number of calories to your daily total. Rather than jettisoning salads during this phase, soup them up by adding some feta cheese, olives, grilled chicken, or sliced ham.

Power Protein

Of the calories you consume, make plenty of them protein. Protein is chock-full of the amino acids re-quired to make the enzymes, hormones, and anti-bodies your body needs for manufacturing red blood cells, buttressing the immune system, and otherwise supporting the proper functioning of the human body. Protein also helps repair muscle tissue that's been temporarily damaged by resistance training. For

PROTEIN POINTERS

FOLLOW THESE POINTERS WITH RESPECT to protein consumption.

■ To make things easy, use 1 gram per pound of body weight as your daily baseline.

■ If you're a strict vegetarian, add 10 percent to your intake to account for the dispropor-tionate amount of "incomplete" protein in your diet.

■ Consume some of your protein before and after you train, when your body can put it to maximum use. In general, spread it throughout the day rather than eating it in a few big globs.

■ If you consume less than 1 gram per pound of body weight, rely heavily on whole foods for your protein. If you follow a high-protein diet, however, use supplements to limit in-take of saturated fats and cholesterol.

■ Don't skimp on carbs if you're eating high amounts of protein in an attempt to gain size. Reducing carbs will cause your body to draw upon branched-chain amino acids, particu-larly during endurance exercise.

■ Drink plenty of water. The more protein you consume, the more fluid you need to avoid dehydration.

■ Steer clear of a high-protein diet if you have kidney problems—or a family history of them.

reasons just discussed, active guys should consume considerably more protein than guys who just sit around all day.

Don't be surprised if it's more than you consume now—exercise increases the need for protein over and above any prescription suitable for a couch potato. The added protein will give you an abundance of the essential amino acids needed for constant muscle growth and repair.

Uncle Sam, with the vast array of scientific resources and billions of dollars at his disposal, suggests in his Recommended Dietary Allowances, or RDAs, that you consume 0.36 grams of protein per pound (or 0.8 grams/kilogram) a day. With a small margin for error baked in, the RDA aims to keep protein synthesis and breakdown more or less in equilibrium for the general population. In other words, the RDA was designed for the average guy who sits at his desk all day long and then comes home and sits on his couch.

You need much more protein than that. You exercise—right?—which highlights the most glar-

VEGETARIAN MUSCLE-BUILDING RECIPES

IF YOU ARE A VEGETARIAN, USE THESE RECIPES to ensure that you consume enough protein.

Breakfast: Granola

Makes 3 servings
1 serving = 306 calories (53 grams carbohydrates, 5 grams fiber, 10 grams fat, 6 grams protein)

   1 cup rolled oats
   1/2 cup Kashi ready-to-eat cereal
   1/8 cup honey
   1 tablespoon canola oil
   1 tablespoon water
   1/4 cup dried, sweetened cranberries
   1/4 cup golden raisins
   2 tablespoons slivered almonds

1. Preheat oven to 300°F.

2. In a large bowl, mix together the oats, Kashi, and honey. In a separate bowl, combine the oil and water; pour over the oat mixture. Blend well.

3. Spread the mixture evenly onto a nonstick cookie sheet and bake for 10 minutes. Stir and return to oven for another 10 minutes. Remove from the oven and add the cranberries, raisins, and almonds while the cereal is still hot. Cool completely before serving.

Snack: Edamame

Makes 2 servings
1 serving = 120 calories (9 grams carbohydrates, 4 grams fiber, 5 grams fat, 10 grams protein)

   10-ounce bag frozen soybeans in the hull
   2 quarts boiling water
   1/2 tablespoon coarse or sea salt

In a large saucepan, cook the soybeans in boiling water for 3 minutes. Drain and rinse under cold running water. Sprinkle with salt to taste. Serve warm or cold in the hull. Remove hull to eat soybeans inside.

Reprinted with permission from *The Be Healthier, Feel Stronger Vegetarian Cookbook,* by Susan M. Kleiner, Ph.D., R.D., and Karen Friedman-Kester, M.S., R.D.

ing problem with the RDAs. Like most government recommendations on nutrition matters, the RDAs address sedentary individuals. How backward. We live in a nation with a pitifully out-of-shape populace, as evidenced by near-epidemic obesity, with a government rhetorically dedicated to getting citizens more physically active, and yet the protein recommendations it makes target couch potatoes who do precisely what the government says they shouldn't be doing: sitting on their butts all day.

For those of you who exercise—and I'm assuming that means everyone reading *Power Food*—you need approximately *two and a half times* what the U.S. government recommends. That may sound radical, but the research is in our corner, not theirs.

Here are some tips for meeting your protein needs.

Consume 1 gram of protein daily per pound of body weight. Guys who lift weights should be consuming 0.8 grams of protein for every pound that you weigh, each and every day. And if you're trying to gain muscle, which is the focus of this chapter, that amount needs to be bumped up to 1 full gram. This higher amount accounts for the energy you expend training, as well as the physiological processes set in motion by exercise. For example, amino acids aren't used as much for fuel during weight training as they are during cardiovascular exercise. Still, you need them to provide raw materials to your muscles to spur growth. Amino acids are not only the building blocks of new muscle, they are the catalysts of the muscle-building process.

Don't go overboard. If twice the RDA for protein is good for guys who work out, might still more be better? Probably not. At a certain point excess protein likely just gets wasted.

Keep in mind that in the context of your everyday diet, some of these numerical differences can be relatively insignificant. For a 200-pounder, the difference between consuming 0.70 and 0.85 grams

per pound of body weight is less than the protein contained in a can of tuna fish.

A final caveat regarding protein amount: When guys consume supplements to push their protein intake above 1 gram per pound of body weight a day, urine output typically doubles. In unusual circumstances, a guy might expel five times his usual amount of urine. If you're consuming heaping amounts of protein, be prepared to double your fluid consumption. Monitor your body weight for a week after switching. If you lose several pounds almost overnight, that's obviously water, so drink up until you erase the deficit.

Opt for real food over fake. No disrespect to protein supplements, which are very useful in certain situations, but a healthy diet always starts with whole foods. Among the best sources are lean meats, fish, low-fat dairy products, and soy products, although all of these contain varying amounts of fat and cholesterol. Therein lies the trick with whole-food sources: balancing the need for high-quality, biologically complete proteins with the negative effects from ingesting too much saturated fat and cholesterol. This is where protein supplements, which I'll discuss momentarily, can play an important role.

Opt for quality protein foods. As long as you consume protein in ample amounts—consistent with the recommendations made here, rather than the RDAs—the form that protein takes seems to have a relatively small effect on the rate at which you gain muscle. (Exceptions include consuming whey protein, which is rapidly absorbed by the body pre- and post-workout.) At a minimum, consuming enough protein gives you a buffer if some of your protein sources for some period of time have low biological values.

In theory, however, if you're really serious about weight training, or if you're an athlete who plays a sport or sports regularly, you want your diet to emphasize proteins that contain large amounts of the essential amino acids. Their exercise-induced depletion has been shown to diminish both adaptations to training and the strength of the immune system. What's more, certain high-quality proteins and essential amino acids have been shown to improve the hormonal and immune responses to exercise. So it makes sense to satisfy most of your daily protein needs from high-quality sources in foods (turkey, chicken, lean red meat and pork, fish, shellfish, eggs, low-fat or fat-free milk, yogurt, cheese), supplements (whey, egg, milk, soy), or both.

Eat a variety of foods. More important, probably, is making sure your diet includes a sufficient range of protein sources. Different types of protein function uniquely, which is why even though egg whites are a great protein source, you don't want to eat only them—or just cans of tuna, or just chicken breast. Mix it up.

This is doubly important for vegetarians: Vegetables, grains, and legumes also contain small amounts of protein, but these are incomplete, lower-quality sources. As a result, to get enough essential amino acids from a predominantly vegetarian or vegan diet, you have to eat a variety of plant-protein sources throughout the day and over a week's time, so that those low in one particular essential amino acid are balanced by ones higher in the same amino acid. Certain cultures have developed traditional dishes that often combine several foods that complement each other to create complete proteins. Combining beans with grains, flour, nuts, or seeds—for example, beans with rice, corn tortillas with refried beans, and pasta with bean soup—creates a fully nutritious protein meal.

Eat every 2 to 3 hours. When you're trying to build muscle, you need to stay anabolic more or less all day by avoiding energy deficits. Should they occur, these prompt your body to start scavenging for energy, resulting in muscle loss.

By consuming protein as part of smaller meals spaced throughout the day, rather than downing large amounts sporadically, you can likely keep your body's pool of amino acids adequate all day, which should lengthen, if not intensify, anabolism. A study published in a German journal found that consuming protein in six small meals versus two large ones leads to improved protein utilization and tissue growth.

Eat protein before your workouts. Consuming a snack containing carbohydrates and protein an hour or so before an intense workout has been shown to increase the availability of carbs toward the end of that session. Not only does this keep your energy levels up, it also increases the availability of amino acids and decreases exercise-induced catabolism of protein. Think of it as an insurance policy for your muscles and the best way to maximize your gym results.

There are a million great carb-protein combinations. Lean turkey on whole-wheat bread, yogurt and a banana, and homemade trail mix consisting of soy nuts, sunflower seeds, raisins, and dried apricots are all great snacks. If you don't have time to prepare or acquire even these simple snacks, eat a sports bar or drink a store-bought energy beverage.

And after your workouts. When it comes to building muscle, eating after your workout is just as important as eating before it. After you finish lifting weights for an hour, the pump you feel raging through your muscles might make you think that they're readying to grow, practically before your eyes. And though you won't blow up like the Incredible Hulk, your muscles are indeed primed after the pump, if only to absorb the nutrients they need to grow over the next few days. Study after study has shown that this post-workout window is the time when your body is most efficient at restocking carbs in their storage form, glycogen. Fed properly, your body also has the potential to be at its most anabolic during this period.

PROTEIN AND FAT CONTENT OF VARIOUS FOODS

WANT TO KNOW HOW MUCH PROTEIN is in your dinner? Consult this chart.

Food	Protein (g)	Fat (g)	Saturated Fat (g)	Monounsaturated Fat (g)	Polyunsaturated Fat (g)	Cholesterol (mg)
MEAT AND POULTRY						
Ground beef (100 grams or 3½ ounces)						
Lean	24	18	7	8	‹1	87
Regular	23	21	8	9	‹1	90
Chicken (100 grams or 3½ ounces)						
Dark (with skin)	26	16	4	6	3	93
Dark (no skin)	27	10	2	3	2	75
Light (with skin)	29	11	2	3	2	84
Light (no skin)	31	4	1	1	‹1	85
Ham (100 grams or 3½ ounces, roasted)						
Lean	21	6	3	4	1	57
Regular	20	15	5	6	2	96
Pork (100 grams or 3½ ounces)	29	22	8	11	3	67
SEAFOOD						
Atlantic salmon (85 grams or 3 ounces)	19	11	2	4	4	54
Shrimp (85 grams or 3 ounces)	17	1.5	‹1	‹1	‹1	129
Sole (1 fillet)	18	1	‹1	‹1	‹1	86
DAIRY PRODUCTS						
Egg (1 large)						
Fried	6	7	2	3	1	211
Boiled	6	5	2	2	‹1	213
Milk (240 milliliters or 8 ounces)						
Fat-free	8	‹1	‹1	‹1	‹1	5
Whole	8	8	5	2	‹1	33
LEGUMES (1 CUP)						
Pinto beans, boiled	14	1	‹1	‹1	‹1	0
Soybeans, green, boiled	22	11	1	2	5	0

Adapted from Pennington, J., Bowes, A. P., and Church, H. N., *Bowes and Churches Food Values of Portions Commonly Used,* 17th edition, Lippincott Williams & Wilkins Publishers, 1997; and Murray, R., "Nutrient requirements for competitive sports," in Wolinsky, I. (Ed.), *Nutrition in Exercise and Sport,* 3rd Edition, Horswill, CA: CRC Press, 1997, pp. 521–558; and *The Food Processor Version 7.5,* ESHA Research, Inc., Salem, OR, 2000.

In fact, one of the best things you can do to gain muscle is to feed your muscles almost as soon as the end of your last rep, if possible, and definitely within 30 minutes of the end of the session. What that does, first and foremost, is trigger a major surge in the release of the anabolic hormone insulin, which will carry other nutrients into muscle cells for muscle building.

This first post-workout feeding should combine protein and carbohydrates. Your body needs both to really hit on all cylinders with glycogen replenishment and muscle-tissue repair. Between 300 and 400 calories should do the trick, consisting of 3 grams of carbs for every 1 gram of protein, preferably whey. Your goal is to take in about 30 to 40 grams of protein, with a high proportion of all the essential amino acids. That's why whey protein is such a great choice.

Then, 2 hours after your training session ends, eat again. This time, feel free to have a more conventional meal, again rich in protein and carbohydrates, because the convenience issue should no longer be pressing. This double-barreled approach—a quick hit after training and a big meal after that—has been found to speed up glycogen reloading and maximize the anabolic effects of your hormones.

Make Friends with Carbohydrates

Often overlooked during a mass-building phase, carbs rank in importance right up there with protein. After all, you need sufficient energy to fuel what will be increasingly intense workouts, and they have a secondary muscle-building effect in that they spare protein from being used as fuel.

But though really good data exist on how much protein the body needs to gain muscle—and even some good data on how much fat the body needs— much less is known about how much carbohydrate guys need to build muscle. Endurance athletes get poked and probed all the time in this regard, but the relationship between men who lift weights and the carbs they eat remains murky.

The way I used to design diets was to figure out how much protein a guy needed, figure out how much healthy fat he could accommodate, and then fill in the remaining calories with carbs. That's okay for some guys, but those who lift weights really need to make sure they're consuming enough carbs. A smaller guy needs at least 300 grams a day; bigger guys can go up to 600 pretty easily. A guy who's seeking more muscle has to have enough energy to push hard in the gym. There's no getting around that. Serious exercisers need serious carbs.

Here's some advice.

Pack on the starch. In the search for growth, avoid simple sugars, but don't be afraid to down 8 to 12 starch servings in a day. Starchy vegetables high in antioxidants, like yams and winter squash, are great here. So are whole-grain breads, whole-wheat couscous, whole-wheat pasta, and Shredded Wheat cereal. Don't forget peas and beans for a unique combo of low-GI carbohydrates and protein.

Match your intake to your exercise level. Where carbs are concerned, it's all about energy output: How much exercise are you really doing? If you're barely training, you can get by with fewer carbs, consuming even more protein and healthy fats to make up for them. That will help you avoid adding too much fat along with your muscle. If you're not exercising, the higher your carb intake, the greater your insulin production, and the more you're enhancing fat metabolism. The tendency, then, will be to store those extra carbs as fats.

Additional Rules for Packing On Size

In addition to eating more protein and carbohydrates, follow these tips for optimal muscle building.

Put fat in its place. You don't want dietary fat to substitute for the muscle-building macronutrients your body needs for growth because protein and carbohydrates both are more vital for lean-tissue development than fat is. But it would be a mistake to marginalize or even exclude fat from your diet. When you are trying to gain muscle, fat can help, particularly by helping you consume enough calories. After all, 1 gram of fat contains 9 calories; protein and carbs have 4 each.

Also, research published recently in the *Journal of Applied Physiology* suggests that diets in which fat contributes 15 percent or less of total calories can actually decrease testosterone production. To keep your *cojones* cranking out the anabolic hormone your muscles crave during this phase, draw about one-fourth to just under one-third of your calories from fat, which shouldn't add up to much more than 0.5 grams of fat per pound of body weight per day. Particularly good are monounsaturated fats such as peanut oil and olive oil, because they're heart-healthy and help push the fat-burning

AMINO AMMO

AMINO ACIDS COME IN 22 VERSIONS. Different proteins contain them in different configurations. Of the 22, 8 are deemed "essential," meaning they can be obtained only from diet—if you couldn't eat or drink, you'd be denied them completely. Another 7 amino acids are deemed conditionally essential, meaning that under certain conditions, they can't be synthesized, either, and must therefore be consumed through your diet. Proteins that contain all of the essential amino acids are said to be complete, in contrast to those missing or low in even one essential amino acid, which are deemed incomplete.

Essential Amino Acids	Conditionally Essential Amino Acids	Nonessential Amino Acids
Isoleucine	Arginine	Alanine
Leucine	Cysteine	Asparagine
Lysine	Glutamine	Aspartic acid
Methionine	Histidine	Citruline
Phenylalanine	Proline	Glutamic acid
Threonine	Taurine	Glycine
Tryptophan	Tyrosine	Serine
Valine		

Adapted from Di Pasquale, M. G., "Proteins and amino acids in exercise and sport," in Driskell, J. A., and Wolinsky, I. (Eds.), *Energy-Yielding Macronutrients and Energy Metabolism in Sports Nutrition*, CRC Press, 2000, pp. 119–162.

machinery along. Fish fats are great here, too.

Be patient. You really don't have any choice in the matter. You're not going to see dramatic changes overnight. In the absence of anabolic steroids and other unethical means, gaining size takes time. And because your body more easily stores calories in your fat cells than using them to build larger muscles, haste makes *waist* if your body has to struggle to assimilate a too-rapid influx of additional fuel. You want to gain slower, rather than faster. The faster you gain body weight, the higher the proportion will be of fat to muscle. Building muscle takes work, and changes can appear only so quickly. As a result, if you pack on the calories too fast, many of them will migrate to your fat cells.

What's more, unrealistic expectations can set you up for a fall. After all, any healthy body has the physical capacity to accommodate more weight, so when you do tumble off the wagon, it's usually headfirst.

Integrate your weight-gain program with the rest of your life gradually, step by step. If your goal is to gain 20 pounds of muscle, break down that rather ambitious goal into smaller, short-term ones that collectively will help you achieve your desired aim. Whereas the bigger goal will seem daunting, gaining one-twelfth of that amount per month for a year will seem much more manageable.

Junk the scale. Although the take-it-slow approach will help you avoid the pitfall of overreaching, it presents a potential problem of its own: Your gradual improvement might seem imperceptible. Watching the scale, which is usually discouraged by weight-loss experts, can be equally counterproductive when you're packing on size. Instead, track your strength gains in the gym. Also, measure the circumference of your biceps, chest, waist, quads, and calves. Those are the real changes you're looking for anyway.

Train, or your effort is in vain. Don't forget that your diet, while absolutely critical for mass gaining, should be pursued in conjunction with weight training and cardiovascular exercise. A good diet provides a lot of kindling and other inflammable material for muscle growth, but weight training is the match needed to ignite it all. Pound down more and more calories without exercising, and next thing you know you'll be squeezing through the doors of one of those weight-loss centers.

Advice for Hardgainers

If you're tall, lanky, and thin—the genetically determined body type called *ectomorph*—building muscle is going to be a bit more challenging than bumping up your calorie and protein consumption. You've been blessed (or cursed, depending on your perspective) with a jackrabbit's metabolism and a frame that's more like a scaffolding than a skeleton, and you're going to have to work twice as hard as the next guy to build on it.

Not to worry: Ectomorphs can indeed build muscle, and those who do manage to pack on size look great (or, at least the ones I know do, as their girlfriends and wives will attest to).

But it takes hard, hard work, in the gym and at

Foods That Pack On Muscle

Here are seven super-foods that you should include in your new diet.

Brown rice	Grilled chicken breast
Fresh fruit (especially berries, oranges, and bananas)	Grilled salmon
	Fat-free milk
Fresh vegetables (especially broccoli, cauliflower, spinach, yams, and winter squash)	Oatmeal

the table. Pretty much everything in this chapter applies to you, only you need to amp it all up even further.

Eat and then eat again. Instead of eating more frequently, you need to eat almost constantly—probably more than you'll feel like eating, at least initially. Skipping meals, which is okay for most guys, is a killer for the hardgainer. The big, heaping plate of lasagna that would make most women run screaming from the dining room? That pile of carb calories is just what the doctor ordered for Joe Hardgainer. Don't worry about getting fat—just eat. The thinnest ectomorph doing the least amount of exercise can stand to eat a good 3,500 calories a day.

Eat even more protein. You'll be eating more of everything, which means you'll be eating more protein as well. Consume 1½ grams of protein per pound of body weight per day. Protein can account for up to 30 percent or so of total calories. You'll probably need to drink a supplement shake or two a day—day in, day out—to reach those protein and calorie numbers.

Combine protein with carbs. Regardless of when you're eating, combine healthy, heaping amounts of protein and carbs. The latter will provide a constant insulin stimulus, but your insulin response won't be overstimulated because you'll have protein to slow digestion and prevent the fat building that pure carbs would promote. Instead, you'll remain anabolic, giving you the best of both worlds.

Hardgainers: Eat Late at Night

The postmidnight snack is frowned upon by most people, and no wonder: We've been conditioned to associate late-night meals with overweight men and women creeping down to the Frigidaire in a furtive search for leftovers.

The inference, of course, is that anyone with a shred of dignity has enough self-control to stay out of the kitchen between the *Tonight* show and the

> ### *Sleep More, Get Bigger*
>
> Sleep deprivation and stress are extremely counterproductive for packing on size. Both trigger the release of cortisol, a catabolic hormone. It's a hardwired response dating back tens of thousands of years, when the major source of stress was famine and starvation. Cortisol's intended effect was, and is, to stop weight loss by helping increase fat. That's unhelpful when you're trying to build muscle, not accommodate fat. So if you go back to chapter 2, all of those nutritional strategies and supplements for stress reduction can help you here as well.

Today show. If you're a hardgainer, however, late-night eating can be a novel way to shift the body into anabolic overdrive by ensuring that the pistons of muscle growth—hormones such as testosterone, insulin, and insulinlike growth factors—are hitting on all cylinders 24/7. After all, sleep, among other things, is an extended fast.

Just because your mind slips from consciousness during sleep doesn't mean a lot isn't happening in your body, including some serious muscle repair and growth. Assuming your body is adequately nourished by the time you doze off, anabolism actually peaks while you're asleep. Soon after the onset of deep sleep, secretions of growth hormone spike way above the steady levels that prevail while you were awake. Those surges continue rhythmically throughout the night, except during rapid-eye-movement (REM) sleep. The most powerful growth stimulus in the human body, growth hormone, also exerts a profound metabolic effect. The net result is a shift toward using fat as a fuel source, which spares amino acids for use in protein synthesis.

Also in high gear is your testosterone secretion. After bottoming out in the late afternoon, that primary muscle-building hormone starts rising as well. By the early-morning hours, your testosterone levels are peaking. Cortisol, a catabolic hormone, follows the reverse pattern.

Here's where your postmidnight snack can help. By eating, you'll maximize the effects of heightened testosterone levels at night. Those effects include decreasing cortisol and boosting the availability of building blocks like branched-chain amino acids and glutamine.

Although it will doubtless involve some trial and error, planning your midnight meal is the easy part; the hard part is getting up in the middle of the night!

If you're a problem sleeper, interrupting your snooze is probably more disruptive than helpful. Sleep deprivation can lead to testicular dysfunction and hence lower testosterone levels, which will more than offset gains from late-night eating. Also, as I warned in chapter 1, eating at night and the digestive process that follows can wreak havoc on some people's sleep. But if you can manage the routine, I highly suggest it. Here are some tips to get you started.

NUTRIENTS THAT PROMOTE MUSCLE BUILDING

THE FOLLOWING MINERALS ARE IMPORTANT in the muscle-building process.

Calcium. Milk does a body good, indeed. The most abundant mineral in the body, calcium does more than just maintain strong bones, although that's certainly important for mass gaining—you need a strong skeletal structure to perform the sorts of lifts you need to be doing to gain size. Calcium is also important every time you flex, as nerves can't send the messages needed for muscle contractions without it.

Iron. Iron combines with protein to make hemoglobin, the special molecule that carries oxygen in the blood from the lungs to the tissues. Iron also helps form myoglobin, the oxygen-transporting molecule found only in muscle tissue. Myoglobin transports oxygen to muscle cells to be used in the chemical reaction that makes muscle cells contract. Iron is also needed for the formation of cytochromes and iron-containing enzymes critical in immune function.

When you strength-train, the tearing down and rebuilding of muscle tissue causes an additional need for iron. When iron stores are low, your tissues become starved for oxygen and you tire easily. Recovery from exercise takes even longer.

The best dietary sources of iron are lean red meats, the dark meat of poultry, clams, oysters, green leafy vegetables, soybeans, dried fruits, and iron-fortified breads and cereals.

Zinc. This antioxidant mineral is involved in hundreds of body processes, including maintaining normal taste and smell, regulating growth and reproduction, and promoting wound healing. Zinc also helps to clear lactic acid buildup from the blood during exercise, increasing the time to fatigue. Foods rich in zinc include lean red meats, dark-meat poultry, eggs, seafood, and whole grains.

Make it a small meal. If you're in search of size, view this predawn feeding as simply another in the sequence of meals you consume over the course of a day. For example, if your target daily calorie consumption is 3,000 and your late-night meal is your sixth one of the day, it should consist of approximately 500 calories. For the sake of convenience, you might want to reduce that slightly and bump up breakfast or dinner to compensate.

Eat something that sits well. Consume foods, liquids, or supplements in a way that doesn't induce sleep-disrupting gastrointestinal discomfort. If your late-night meal takes the form of a supplement—whether powder, or drink—avoid products whose labels list stimulants such as caffeine, ephedrine, or ma huang. Taking a supplement that includes 250 milligrams of caffeine is equivalent to drinking a "tall" cup of Starbucks coffee. If you down that along with your protein, carbs, or creatine, don't plan on going back to sleep anytime soon.

Aim for fast-absorbing protein. Not all proteins are created equal, and in the middle of the night, the best alternative for promoting muscle growth is an easily absorbed form, like egg whites or skim milk. Or try a powder form that combines a fast-absorbing dietary protein, such as whey, with a slower-releasing alternative, such as casein. The timed-release effect of such combinations can improve muscle gains and limit muscle damage, according to a study published in the *Proceedings of the National Academy of Science*.

Allow for some fat. Although late-night fat consumption should be limited, small amounts can complement your protein intake by helping to boost the output of testosterone and growth hormone. For example, a meal that includes cottage cheese (4.5 percent fat), salmon or turkey, and avocado would contain the right amount of fat.

Keep carbs low. Again, this is specifically for nighttime eating. Carbohydrate management can be tough for hardgainers. Small amounts help shuttle protein into muscle cells. However, a large influx of carbs, particularly simple sugars, will prompt your body to produce higher levels of insulin, which compensates for a rise in blood sugar by taking a corresponding amount of glucose out of the bloodstream and into cells. If you're eating a well-balanced diet during the day, those cells should already be sufficiently filled with glycogen, and unneeded carbs will be deposited as fat. Although insulin is an important anabolic hormone, unless you're a young, hard-training bodybuilder trying to fill out a big frame, that's probably an unacceptable price to pay.

Advice for Vegans

Building muscle as a vegan presents a unique set of challenges. Let's face it: Other than where Popeye is concerned, vegetables have never been synonymous with muscle growth. Even the most die-hard carnivore would probably concede the various health benefits of vegetarianism, but gaining size? Veggies are fuel, the reasoning goes, and to pack on slabs of beef—well, you're going to have to start by *eating* slabs of beef.

That's a myth, of course. In theory, it shouldn't be any more difficult for vegans, who abstain from all animal products including dairy, to gain muscle than it is for carnivores. Even the strictest vegetarian can pack on some serious muscle by adhering to some basic nutritional strategies.

Eat even more protein. Vegetarians have to pay greater heed to making sure they get enough protein—in the right combinations—during the day. To make up for a lack of high-quality protein, vegetarians should eat 10 percent more than the 1 gram of protein per pound of body weight per day benchmark for meat-eating athletes trying to gain size. That's a challenge: Along with all that fat and cholesterol in red meat, whole milk, and eggs comes a lot of protein.

Eat a variety of proteins. Animal proteins tend to be complete, meaning they have all of the essential amino acids, and in the correct proportions. As I've discussed, your muscles can't grow without the full array. Plant proteins almost always are low in at least one essential amino acid, so you have to combine two or more sources. Luckily, this isn't rocket science. Alone, ½ cup of kidney beans, 1 cup of rice, a piece of bread, and a knifefull of peanut butter are incomplete. Dump the beans on the rice and slather the bread with peanut butter, however, and you have two complete sources. Moreover, you don't have to combine complementary proteins during each sitting but over the course of a day, which shouldn't be a problem if you eat a variety of fruits, vegetables, grains, nuts, legumes (dried beans and peas), and seeds. Your body's amino-acid pool can compensate for temporary imbalances.

Include soy in your diet. When mixed into a diet that may or may not include animal protein, soy has merits. The results of a study published recently in the *American Journal of Clinical Nutrition* confirm that soy protein and isoflavones can help increase muscle-protein synthesis and fat burning, and dramatically so. Soy does not promote muscle growth as well as animal protein does; however, it still promotes muscle growth. So if you exclude all animal products from your diet, make sure to include soy as a primary protein source. And unless you are a very strict vegetarian or vegan, try to include at least dairy and some kind of animal protein in your diet. You can still gain muscle, just not as quickly.

Cook your food. To get the most out of vegetable proteins, make sure you cook them first. Most plant food is difficult to digest because of the starch cellulose that forms part of the cell wall. Cooking changes the structure of the cellulose, making it easier for the digestive enzymes to get to the protein in the plant cell.

Foods That Hinder Muscle Building

Give these foods the old heave-ho, save for an occasional indulgence.

Chips	Nachos with the works
French fries	Soda
Fried doughnuts	Sugar-loaded
Fried sandwiches	desserts

Eat more food more often. Plant foods typically offer fewer calories and less protein per unit than meat does, so strict vegetarians and vegans need to consume a higher volume of food to obtain the amount they need to pack on muscle, which varies from individual to individual. Getting enough calories is a big issue. Vegan diets, especially, are unusually high in fiber, so you get really full. Your calorie needs may very well exceed your appetite. As a result, vegans need to avoid the empty calories found in sweets and fatty foods, particularly junk food.

To maximize the intake of calories and protein, hard-training vegans should space five or six nutritious, well-balanced meals (including protein) throughout the day—which probably means planning ahead and taking some meals with you. Eating and drinking correctly before and after workouts is also crucial.

Protein Supplements

Although many guys satisfy all of their protein needs from foods, an increasingly large number augment that intake with supplements that contain protein, including traditional protein powders, meal-replacement powders, and sports bars. Protein supplements, once the province of recreational bodybuilders and serious athletes, are now commonplace among guys from construction workers to architects.

Advances in food technology have simultaneously met and fueled this growing demand. In this instance, progress has been positive: The lab-coat set have now isolated very high quality protein from a range of animal and plant sources, yielding casein, bovine colostrums, ovalbumin, soy, and whey. Many of these newfangled proteins have been used to develop low-fat and nutrient-dense dietary supplements.

Augmenting a diet rich in whole foods with high-quality protein supplements is a great way to muscle it up. For one, protein powder is a great way to consume a lot of protein and a lot of calories without feeling full as quickly as you would when eating whole foods. What's more, because they travel easily and don't spoil easily, these supplements are especially useful immediately after you train, when whole foods might not be readily available and your appetite for them will likely be suppressed anyway.

Beyond the critically important post-workout window, protein supplements are great for conveniently filling the gaps in your diet once you start eating more frequently. Best of all, they give you

WHO CAN YOU TRUST?

Not the food industry

REGARDLESS OF ITS SHORTCOMINGS AND BAD APPLES, the medical establishment is far more interested in your health than the U.S. food industry is. It's not that food makers don't deserve some credit. Going to a supermarket and having to sift through a bunch of prepackaged, overly processed junk to find the nutritious foods hiding among them isn't ideal, but it beats the hell out of spending hours waiting in food lines or trying to coax some grain to emerge through cracks in a parched desert.

Nor is this intended as a Pollyanna broadside against big, bad food corporations that conspire to exploit helpless consumers while making loads of money, although many of them do (make lots of money, that is). That underlying motive, profit, is how things work in a free market. This should be stating the obvious, but here goes: In an incredibly competitive market, with few exceptions, food companies are far more concerned with getting you to buy their products than they are with the nutritional value of those products. The fiduciary responsibility of food makers—at least the publicly owned ones—is to their shareholders, not to you, the consumer. If Food Company XYZ can put out a product legally and make lots of money on it, they will.

The U.S. Food and Drug Administration levels the playing field to some extent by requiring manufacturers to print detailed nutritional information on their labels. So if you buy a product that's obviously bad for you, don't blame the company or the government for your ignorance—it's on you, dude. Get informed. Take the information in this book seriously. Learn how to read a food label. It's not rocket science, although I will alert you to some "stealth" ingredients as you proceed through *Power Food*.

what you want—lots of protein—without much, if any, of the saturated fat or cholesterol included in protein-rich whole foods such as eggs and red meat.

Supplements typically differ according to the protein's primary source, its amino-acid profile, and the methods by which it was processed or isolated. At the low end of the quality scales sit wheat proteins and gelatin (collagen); meat and fish rank higher up. Soy rates pretty high, too. Although it has comparatively low levels of the essential amino acid methionine, it has high concentrations of remaining essential amino acids, making it complete, technically.

Here's how a few common types of protein fare.

Egg whites. At the top of the heap sit egg whites, the reference standard against which other proteins are compared. That's why egg whites are often used in protein supplements, even though they are a relatively expensive ingredient.

Dairy. Another heavyweight among proteins is milk, consisting of 80 percent casein and 20 percent whey (the "liquid fraction"). High quality but less expensive than egg protein, milk proteins are ubiquitous in the supplement world.

Whey protein. The darling of the moment is

HOW GOOD IS YOUR PROTEIN SUPPLEMENT?

CHECK THE LIST OF INGREDIENTS ON YOUR SUPPLEMENT label, and then consult this chart to see where your supplement stands.

Protein	PDCAAS*	PER**	Comment
Whey	1.00	3.0–3.2	A high-quality protein source, whey protein is digested rapidly, allowing fast uptake of amino acids (a.k.a. whey protein hydrolysate, ion exchange whey protein isolate, and cross-flow microfiltration whey protein isolate). Although whey protein is a more expensive form of quality protein, it is currently the most poplar protein supplement used by resistance-trained athletes.
Bovine Colostrum (BC)	1.00	3.0	A high-quality protein source, BC may have some added benefit compared with other forms of protein due to a high concentration of growth factors, immunoglobulins, and antibacterial compounds. Although higher in cost than most protein supplements, preliminary evidence indicates that BC may promote greater gains in strength and muscle mass during training than whey protein. More research is needed before definitive conclusions can be made.
Casein	1.00	2.9	Caseinates are extracted from skim milk (a.k.a. sodium caseinate, potassium caseinate, and calcium caseinate). The protein quality of casein is high, and it is relatively inexpensive. Compared with whey protein, the amino-acid release is generally more delayed.
Milk Protein	1.00	2.8	Milk protein contains about 80 percent casein and 20 percent whey protein. Milk protein is available in concentrated and isolated forms and contains about 90 percent protein. It's commonly used in supplements due to its high quality and relatively low cost.

whey protein, which is also fairly expensive. It comes in three forms: hydrolysate, ion-exchange isolate, and cross-flow micro-filtrated isolate. That probably sounds like so much pseudoscientific jibber-jabber, but the terms merely refer to different methods of processing, fat and lactose content, amino-acid profiles, and ability to preserve glutamine residues. Compared with milk protein, which is a combination of whey and casein, pure whey protein is more rapidly absorbed by the body. Whey is high in branched-chain amino acids (BCAAs), especially leucine, which makes it a perfect supplement before and after exercise.

Bovine colostrum. Equal in quality to whey are proteins collected from bovine colostrum, the milk produced by cows during the first few days after calving. Along with higher nutrient density than ordinary dairy milk, bovine colostrum also contains high concentrations of growth factors, immunoglobulins, and antibacterials not found in other proteins.

In theory, ingesting these undeniably bioactive compounds could strengthen the immune system and promote muscle growth triggered by weight training. Whether ingestions of these compounds raise serum levels of growth factors and immuno-

Protein	PDCAAS*	PER**	Comment
Ovalbumin (Egg)	1.00	2.8	Protein from egg whites is considered the reference standard for comparing protein quality. Egg protein powders were once considered the best source of protein for supplements. However, egg protein is fairly expensive compared with other forms of quality protein, and has decreased in recent years.
Soy	1.00	1.8–2.3	Soy is a high-quality protein extracted from soybeans. Soy protein concentrate (70 percent protein) and isolate (90 percent protein) are particularly good protein sources for vegetarians. Soy protein also contains isoflavone glucasides, which have a number of potential health benefits.
Beef/Poultry/Fish	0.8–0.92	2.0–2.3	Fairly good sources of quality protein. However, some types contain relatively high amounts of fat, which reduces the utility of using some animal meats as a primary means of obtaining protein in the diet.
Wheat	0.43	1.5	Wheat protein is relatively poor in quality. However, wheat serves as the starting material for glutamine peptide, which is a protein hydrolysate that contains high amounts of glutamine (see page 160).
Gelatin (Collagen)	0.08	—	Inexpensive but poor-quality protein that was popular as a nutritional supplement in the 1970s and 1980s. Gelatin is still found in some liquid protein supplements.

*Protein Digestibility Corrected Amino Acid Score
**Protein Evaluation Ratio

globulins remains to be seen. To date, the research published on this supplement hasn't produced definitive results.

Others. Some of the new powders combine proteins with different absorption rates (normally whey and casein), producing what amounts to a time-release effect. In theory, this could give you an anabolic edge while you sleep.

For any protein supplement to be effective, you have to use it more than once or twice, making *palatability* and *digestibility* more than just pompous, awkward-sounding word choices for this sentence. You can have reams of studies showing that a protein powder, bar, or drink is the greatest thing since the return of hip-huggers, but if the stuff makes you gag on its way down and then causes gastrointestinal distress once it reaches its destination, you're not going to stick with it.

In that case, switch to a product whose label lists protein isolates rather than concentrates. Whey protein concentrate, for example, can contain anywhere from 20 to 80 percent lactose—that is, the sugar found in milk—whereas isolates should be at least 90 percent pure. Isolate-based products generally mix up like juice, rather than liquid cement, and slide down your throat, rather than sticking in it.

Additional Muscle-Building Supplements

Fat-loss supplements have a grand history that runs from the days of the snake-oil salesmen up to their present-day inheritors, some of whom you've seen on C-SPAN, if you've witnessed any of the hearings Congress has held on ephedra and other thermogenic supplements. But in reality, supplements are more useful for gaining weight. Because most are convenient, cost-effective ways to add calories, these protein powders, meal-replacement products, liquid-carb drinks, and, yes, even weight-gain pow-

ders can help you add size much more effectively than a pill laced with some caffeine and ma huang can help you lose it.

Bear in mind that these are supplements—meant to augment, not replace, food. To reiterate a point made throughout this chapter, you can stay anabolic through whole foods alone if you manage your diet correctly.

Weight-gainers. Remember at the start of the chapter when I talked about supplements that "taste like liquid cement"? Welcome to the world of weight-gain shakes.

These products throw everything but the kitchen sink into a mix that contains lots of protein, lots of carbs, lots of fat, and lots of calories. Not for the faint of heart, a single serving of a typical weight-gainer gives you 1,000 calories or more.

Dose: Follow label instructions.

Meal-replacement powders (MRPs). These can be more effective than straight-ahead protein shakes for gaining mass. One advantage is that they contain carbs, which produce an anabolic insulin response. Those carbs also give you more calories than a protein shake would contain. A single serving typically offers 400 to 550 calories, with some going as high as 600. That's exactly the sort of energy influx you need for getting bigger.

Avoid the ones loaded with sugars, however. If you need to sweeten up your MRP, try adding fruit or honey instead. Also, be wary of MRPs that throw so much extra stuff into the mix that they verge on becoming weight-gainers. In doing so, these products are typically trying to carve out a unique niche, allowing the manufacturer to say, "Look—I've got something special here." Many of them have creatine added, for example.

My recommendation is not to buy an MRP with everything already mixed into it because it robs you of the ability to individualize it. You may have this 5-pound bucket of something with creatine, and if you decide that you don't want creatine, you're stuck. Aim for a basic mix of protein and carbs instead, and add in more goodies as needed.

Dose: Follow label instructions.

Branched-chain amino acids (BCAAs). The amino acids leucine, isoleucine, and valine, a.k.a. BCAAs, so named because of their bifurcated chemical structure, make up one-third of all the amino acids in muscle. Because they're so widespread in muscle, they deplete rapidly in response to exercise.

Not surprisingly, then, various studies have shown that taking BCAAs as a supplement before or after training can simultaneously elevate the rate of protein synthesis and downshift the rate of tissue breakdown in muscle. Under times of physical stress, BCAAs appear to be one of the most effective ways, where nutrition is concerned, for sparing protein.

Leucine in particular appears to play a key role in promoting protein synthesis. It gets the ball rolling, so to speak, before other amino acids lend a helping hand. This effect seems to be negated when insulin levels are low, however, so take leucine with carbs.

Dose: 5 to 20 grams daily, divided among several doses. Don't exceed 20 grams daily.

Creatine monohydrate. This is the mother of all muscle-building supplements and a great alternative to anabolic steroids. No nutritional supplement has more research standing behind it, and the studies consistently show that creatine enhances physical exercise, particularly high-intensity, short-burst activities such as strength training.

In addition to that indirect influence on muscle growth, creatine appears to act more directly, perhaps through cell volumization. Water has the same effect, and you want to drink plenty of it when taking creatine. The combined effect will further enhance protein metabolism and muscle building.

The only real caveat with creatine is to abstain from taking it if you've been diagnosed with kidney disease or have a family history of the same. The re-

---

Anabolic Foods

Anabolic—muscle building—foods include the following.

■ High-quality proteins of all kinds, especially meat, chicken, fish, dairy, eggs, and soy (no special order here).

■ Carbohydrates of all kinds, but the most healthful are those from whole foods such as whole grains and cereals, fruits, vegetables, nuts, and seeds. Simple carbs such as those found in sugar, honey, jams, jellies, syrups, etc., are best used only for recovery after exercise.

■ Essential fats, omega-3 fats, and fish oils, such as those found in vegetable oils, nuts, seeds, nut and seed butters, and fatty fish (salmon, mackerel, tuna, black cod, halibut).

Your best anabolic combination is 0.5 gram of protein per kilogram of body weight (0.23 gram per pound), plus 1 to 1.5 grams of carbohydrates per kilogram (0.45 to 0.68 grams per pound).

---

ports about creatine leading to athletes collapsing on playing fields have been sensationalized in the media and undercut by research. After nearly 500 studies on the supplement, no results—zilch—link creatine with dehydration.

To cite one example, a researcher in New Mexico presented an abstract on creatine at a meeting of the American College of Sports Medicine in 2003. In his experiment, athletes were made to exercise without fluids in hot weather. Some athletes were given creatine; others were not. Lo and behold, at the end of the exercise session, those who had taken creatine were better hydrated than those who hadn't.

Dose: 5 grams daily, or a loading dose phase using 5 grams, 4 times a day for 5 to 7 days, fol-

The Importance of Water

You're probably aware of the myriad health benefits of water, but it isn't the first thing that leaps to mind when you think of gaining size. Yet if you want to gain size, it's important that you drink at least eight glasses of water a day. Water helps maintain the normal cell volume levels, which contributes to the maintenance of muscle-protein levels.

lowed by 5 grams daily. (If you want to save yourself some money, ignore the loading phase. Research shows that you will have "caught up" in a month or so anyway without it.) To further creatine's uptake into muscle cells, take it on an empty stomach with liquid carbs a half-hour before a meal. You can also add it to your postexercise recovery shake, when your muscles are eager to absorb just about everything.

Glutamine. This is one of six amino acids the body breaks down and uses for fuel. Among its myriad roles is that of muscle builder, which shouldn't come as a surprise—glutamine constitutes 60 percent or so of the free pool of amino acids inside lean tissue. There's likely a connection between that and rat-based studies in which extra glutamine stoked protein synthesis even without a rise in insulin.

Glutamine also appears to diminish the breakdown of protein in muscles, perhaps because it, too, is a cell volumizer. The better hydrated a cell is, the more efficiently protein is synthesized, and the more muscle that gets made, the reasoning goes.

Last but not least, glutamine supports the immune system, which has an indirect but major effect on muscle growth. If you're feeling less than 100 percent, your workouts will inevitably suffer as a result. You won't stimulate as many muscle fibers as you will going full bore.

Dose: 2 to 14 grams daily; 5 grams added to a drink twice daily should do the trick for most guys.

Beta-hydroxy beta-methylbutyrate (HMB). The research on this for muscle building is equivocal—not many studies have been done, and not much data exist. But the primary mechanism seems to be interference with the breakdown of muscle protein, which in theory should help with hypertrophy. The data at this point show that HMB is most effective in guys just beginning a weight-training program or returning to it after a hiatus. It doesn't seem to do much for experienced strength trainers.

Dose: 3 grams daily. Most effective when taken between meals.

Multivitamin/mineral: If you haven't been taking one of these containing the full nine yards of antioxidants and B vitamins, each and every day, start now. Consider it an insurance policy, like wearing a seat belt and a condom—except you're not driving or having sex. Because you're already eating like a horse to gain muscle, there's no need to go crazy with megadoses of anything. Choose one with about 100 percent of the daily value for most of the nutrients listed on the label.

Hey, if nothing else, at least your mom will be happy.

Dose: Follow labels.

Zinc magnesium asparatate (ZMA): Zinc and magnesium are involved in more than 400 metabolic reactions in the body—some of which are undoubtedly related to exercise and muscle building. Given that, and given that both nutrients are commonly in short supply in the body, it's not surprising that a study using college football players found that a zinc-magnesium supplement enhanced strength and functional power. But more research needs to done.

Dose: Three capsules daily, providing 450 milligrams of magnesium, 30 milligrams of zinc, and 10.5 milligrams of vitamin B_6.

"Vegetarian" supplements. Normally, strict vegetarians and vegans have depleted stores of creatine inside their muscles, but that problem is now easily rectified with supplemental creatine, which is chemically synthesized rather than derived from animals. In fact, when you consider supplementing a vegan diet with glutamine, BCAAs, and glucosamine, it can be souped up considerably to handle intense exercise and muscle building pretty easily.

Depending on their food choices, vegans may also need to consume supplemental amounts of iron, calcium, zinc, and vitamin B_{12}. Although these substances may not have the direct connection to muscle building that protein does, being deficient in them could eventually diminish your workouts. You can probably get enough calcium from fortified soy and leafy green vegetables; for the rest, explore supplements, as well as fortified soy milk and cereals.

Soy protein powders are a good alternative for vegans because most protein powders are extracts of eggs or milk. Also keep in mind that some amino-acid capsules and tablets are actually hydrolysates of whey protein, which is derived from milk, and that some supplement capsules have a gelatin base. Any information not on the package can likely be gotten from the manufacturer.

One other caveat, though self-evident, bears repeating: None of these vegetarian muscle-building strategies will amount to a hill of beans if you don't lift weights and do regular cardio.

THE HARDGAINER'S MEAL PLAN

THE HARDGAINER DOESN'T CONSUME ENOUGH CALORIES, has an above-average metabolic rate, and carries a large frame that makes it hard to see visible progress. If you're a hardgainer, you'll need to think about food more than most people do, eat more of almost everything, and learn to eat even when you're not hungry. To add calories and make eating more convenient, throw in a 500-calorie MRP shake once a day.

Daily Assumptions*†

4,870 calories
664 grams carbohydrates‡
199 grams protein‡
102 grams fat‡

Daily Breakdown*†

14 bread
12 fruit
4 milk
44 teaspoons added sugar
11 vegetable
9 very lean protein
5 lean protein
1 medium-fat protein
12 fat

Note: Occasionally, a fat-free product, like mustard or cooking spray, is included on the menus. These do not count toward your daily breakdown but should not be overused.

*Use every day.

† Based on a 185-pound man.

‡Any 500-calorie commercial meal-replacement shake will change these values depending on the MRP you choose.

THE MENU

DAY 1

Breakfast

3 bread	3 slices whole-grain bread
1 milk	1 cup fat-free milk
2 fruit	1 cup cubed cantaloupe
	1/2 cup fresh raspberries
11 teaspoons added sugar	3 1/2 tablespoons 100% fruit spread
2 vegetable	1 small tomato, diced (add to egg)
	1/2 cup diced onion
1 medium-fat protein	1 egg, scrambled in a nonstick pan
3 very lean protein	6 egg whites, scrambled with whole egg
3 fat	1/4 avocado, diced (add to egg)
	1 1/2 tablespoons ground flaxseed
	Water
	Oil-free cooking spray (for eggs)

Snack

2 bread	8 whole-wheat crackers
3 vegetable	3 cups celery sticks
3 teaspoons added sugar	Tea with 1 tablespoon honey
4 fat	2 tablespoons natural peanut butter

Lunch

5 bread	Foot-long Subway sandwich with extra meat (choose from "6 grams fat or less" list)
1 milk	1 cup fat-free milk
2 vegetable	Lettuce, tomato
2 fruit	1 small banana
	1 apple
4 very lean protein	Included (in sandwich)
2 fat	2 teaspoons olive oil or 2 tablespoons salad dressing

Snack

1 bread	1 serving Grape Nuts cereal
2 fruit	2 cups blueberries
6 teaspoons added sugar	2 tablespoons honey
1 milk	1 cup plain nonfat yogurt
1 MRP	1 meal replacement shake

Dinner

3 bread	1 large sweet potato, baked
	1 small ear corn on the cob
2 fruit	2 slices watermelon
8 teaspoons added sugar	1½ cups frozen yogurt
4 vegetable	3 cups salad with lettuce, tomato, cucumber, pepper
	1 cup broccoli
5 lean protein	5 ounces salmon, grilled
3 fat	3 tablespoons olive oil (for dressing)
	Vinegar (for dressing)

Pre-Workout Snack

SMOOTHIE

Blend until smooth.

1 milk	1 cup fat-free milk
4 fruit	1 cup orange juice
	1 small banana
2 very lean protein	14 grams whey protein powder
	Ice cubes

Workout

16 teaspoons added sugar	32-ounce sports drink
	Water

DAY 2

Breakfast

Combine yogurt, fruit, and honey. Combine mayo, mustard on muffin.

3 bread	1½ whole-wheat English muffins
1 milk	1 cup fat-free unsweetened yogurt
2 fruit	2½ cups fresh strawberries
11 teaspoons added sugar	3½ tablespoons honey
2 vegetable	1 cup tomato juice
1 medium-fat protein	1 egg, hard-cooked
3 very lean protein	6 eggs, hard-cooked (discard yolks)
3 fat	1½ tablespoons ground flaxseed
	2 teaspoons mayonnaise and mustard (for egg salad)
	Water

Snack

2 bread	4 rice cakes
3 vegetable	3 cups vegetable sticks
3 teaspoons added sugar	1 tablespoon 100% fruit spread
4 fat	4 tablespoons salad dressing (for dipping)

Lunch

5 bread	2 slices whole-grain bread
	1 ounce croutons
	1 cup brown rice
1 milk	1 cup fat-free milk
2 vegetable	Salad with romaine lettuce, tomato, grilled eggplant, roasted red pepper
2 fruit	2 kiwis, sliced
4 very lean protein	4 ounces skinless white-meat chicken, grilled with lime juice
2 fat	2 tablespoons reduced-fat dressing
	1 teaspoon olive oil (for roasted vegetables)

Snack

1 bread	5 melba toast
2 fruit	1 large peach
6 teaspoons added sugar	2 tablespoons honey
1 milk	1 cup fat-free milk
1 MRP	1 meal replacement shake

Dinner

3 bread	1 cup cooked pasta
	1 slice garlic bread
2 fruit	2^1/$_2$ cups strawberries
8 teaspoons added sugar	1^1/$_2$ cups flavored gelatin dessert
4 vegetable	2 cups ratatouille (over pasta)
	Salad with 2 cups romaine lettuce, ^{1}/$_2$ cup tomato, ^{1}/$_2$ cup cucumber
5 lean protein	5 ounces lean ground beef (add to ratatouille)
3 fat	3 tablespoons salad dressing

Pre-Workout Snack

SMOOTHIE
Blend until smooth.

1 milk	1 cup fat-free milk
4 fruit	1 cup orange juice
	1 small banana
2 very lean protein	14 grams whey protein powder
	Ice cubes

Workout

16 teaspoons added sugar	32-ounce sports drink
	Water

DAY 3

Breakfast

3 bread	3 slices whole-wheat bread
1 milk	1 cup fat-free cottage cheese (on bread; sprinkle with sugar and cinnamon)
2 fruit	4 ounces freshly squeezed orange juice (with pulp)
	^{1}/$_2$ cup sliced pineapple
11 teaspoons added sugar	3^1/$_2$ tablespoons sugar
2 vegetable	1 cup V8 juice
1 medium-fat protein	1 egg, cooked sunny-side up in a nonstick pan
3 very lean protein	6 egg whites, cooked with sunny-side up egg
3 fat	1^1/$_2$ tablespoons ground flaxseed
	2 teaspoons oil (for cooking)
	Water

Snack

2 bread	1 bagel
3 vegetable	1 small tomato
	1 cup sprouts
	6 cucumber slices
3 teaspoons added sugar	Tea with 1 tablespoon honey
4 fat	2 tablespoons cream cheese
	2 tablespoons pumpkin seeds

Lunch

5 bread	2½ cups rice
1 milk	1 cup fat-free milk
2 vegetable	1 cup Chinese vegetables, stir-fried with garlic, onion, fresh ginger
2 fruit	1 cup citrus sections
4 very lean protein	4 ounces scallops, stir-fried
2 fat	2 teaspoons oil (for stir-frying)

Snack

1 bread	2 squares graham cracker
2 fruit	2 apples, diced
6 teaspoons added sugar	2 tablespoons brown sugar
1 milk	½ cup fat-free cottage cheese
1 MRP	1 meal replacement shake

Dinner

3 bread	2-inch square of corn bread
	1 cup kidney beans (add to chili)
2 fruit	2 pears
8 teaspoons added sugar	1½ cups frozen yogurt
4 vegetable	1 cup chopped cooked tomatoes with chili seasoning
	½ onion, garlic (for seasoning)
	Salad with 1 cup lettuce, ¼ cup tomato, ¼ cup cucumber
5 lean protein	Included (in beans)
	3 ounces soy crumbles (for chili)
3 fat	2 slices bacon, cooked very crisp (crumble into chili)
	2 tablespoons reduced-fat dressing
	Included (in corn bread)

Pre-Workout Snack

SMOOTHIE

Blend until smooth.

1 milk	1 cup fat-free milk
4 fruit	1 cup orange juice
	1 small banana
2 very lean protein	14 grams whey protein powder
	Ice cubes

Workout

16 teaspoons added sugar	32-ounce sports drink
	Water

DAY 4

Breakfast

2 fruit	2 cups raspberries
1 milk	1 cup fat-free milk ($^1/_2$ cup for French toast)
2 vegetable	1 cup tomato juice

FRENCH TOAST *(See recipe directions on page 44.)*

3 bread	3 slices whole-wheat bread
1 medium-fat protein	1 egg
3 very lean protein	6 egg whites
3 fat	1$^1/_2$ tablespoon ground flaxseed
	2 teaspoons oil (for cooking)
11 teaspoons added sugar	3$^1/_2$ tablespoons no-calorie sweetener
	Water

Snack

2 bread	24 Wheat Thins
3 vegetable	Sliced bell peppers, radishes, mini-carrots
3 teaspoons added sugar	1 tablespoon 100% fruit spread
4 fat	2 tablespoons salad dressing (for dipping)
	12 almonds

Lunch

2 fruit	2 cups blueberries
1 milk	1 cup fat-free milk

FAJITAS

Combine ingredients.

5 bread	1½ cups Spanish rice
	2 tortillas
2 vegetable	1 cup sautéed onions, peppers
	2 tablespoons salsa
4 very lean protein	4 ounces skinless white-meat chicken, grilled with lime juice
2 fat	2 teaspoons olive oil (for cooking)

Snack

1 bread	2 rice cakes
2 fruit	2½ cups strawberries
6 teaspoons added sugar	2 tablespoons sugar (for berries)
1 milk	1 cup fat-free milk
	1 meal replacement shake

Dinner

3 bread	1 ounce croutons (for salad)
	1 cup chicken noodle soup
	4 crackers
2 fruit	2 nectarines
8 teaspoons added sugar	1½ cups cranberry juice cocktail
4 vegetable	4 cups large mixed salad with lettuce, tomato, cucumber, pepper
5 lean protein	5 ounces swordfish, grilled with ginger and scallions
3 fat	3 tablespoons salad dressing

Pre-Workout Snack

SMOOTHIE

Blend until smooth.

1 milk	1 cup fat-free milk
4 fruit	1 cup orange juice
	1 small banana
2 very lean protein	14 grams whey protein powder
	Ice cubes

Workout

16 teaspoons added sugar	32-ounce sports drink
	Water

DAY 5

Breakfast

3 bread	1½ cups quick oats (not instant)
1 milk	1 cup fat-free milk
2 fruit	1 cup apples, diced (for carrot-apple salad)
	½ tablespoon raisins
11 teaspoons added sugar	½ tablespoon brown sugar
2 vegetable	4 large carrots, shredded (add some cinnamon and ½ of the brown sugar)
1 medium-fat protein	1 egg, hard-cooked
3 very lean protein	6 eggs, hard-cooked (discard yolks)
3 fat	1½ tablespoons ground flaxseed
	2 teaspoons sesame, hazelnut, or almond oil (for oatmeal)
	Water

Snack

2 bread	1½ ounces baked tortilla chips
3 vegetable	½ cup salsa
	1 cup chopped vegetables
3 teaspoons added sugar	½ cup pineapple juice
4 fat	16 black olives
	¼ avocado, cubed

Lunch

5 bread	1½ cups minestrone soup
	1½ cups cooked linguini
1 milk	1 cup fat-free milk
2 vegetable	Salad with 1 cup lettuce, ¼ cup tomato, ¼ cup cucumber
	½ cup marinara sauce
2 fruit	1 grapefruit, sectioned
4 very lean protein	4 ounces shrimp, grilled
2 fat	2 teaspoons olive oil (for cooking)

Snack

1 bread	1 serving Grape Nuts cereal
2 fruit	2 cups blueberries
6 teaspoons added sugar	2 tablespoons honey
1 milk	1 cup plain nonfat yogurt
1 MRP	1 meal replacement shake

Dinner

3 bread	1 large pita
	¹/₂ cup couscous
2 fruit	4 large figs
8 teaspoons added sugar	12 ounces apricot nectar
4 vegetable	4 cups tossed salad with cucumber, tomato, sprouts
5 lean protein	5 ounces lean lamb, grilled with lime juice
3 fat	3 tablespoons vinaigrette

Pre-Workout Snack

SMOOTHIE

Blend until smooth.

1 milk	1 cup fat-free milk
4 fruit	1 cup orange juice
	1 small banana
2 very lean protein	14 grams whey protein powder
	Ice cubes

Workout

16 teaspoons added sugar	32-ounce sports drink
	Water

DAY 6

Breakfast

3 bread	3 slices multigrain toast
1 medium-fat protein	1 egg, scrambled in a nonstick pan
3 very lean protein	6 egg whites, scrambled with whole egg
2 vegetable	1 cup sliced mushrooms (for omelet)
	¹/₂ cup V8 juice
3 fat	1¹/₂ tablespoons ground flaxseed
	2 teaspoons oil (for cooking)
	Water

SMOOTHIE

Blend until smooth.

1 milk	1 cup fat-free milk
2 fruit	¹/₂ cup orange juice
	1 fresh peach
11 teaspoons added sugar	3¹/₂ tablespoons honey

Snack

2 bread	2 slices whole-wheat bread
3 vegetable	3 cups salad with lettuce, tomato, cucumber, pepper
3 teaspoons added sugar	2 tablespoons raisins (for salad)
4 fat	3 slices bacon
	1 tablespoon reduced-fat mayonnaise

Lunch

5 bread	1 whole-wheat bagel
	1 cup potato salad, made with reduced-fat mayonnaise
	$3/4$ cup vegetable noodle soup
1 milk	1 cup fat-free milk
2 vegetable	1 cup carrot sticks
	Onion, tomato
2 fruit	2 cups honeydew
4 very lean protein	4 ounces smoked salmon
2 fat	2 tablespoons reduced-fat cream cheese

Snack

1 bread	$1/2$ cup granola
2 fruit	2 kiwis, diced
6 teaspoons added sugar	1 tablespoon honey
1 milk	1 cup plain fat-free yogurt
	1 meal replacement shake

Dinner

3 bread	2 slices rye bread
	$1/2$ cup pasta salad
2 fruit	24 grapes (slice grapes in half, add to gelatin)
8 teaspoons added sugar	$1^1/2$ cups flavored gelatin dessert
4 vegetable	1 cup coleslaw
	1 cup chopped vegetables (cucumbers, carrots, onions; mix into tuna)
5 lean protein	5 ounces tuna in olive oil, drained
3 fat	2 tablespoons mayonnaise (for tuna)
	Included (in coleslaw and pasta salad)

Pre-Workout Snack

SMOOTHIE

Blend until smooth.

1 milk	1 cup fat-free milk
4 fruit	1 cup orange juice
	1 small banana
2 very lean protein	14 grams whey protein powder
	Ice cubes

Workout

16 teaspoons added sugar	32-ounce sports drink
	Water

DAY 7

Breakfast

3 bread	$1^{1}/_{2}$ cups Shredded Wheat
1 milk	1 cup fat-free milk
2 fruit	2 cups raspberries
11 teaspoons added sugar	$3^{1}/_{2}$ tablespoons sugar
2 vegetable	1 cup V8 juice
1 medium-fat protein	1 egg, hard-cooked
3 very lean protein	6 eggs, hard-cooked (discard yolks)
3 fat	$1^{1}/_{2}$ tablespoons ground flaxseed
	2 teaspoons oil (for cooking)
	Water

Snack

2 bread	2 tortillas
3 vegetable	$2^{1}/_{2}$ cups sliced vegetables
	$^{1}/_{2}$ cup salsa
3 teaspoons added sugar	$^{1}/_{2}$ cup lemonade
4 fat	16 black olives, chopped
	$^{1}/_{4}$ avocado, diced

Lunch

5 bread	1 large multigrain roll
	6 ounces baked yam
1 milk	1 cup fat-free milk
2 vegetable	Sliced tomato, lettuce for sandwich
	1 cup radishes, celery, carrots
2 fruit	2 nectarines
4 very lean protein	4 ounces skinless white-meat chicken, grilled with lime juice
2 fat	4 tablespoons low-fat ranch dressing (for dipping)

Snack

1 bread	1 slice whole-grain bread

SMOOTHIE

Blend until smooth.

2 fruit	1¼ cups strawberries
	½ large banana
6 teaspoons added sugar	2 tablespoons honey
1 milk	1 cup fat-free milk
	1 meal replacement shake

Dinner

3 bread	2-inch square of corn bread
	1 ounce croutons
2 fruit	2 tangerines
	4 tablespoons dried fruit
8 teaspoons added sugar	1 cup applesauce
4 vegetable	4 cups salad and vegetables
5 lean protein	4 ounces salmon, poached
	1 ounce shredded cheese
3 fat	2 tablespoons Caesar dressing

Pre-Workout Snack

SMOOTHIE

Blend until smooth.

1 milk	1 cup fat-free milk
4 fruit	1 cup orange juice
	1 small banana
2 very lean protein	14 grams whey protein powder
	Ice cubes

Workout

16 teaspoons added sugar	32-ounce sports drink
	Water

THE WANTS-MUSCLE-YESTERDAY MEAL PLAN

YOU WANT TO GAIN MUSCLE FAST, BUT YOU DON'T WANT to add too much fat along with the muscle. To do so, you'll need to consume enough calories, relying heavily on lean proteins, good fats, and homemade smoothies.

Daily Assumptions*†

4,259 calories
630 grams carbohydrates
185 grams protein
110 grams fat

Daily Breakdown*†

14 bread
11 fruit
4 milk
40 teaspoons added sugar
9 vegetable
9 very lean protein
5 lean protein
1 medium-fat protein
12 fat

Note: Occasionally, a fat-free product, like mustard or cooking spray, is included on the menus. These do not count toward your daily breakdown but should not be overused.

*Use every day.

† Based on a 185-pound man.

THE MENU

DAY 1

Pre-Workout Snack

SMOOTHIE
Blend until smooth.

1 milk	1 cup fat-free milk
3 fruit	1 cup orange juice
	½ large banana
2 very lean protein	14 grams whey protein powder
	Ice cubes

Workout

16 teaspoons added sugar	32-ounce sports drink
	Water

Breakfast

3 bread	3 slices whole-grain bread
1 milk	1 cup fat-free milk
2 fruit	1 cup cubed cantaloupe
	1 cup fresh raspberries
1 vegetable	1 small tomato, diced (add to egg)
7 teaspoons added sugar	2½ tablespoons 100% fruit spread
1 medium-fat protein	1 egg, scrambled in a nonstick pan
3 very lean protein	6 egg whites, scrambled with whole egg
3 fat	⅓ avocado, diced (add to egg)
	Water
	Oil-free cooking spray (for eggs)

Snack

2 bread	8 whole-wheat crackers
3 vegetable	3 cups celery sticks
3 teaspoons added sugar	Tea with 1 tablespoon honey
4 fat	2 tablespoons natural peanut butter

Lunch

5 bread	Foot-long Subway sandwich with extra meat (choose from "6 grams fat or less" list)
2 vegetable	Lettuce, tomato
2 fruit	1 small banana
	1 apple
1 milk	1 cup fat-free milk
4 very lean protein	Included (in sandwich)
2 fat	2 tablespoons olive oil or 2 tablespoons salad dressing

Snack

1 bread	$1/4$ cup Grape Nuts cereal
2 fruit	$1^1/_2$ cups blueberries
6 teaspoons added sugar	2 tablespoons honey
1 milk	1 cup plain nonfat yogurt

Dinner

3 bread	1 large baked sweet potato
	1 small ear corn on the cob
2 fruit	2 slices watermelon
8 teaspoons added sugar	$1^1/_2$ cups frozen yogurt
3 vegetable	Salad with 2 cups romaine lettuce, $1/2$ cup tomato, $1/2$ cup cucumber
	$1/2$ cup broccoli
5 lean protein	5 ounces salmon, grilled
3 fat	3 tablespoons olive oil (for dressing)
	Vinegar (for dressing)

DAY 2

Pre-Workout Snack

SMOOTHIE

Blend until smooth.

1 milk	1 cup fat-free milk
3 fruit	1 cup orange juice
	$1/2$ large banana
2 very lean protein	14 grams whey protein powder
	Ice cubes

Workout

16 teaspoons added sugar | 32-ounce sports drink

Water

Breakfast

Combine yogurt, fruit, and honey. Combine muffin and egg for sandwich.

3 bread | 1½ whole-wheat English muffins

1 milk | 1 cup fat-free, unsweetened yogurt

2 fruit | 2½ cups fresh strawberries

1 vegetable | ½ cup tomato juice

7 teaspoons added sugar | 2½ tablespoons honey

1 medium-fat protein | 1 egg, hard-cooked

3 very lean protein | 6 eggs, hard-cooked (discard yolks)

3 fat | 1½ tablespoon ground flaxseed

2 teaspoons oil (for cooking)

Water

Snack

2 bread | 2 rice cakes

3 vegetable | 3 cups vegetable sticks

3 teaspoons added sugar | 1 tablespoon 100% fruit spread

4 fat | 4 tablespoons salad dressing (for dipping)

Lunch

5 bread | 2 slices whole-grain bread

1 ounce croutons

1 cup brown rice

2 vegetable | Large salad with romaine lettuce, tomato, grilled eggplant, roasted red pepper

2 fruit | 2 kiwis, sliced

1 milk | 1 cup fat-free milk

4 very lean protein | 4 ounces skinless white-meat chicken, grilled with lime juice

2 fat | 2 tablespoons low-fat salad dressing

1 teaspoon olive oil (for roasted vegetables)

Snack

1 bread | 5 melba toast

SMOOTHIE

Blend until smooth.

2 fruit | 1 cup sliced peaches

6 teaspoons added sugar | 2 tablespoons honey

1 milk | 1 cup fat-free milk

Ice cubes

Dinner

3 bread	1 cup cooked pasta
	1 slice garlic bread
2 fruit	2$\frac{1}{2}$ cups whole strawberries
8 teaspoons added sugar	1$\frac{1}{2}$ cups flavored gelatin dessert
3 vegetable	2 cups ratatouille (over pasta)
	Salad with 1 cup lettuce, $\frac{1}{4}$ cup tomato, $\frac{1}{4}$ cup cucumber
5 lean protein	5 ounces lean ground beef (add to ratatouille)
3 fat	2 tablespoons salad dressing
	1 teaspoon butter (for garlic bread)

DAY 3

Pre-Workout Snack

SMOOTHIE

Blend until smooth.

1 milk	1 cup fat-free milk
3 fruit	1 cup orange juice
	$\frac{1}{2}$ large banana
2 very lean protein	14 grams whey protein powder
	Ice cubes

Workout

16 teaspoons added sugar	32-ounce sports drink
	Water

Breakfast

3 bread	3 slices whole-wheat bread
1 milk	1 cup fat-free cottage cheese (on bread; sprinkle with no-calorie sweetener and cinnamon)
2 fruit	4 ounces freshly squeezed orange juice (with pulp)
	$\frac{1}{2}$ cup sliced pineapple
1 vegetable	$\frac{1}{2}$ cup V8 juice
7 teaspoons added sugar	2$\frac{1}{2}$ tablespoons sugar (for tea or coffee and cottage cheese)
1 medium-fat protein	1 egg, cooked sunny-side up in a nonstick pan
3 very lean protein	6 egg whites, cooked with sunny-side up egg
3 fat	1$\frac{1}{2}$ tablespoons ground flaxseed
	2 teaspoons oil (for cooking)
	Water

Snack

2 bread	1 bagel
3 vegetable	3 cups tomato and sprout salad
3 teaspoons added sugar	1 tablespoon 100% fruit spread
4 fat	2 tablespoons cream cheese
	1 tablespoon sunflower seeds
	1 tablespoon vinaigrette

Lunch

5 bread	2$^1/_2$ cups rice
2 vegetable	1 cup Chinese vegetables, stir-fried with garlic, onion, fresh ginger
2 fruit	1 cup citrus sections
1 milk	1 cup fat-free milk
4 very lean protein	4 ounces scallops, stir-fried
2 fat	2 teaspoons oil (for stir-frying)

Snack

1 bread	2 squares graham crackers
2 fruit	2 apples, diced
6 teaspoons added sugar	2 tablespoons brown sugar
1 milk	1 cup fat-free cottage cheese

Dinner

3 bread	2-inch square of corn bread
	1 cup kidney beans (add to chili)
2 fruit	2 pears
8 teaspoons added sugar	1$^1/_2$ cups frozen yogurt
3 vegetable	1 cup chopped cooked tomatoes with chili seasoning
	$^1/_2$ onion, garlic (for seasoning)
	Salad with 1 cup lettuce, $^1/_4$ cup tomato, $^1/_4$ cup cucumber
5 lean protein	Included (in beans)
	3 ounces soy crumbles (for chili)
3 fat	2 slices bacon, cooked very crisp (crumble into chili)
	2 tablespoons reduced-fat dressing
	Included (in corn bread)

DAY 4

Pre-Workout Snack

SMOOTHIE

Blend until smooth.

1 milk	1 cup fat-free milk
3 fruit	1 cup orange juice
	$^1/_2$ large banana
2 very lean protein	14 grams whey protein powder
	Ice cubes

Workout

16 teaspoons added sugar	32-ounce sports drink
	Water

Breakfast

2 fruit	1 cup raspberries
	$^1/_2$ cup grapefruit juice
1 milk	1 cup fat-free milk ($^1/_2$ cup for French toast)
1 vegetable	Sliced tomato, cucumber

FRENCH TOAST *(See recipe directions on page 44.)*

3 bread	3 slices whole-wheat bread
7 teaspoons added sugar	2$^1/_2$ tablespoons maple syrup
1 medium-fat protein	1 egg
3 very lean protein	6 egg whites
3 fat	1$^1/_2$ tablespoons ground flaxseed
	2 teaspoons oil (for cooking)
	Water

Snack

2 bread	24 Wheat Thins
3 vegetable	3 cups bell peppers and other vegetables, sliced
3 teaspoons added sugar	1 tablespoon 100% fruit spread (for crackers)
4 fat	4 tablespoons salad dressing (for dipping)

Lunch

2 fruit	1$^1/_2$ cups blueberries
1 milk	1 cup fat-free milk

FAJITAS

Combine ingredients.

5 bread	1 cup Spanish rice
	2 tortillas
2 vegetable	1 cup sautéed onions, peppers
	2 tablespoons salsa
4 very lean protein	4 ounces skinless white-meat chicken, grilled with lime juice
2 fat	2 teaspoons olive oil (for cooking)

Snack

1 bread	2 rice cakes
2 fruit	2½ cups strawberries
6 teaspoons added sugar	2 tablespoons sugar (for berries)
1 milk	1 cup fat-free milk

Dinner

3 bread	1 ounce croutons (for salad)
	1 cup chicken noodle soup
	4 crackers
2 fruit	2 nectarines
8 teaspoons added sugar	1½ cups cranberry juice cocktail
3 vegetable	3 cups salad with lettuce, tomato, cucumber, pepper
5 lean protein	5 ounces swordfish, grilled with ginger and scallions
3 fat	3 tablespoons salad dressing

DAY 5

Pre-Workout Snack

SMOOTHIE

Blend until smooth.

1 milk	1 cup fat-free milk
3 fruit	1 cup orange juice
	½ large banana
2 very lean protein	14 grams whey protein powder
	Ice cubes

Workout

16 teaspoons added sugar	32-ounce sports drink
	Water

Breakfast

3 bread	1½ cups quick oats (not instant)
1 milk	1 cup fat-free milk
2 fruit	½ cup apples, diced (for apple-carrot salad)
	¾ cup sliced strawberries (for oatmeal)
	¼ cup raisins (for apple-carrot salad)
1 vegetable	2 large carrots, shredded (add some cinnamon and ¼ of the brown sugar)
7 teaspoons added sugar	3 tablespoons brown sugar
1 medium-fat protein	1 egg, hard-cooked
3 very lean protein	6 eggs, hard-cooked (discard yolks)
3 fat	1½ tablespoons ground flaxseed
	2 teaspoons sesame, hazelnut, or almond oil (for oatmeal)
	Water

Snack

2 bread	1½ ounces baked tortilla chips
3 vegetable	2 cups raw vegetables
	½ cup salsa
3 teaspoons added sugar	½ cup cranberry-apple juice
4 fat	8 olives
	⅓ avocado, cubed

Lunch

5 bread	1½ cups minestrone soup
	1½ cups cooked linguini
2 vegetable	1 cup marinara sauce
2 fruit	1 mango, sliced
1 milk	1 cup fat-free milk
4 very lean protein	4 ounces shrimp, grilled
2 fat	2 teaspoons olive oil (for cooking)

Snack

1 bread	2 squares graham crackers

SMOOTHIE

Blend until smooth.

2 fruit	1 cup sliced mango
6 teaspoons added sugar	2 tablespoons honey
1 milk	1 cup fat-free milk
	Ice cubes

Dinner

3 bread	1 large pita
	1 ounce croutons
2 fruit	4 large figs
8 teaspoons added sugar	8 ounces apricot nectar
3 vegetable	3 cups salad with lettuce, tomato, cucumber, pepper
5 lean protein	5 ounces lean lamb, grilled with lime juice
3 fat	3 tablespoons vinaigrette

DAY 6

Pre-Workout Snack

SMOOTHIE

Blend until smooth.

1 milk	1 cup fat-free milk
3 fruit	1 cup orange juice
	1/2 large banana
2 very lean protein	14 grams whey protein powder
	Ice cubes

Workout

16 teaspoons added sugar	32-ounce sports drink
	Water

Breakfast

3 bread	3 slices multigrain bread, toasted
1 vegetable	Small tomato, diced (add to eggs)
1 medium-fat protein	1 egg, scrambled in a nonstick pan
3 very lean protein	6 egg whites, scrambled with whole egg
3 fat	1 1/2 tablespoons ground flaxseed
	2 teaspoons oil (for cooking eggs)
	Water

SMOOTHIE

Blend until smooth.

1 milk	1 cup fat-free milk
2 fruit	3/4 cup orange juice
	3/4 cup fresh peaches
11 teaspoons added sugar	3 tablespoons honey

Snack

2 bread	2 slices whole-wheat bread
3 vegetable	Tomato, lettuce
	2 cups vegetable sticks
3 teaspoons added sugar	1/2 cup grapefruit juice
4 fat	4 slices bacon
	1 tablespoon fat-free mayonnaise

Lunch

5 bread	1 whole-wheat bagel
	1 cup potato salad, made with reduced-fat mayonnaise
	1/2 cup vegetable noodle soup
2 vegetable	1/2 cup carrot sticks
	Onion, tomato
2 fruit	1/4 honeydew
1 milk	1 cup fat-free milk
4 very lean protein	4 ounces smoked salmon
2 fat	2 tablespoons cream cheese

Snack

1 bread	1/2 cup granola
2 fruit	2 kiwis, diced
6 teaspoons added sugar	2 tablespoons honey
1 milk	1 cup plain fat-free yogurt
1 MRP	1 meal replacement shake

Dinner

3 bread	2 slices rye bread
	1/2 cup pasta salad
2 fruit	34 grapes
8 teaspoons added sugar	1 1/2 cups flavored gelatin dessert
3 vegetable	1 cup coleslaw
	1/2 cup chopped vegetables (cucumbers, carrots, onions; mix into tuna)
5 lean protein	5 ounces tuna in olive oil, drained
3 fat	2 tablespoons mayonnaise
	Included (in coleslaw and pasta salad)

DAY 7

Pre-Workout Snack

SMOOTHIE

Blend until smooth.

1 milk	1 cup fat-free milk
3 fruit	1 cup orange juice
	$^1/_2$ large banana
2 very lean protein	14 grams whey protein powder
	Ice cubes

Workout

16 teaspoons added sugar	32-ounce sports drink
	Water

Breakfast

3 bread	$1^1/_2$ cups Shredded Wheat
1 milk	1 cup fat-free milk
2 fruit	1 cup raspberries
	$^3/_4$ cup blueberries
1 vegetable	2 pickles, chopped (for egg salad)
7 teaspoons added sugar	$2^1/_2$ tablespoons sugar
1 medium-fat protein	1 egg, hard-cooked (for egg salad)
3 very lean protein	6 eggs, hard-cooked (discard yolks)
3 fat	$1^1/_2$ tablespoons ground flaxseed
	2 tablespoons reduced-fat mayonnaise (for egg salad)
	Water

Snack

2 bread	2 tortillas
3 vegetable	2 cups sliced vegetables
	$^1/_2$ cup salsa
3 teaspoons added sugar	$^1/_2$ cup pineapple juice
4 fat	16 black olives, chopped
	$^1/_4$ avocado, diced

Lunch

5 bread	1 large multigrain roll
	6 ounces baked yam
2 vegetable	Sliced tomato, lettuce (for sandwich)
	1/2 cup radishes, celery, carrots
2 fruit	1 large nectarine
1 milk	1 cup fat-free milk
4 very lean protein	4 ounces skinless white-meat chicken, grilled with lime juice
2 fat	4 tablespoons low-fat ranch dressing (for dipping)

Snack

1 bread	3 cups popcorn

SMOOTHIE

Blend until smooth.

2 fruit	1 1/4 cups strawberries
	1/2 banana
6 teaspoons added sugar	2 tablespoons honey
1 milk	1 cup fat-free milk
	Ice

Dinner

3 bread	3-inch square of corn bread
	1 ounce croutons
2 fruit	2 large tangerines
8 teaspoons added sugar	1 1/2 cups fruit juice
3 vegetable	3 cups salad with lettuce, tomato, cucumber, pepper
5 lean protein	4 ounces salmon, poached
	1 ounce reduced-fat shredded cheese
3 fat	6 tablespoons low-fat Caesar dressing
	Included (in corn bread)

CHAPTER FIVE

Food and Athletic Performance

USE FOOD TO UNLEASH THE WINNER INSIDE YOU

When it comes to sports and performance, eating is just as important as how you train or what you wear—it's the key to building a lean, agile, action-ready body that can handle hours of competition. Food can guarantee that your mind will stay nimble and your body charged. On the flip side, the wrong foods can sabotage even the most-natural athletes, slowing and weakening their games and allowing other, more nutrition-savvy competitors to take home the gold.

This chapter is devoted to making food a partner in your quest for athletic glory. Follow my advice here, and you'll not only build a sports-ready body, but you'll also know exactly what to feed that body when it's time to play.

If you're a competitive guy, look at it this way: What separates you from the next guy, over time, are the little things. Something like nutrition, which your opponent may overlook, provides the perfect chance for you to get a leg up. Even elite athletes will often say, "Hey, I've gotten this far without worrying about what I eat. Why should I bother now?" If

that's how some guys in the NFL or NBA approach nutrition, imagine how your opponent in the club tennis tournament is thinking about it. If you become an athlete who genuinely cares about what he puts into his body and pays attention to what he eats before he goes out to play three sets, you'll be able to wipe the court with your opponents—even ones you once thought were unbeatable.

If you don't believe me, ask NFL coach Bill Belichik, whose New England Patriots won the Super Bowl in 2002 and 2004. I worked with him a decade or so ago, when he coached the Cleveland Browns and I was the team's consulting nutritionist. Belichik was incredibly focused on details. In fact, he was so detail-oriented that many observers at that time considered it potentially negative. They asked how any coach could pay so much attention to so many small details and still remain focused on winning the big one. He told me that the details were precisely what would make the difference between the one team that wins it all and the many teams that don't. He was ahead of his time in having a nutritionist work with his players, and I would suggest that's a major reason that he has those Super Bowl rings today.

What I've found is that athletes need their nutrition plan to be as regimented as their training and recuperation. You can't think of it haphazardly, like, "Oh, yeah, I know I'm supposed to eat a little more protein, so I'll throw some of that in." Guys at the top of their game know exactly what they need to eat, and they plan their menus accordingly. They shop for the right foods, and, when necessary, they take the time to prepare their meals. When they leave home, they make sure they have what they need in their backpack or carrying case, whether it's turkey jerky, fruit, dried nuts, a peanut-butter-and-jelly sandwich, a sports bar, or a ready-to-drink protein shake. That way, they have access to the right foods at the right times.

The successful athletes I've worked with never go anywhere without taking some food along with them. These guys never travel without a cooler of food in the car, and once they reach a destination, they exploit whatever refrigerators, blenders, and kitchen facilities they can find. These athletes pay attention to what they eat and when they eat, and they never risk missing a meal. That meal, they know, may be the one that makes the difference between recovering adequately between workouts or not recovering at all.

You probably aren't a professional athlete, but it doesn't matter. Exciting new research shows the importance of eating the right foods at the right times to build as much strength and endurance as possible from your workouts. In other words, no matter what you do, the more you focus on nutrition, the better you'll do.

You'll find two meal plans in this chapter. The first is for guys mostly interested in increasing sports-related strength in the gym. The second is for guys who are mostly interested in game-day endurance. (Incidentally, the strength program should also improve your endurance, and vice versa, al-

though to a lesser degree.) I envision these plans being used one of three ways.

1. Some of you will want to follow the strength meal plan exclusively. For you, I recommend going back to the last chapter and reading about muscle growth. Much of what you need to know is there. Then, use the information and the meal plan for strength to get stronger without putting on too much bulk.

2. Some of you will want to use the endurance meal plan exclusively. Those of you who focus primarily on running long distance year-round, for example, might not be interested in a strength plan.

3. A good number of you, especially those who play organized sports, will want to make significant gains in both strength and endurance. For you, I suggest treating the strength meal plan as an off-season cross-training program. When your season arrives, switch to the endurance meal plan.

Fat Tricks

Before I get to the meal plans, I want to talk about an important topic: guys who want to not only perform better but also lose fat. It's surprisingly difficult to get the most out of the former when you're primarily concerned with the latter. Sports nutrition is a catch-22 that way: You try to lose fat so you look and feel more like an athlete. That means, among other things, cutting calories. But when you cut calories, you also cut the amount of energy you have available for strenuous activities. That means you won't have enough in the tank to get you through any sport more vigorous than chess.

There is a way to do both—to lose fat and to have enough food to fuel your favorite pastime. You just have to give up on the idea of doing them at the same time.

Let's say you're trying to lose a little fat. You hope to look better, of course, but you also hope your streamlined physique will help you get around the bases a little faster, or maybe get up and down the court a few more times before you wave in a substitute off the bench.

Your goal is—or should be—to lose that fat before your competitive season begins. Aside from the energy issue, you want your body to be used to its new weight before the games begin. (The same, of course, would apply to a serious body-building program, which will also lead to weight gain. You don't want to be in the middle of that when your season begins.) Your sense of balance, your center of gravity, your muscles, your inner ear—these have all calibrated themselves to a specific body weight and certain distribution of body fat. Even if you look in the mirror and hate the extra fat you see, you should remember that your body has learned to operate efficiently with that fat just where it is. (This assumes, of course, that you've been practicing and playing your sport at this weight.)

If you want to lose weight, try this: Use the fat-loss meal plans in chapter 3, starting during the off-season and continuing for as long as it takes to shed the fat—or up until a month or two before you want to begin competing. Then, transition to one of the meal plans I outline in this chapter.

General Guidelines for Sports Nutrition

Regardless of which meal plan from this chapter you go with—the strength plan or the cardio endurance plan—there are going to be some general rules to follow.

Eat more food. This is something you've heard before if you've read the last two chapters: You need to eat a lot of calories, probably more than you've been eating if you've been a couch potato. You're going to be expending more energy as an athlete, and you'll need to consume more to account for it. You also need to fuel your workouts and have enough raw materials to help heal and build your muscles during your recovery periods.

How many more calories you need is hard to say, precisely because everyone is different. But I'll give you some ballpark numbers to shoot for in the individual plans.

Eat more often. Eat five meals daily. Better yet, eat six or seven. Because you'll be training harder than before, you'll need to chow down every 3 hours or so, and you can't afford to skip meals. If you do, you're liable to run out of fuel when you need it most: mid-workout. What's more, if your meals are spaced too far apart, your body will adapt by slowing down its metabolism, which will promote fat storage. If it's time for one of those five meals and you're not hungry, don't force-feed yourself. However, don't overcompensate by eating excessively at your next meal.

Eat simple and natural. It's this simple: If you eat junk, you'll probably turn in junk-worthy performances. I'm not saying you can never eat processed food, but keep in mind that processed food is usually nowhere near as nutritious as whole foods. It's been stripped of much of the stuff that will boost your energy, not to mention valuable components such as fiber. The easiest way to avoid processed food is to focus your shopping on the periphery of the supermarket, avoiding the aisles. On the fringe, you'll find good things like fresh fruits and vegetables, fish, low-fat milk, and fresh farm eggs. In the belly of the beast, you'll find junk food, TV dinners, and shopping carts stuffed with the *National Enquirer* and screaming kids. Steer clear.

Here are some of the foods you should be looking for.

Healthy, energy-packed carbs, including brown rice, buckwheat, whole-wheat pasta and couscous, potatoes with skin, fruit, sweet potatoes, winter squash, beans, peas, and assorted fruits. Keep your bread consumption to a minimum. If you do eat bread, choose a sprouted-grain high-protein variety, which can be found at most regular grocery stores these days, as well as at whole-foods stores. Also, go for the so-called "free" vegetables (tomatoes, peppers, celery, jicama, radishes). These make great snacks because they're completely or nearly calorie-free and loaded with fiber.

Assorted lean proteins, with an emphasis on fish that are high in omega-3 fatty acids, eggs, chicken, turkey, dairy, vegetable proteins, protein powder, and red meat, the latter eaten sparingly.

Selected healthy unsaturated fats, such as canola oil, olive oil, avocados, nuts, peanut butter, and olives.

Eat meals that smartly combine protein and carbs. If you can, get protein and carbs at every meal. One of your main sports-nutrition goals is to get more carbs stored in your muscles, where you can access it fairly easily. I'll get into this more later, but for now, understand that a mix of protein and carbs is one of the best ways to make sure this happens. Carb consumption causes your body to secrete insulin, which transports sugar out of the blood into the muscles. Protein consumption enhances this process, first by making insulin more efficient, and second by slowing the release of glucose into the bloodstream. If too much glucose is released at once, your insulin won't be able to shuttle it into your muscles fast enough and the glucose will ultimately become fat. Of course, getting more athletic and getting fatter are contradictory goals, so it's best to avoid this.

Steadily eating protein throughout the day has its advantages, beyond helping with carb utilization.

■ The body can absorb only a certain percentage of the protein you eat at each sitting, and no one is entirely sure what that percentage is. Because the body doesn't store protein except in very small pools, it makes sense to replenish it throughout the day.

■ Probably most important for the athlete in you, protein is an important anabolic driver. You want to make sure your body has what it needs to

KITCHEN SURVIVAL GUIDE

IF YOU'RE LIKE MOST GUYS, your cue to head to the supermarket is rooting around for a "sell by" date that postdates the new millenium. To be primed for the pump before you hit the gym, however, you'll probably need to do a better job of keeping healthy foods at arm's reach. You'll also want to make sure that you have these six things in your kitchen at all times.

■ A variety of fresh fruits. *Tip:* Each time you shop, buy three each of several kinds of portable fruits, such as apples, bananas, pears, grapes, and oranges.

■ Whole-grain breads. *Tip:* Look for brands with at least 2 grams of fiber per slice.

■ Lean meats for making quick sandwiches. *Tip:* Try turkey, chicken breast, lean roast beef, or lean ham.

■ Fresh greens and salad fixings. *Tip:* Buy precut veggies from the supermarket's produce section. Keep them well wrapped and sealed.

■ Frozen chicken breasts and healthy "create-a-meal" frozen entrées. *Tip:* Opt for these instead of fast food when you're pressed for time.

■ Fat-free or low-fat dairy sources. *Tip:* When in doubt, rely on milk and yogurt.

build muscle throughout the day in response to your workouts. Remember that your body breaks down and rebuilds protein in your muscles constantly, and that this process is in overdrive in the 48 hours after a workout.

Aim for variety. Different foods within different groups contain different combinations of nutrients. Nutritionists are only now discovering how important that is, mainly due to technology-driven changes in our ability to measure things in smaller and smaller amounts. We can now get a much clearer picture of why foods affect us, often dramatically, in specific ways. That's how we now know why you need a variety of animal products, fruits, vegetables, and other foods in your diet.

To ensure dietary variety, set aside two-thirds to three-quarters of your plate for plant-based foods. That will help you eat enough fruits, veggies, grains, beans, nuts, and seeds at every meal. Then put differently colored plant foods on your plate, aiming for at least one green food, one yellow, one red, one orange, one white, and one brown during the course of the day. Stay away from single-color meals. The all-white meal is famous among dietitians: It's usually some combination like potatoes or rice, white fish, milk, and a banana. Although these foods aren't bad choices, too many of them may mean you're not getting enough variety.

Steer clear of beer. All it offers is empty calories and more fat storage, along with a short buzz and, perhaps, a long hangover. Obviously, it's hard to play your best when you're nursing a headache, sore limbs, and woozy eyesight. Alcohol consumption in general should be minimized, although an occasional glass of wine or whiskey is fine.

Hydrate, hydrate, hydrate. I saved this one for last because I want to emphasize this: When it comes to athletic performance, no nutrient is more important than water. It will trump carbs and protein in a heartbeat. Loss of just 2 percent of your body weight as fluid will diminish your physical and cognitive performance by 20 percent. Once you become 3 to 4 percent dehydrated, your health is at risk.

SYMPTOMS OF DEHYDRATION

MILD HYDRATION AND CHRONIC DEHYDRATION HAVE SPECIFIC SIGNS. Stay alert for the first set, and you will never need to worry about the second.

Early Signs	Severe Signs
Fatigue	Difficulty swallowing
Loss of appetite	Stumbling
Flushed skin	Clumsiness
Burning in stomach	Shriveled skin
Light-headedness	Sunken eyes and dim vision
Headache	Painful urination
Dry mouth	Numb skin
Dry cough	Muscle spasm
Heat intolerance	Delirium

How quickly can you lose that much fluid? Contrary to our drive to eat, our drive to drink is not as keen. Our thirst mechanism doesn't kick in until we are already mildly dehydrated. When you're working out moderately in a mild climate, you are probably losing 1 to 2 quarts (2 to 4 pounds) of fluid per hour through perspiration. That means that a 150-pound person can easily lose 2 percent (3 pounds) of his body weight in fluid within an hour. If exercise is more intense or the environment is more extreme, fluid losses will be greater. You can see how easily you become dehydrated. If you don't replenish your fluid losses during exercise, you will fatigue early and your performance will be diminished.

Design a fluid plan just as you create a food plan (see "The Dehydrated-Guy Fluid Plan" in chapter 6). In addition to replacing the fluids that you lose just because you're alive and walking around, you need to replace the fluid that you lose during exercise. This has to happen every day: a couple cups when you get up in the morning, a few more mid-morning, a couple at lunch, again in the mid-afternoon, and then at dinner. That covers your minimum intake.

Make sure that these are nonalcoholic (because alcohol can promote water loss), and make at least five of them water. If you drink more than three caffeinated beverages daily, then you'll need to drink a few extra cups of noncaffeinated fluid to make up for the diuretic effects of caffeine. Then add what you need to be well hydrated before, during, and after exercise.

Dehydration is cumulative. If you work out on Monday and lose 2 percent of your fluids but replace only 1 percent, then the following day you are already beginning your workout slightly dehydrated and probably a little fatigued.

Monitor your hydration status. One of the easiest ways is to check your urine—it should be relatively odorless and no darker in color than straw. Anything more and it is a good sign that you are dehydrated and need to be drinking more.

These are all general goals for a general training diet. Now, let's get to specific advice that will help you eat to maximize specific types of workouts and goals.

FLUID GUIDELINES

HERE ARE SOME BASIC GUIDELINES TO STAYING HYDRATED and healthy.

- Drink a minimum of 1 quart (4 cups) of fluid for every 1,000 calories you eat every day.
- Drink at least 5 cups of water every day.
- Drink cool fluids.
- Drink water after moderate exercise that lasts 1 hour or less. (If you like flavored drinks better, then use flavored beverages.)
- Drink carbohydrate-electrolyte sports drinks after intense exercise that lasts less than 1 hour and for any exercise lasting more than 1 hour.
- Drink 2 cups of fluid 2 hours before exercise.
- Drink 4 to 6 ounces every 15 to 20 minutes during exercise.

After exercise, drink 16 to 24 ounces (2 to 3 cups) of fluid for every pound of body weight lost during exercise.

Fueling for Strength

Strength training is the bread and butter of most elite athletes, and it is probably the number-one issue I address with my private clients. Many, including some undersize football players, want to get both bigger and stronger. (If that is your goal, I again recommend looking back at chapter 4.) Others want to stay about the same size and simply teach their bodies to become more powerful, resilient machines. If that is your goal—if you want to sprint faster, be able to box out on the b-ball court, or have more power in your bat swing—this eating plan is for you.

As with the previous chapters, I'm not going to prescribe your weight-lifting plan or the other techniques you'll use to build strength—your programs will vary widely depending on your sport, your goals, your skill level, and the amount of time you can dedicate to your training. What I will do is give you the tools to ensure you train efficiently and effectively, no matter what your program is. Everyone who lifts weights, at some level, is after the same thing: more lean tissue, better known as muscle. The plan I'll lay out in this section satisfies most every muscle-building plan, provided you remember to tweak it for your goals. You can use it 7 days a week, regardless of whether you are exercising or competing.

Here are the general rules you need to remember if you are eating to build strength for sports.

Consume 2 to 4 grams of carbs for every pound of body weight each day. When you lift weights, your primary energy source is carbohydrates. You may associate carbs with endurance exercises, and protein with strength training, but you can't confuse the building materials with the fuel. Eat a healthy

---

PROACTIVE AGING

GIVEN MUSCLE'S SEMINAL ROLE IN ENERGY PRODUCTION, it doesn't take Dick Tracy to figure out that sustaining muscle mass over time is one of the most effective ways to manage the aging process. Among numerous other wonderful benefits, a body composition heavy on muscle and light on fat can help you maintain healthy blood-sugar levels and cholesterol levels, with all of the health benefits those confer. Next time you go in for a checkup, ask your primary-care doc how important these yardsticks are.

What's the alternative? How about reaching 50 or 55 and, instead of still being a stud in the gym and the bedroom, being that guy who seemingly needs 10 minutes to navigate his broken-down body into an elevator, while the old lady in front of him holds the door. That's not to say that injuries and diseases don't slow some men down prematurely, and they are of course excluded from this broadside. Yet many men become dysfunctional physically simply through poor eating and inactivity. When a guy's sloth during his 20s, 30s, and 40s makes him a burden to others when he reaches his 50s, it's a problem.

Speaking of diseases, here's one for you to ponder: sarcopenia. It refers to a loss of muscle, and its leading cause is inactivity. It's one of the biggest precursors to another disease you're probably more familiar with—osteoporosis—as well as a host of other problems. When you lose muscle, a lot of other stuff heads south, too. Your body basically goes to hell in a handbasket.

dose of carbs daily and you'll get the energy you need during training cycles, when the intensity and volume of your training are high. The greater your training volume, the more carbs you'll need. If you really are training mainly for fitness and health and not to gain much mass, then keep your carbs in the 2-gram-per-day range. Otherwise, you'll start to bulge rather than burn. Our meal plan for strength-building days uses 2.6 grams of carbohydrate per pound as a midpoint, putting a 185-pound guy close to a 55 percent carb diet, which is ideal for starting or maintaining a hard training program.

Something to remember here: Most weight lifting taps the carbs stored physically in the working muscles. To fuel the short bursts of activity that weight lifting entails, you need good fuel stores in the muscles that you're exercising. It doesn't matter how much glycogen is in your legs if you're banging out reps on the bench press. If you did a heavy upper-body workout two days ago and now you're about to train upper body again, you won't be able to maximize your performance in the gym if you haven't recovered from the preceding workout. And recovering fully requires eating carbs between then and now.

A key replenishment window opens up for the few hours after you train, but the process of replenishing glycogen stores in the liver and muscles will continue, albeit at a less intense rate, from one workout to the next. Assuming an ideal intake of carbs, glycogen stores are replenished at a rate of 5 to 7 percent per hour, meaning that it takes pretty much a full day to restore muscle-glycogen levels to what they were before you started training.

The goal, then, is to keep stoking the glycogen replenishment and tissue building from one training session to the next. That's something you'll want to keep in mind when designing your training routine. It's one of several reasons that heavy lifting sessions for the same muscle groups are best avoided on consecutive days.

Consume 0.8 grams of protein for every

Calorie Concerns

How many calories you need varies from person to person and is influenced heavily by body composition, activity level, and numerous other factors. To give you a yardstick, the bodybuilders that I've worked with over the years have needed 19 to 20 calories per pound every day just to maintain their way-above-average muscle mass. To build, they would need 24 or more; to taper, 17; and to prepare for a contest, 15. The average guy needs to drop a whole category to achieve similar results. In other words, that maintenance figure for bodybuilders, 19 to 20, is basically what most guys need to gain size. When you try to taper, you need the cutting-level calories, and so on.

pound of body weight every day. This is the no-brainer. As discussed in the last chapter, protein is the key between training sessions for muscle repair, protein synthesis, and maintaining hormone balance. In this plan, you're going for strength, not size, so you'll need a little less. If you want to see some size gains, bumping up your calories by adding extra protein around your exercise sessions, in addition to what you've calculated for the day, is a good strategy.

Allow the rest of your calories to come from fat. We know quite a bit about how much protein and carbohydrates you need to fuel your exercising body. We know a lot less about fat. Here's a good guideline: After you meet your needs for protein and carbs, you can allow the rest of your calories to come from fat. Choose healthful sources, such as fish, nuts, and olive oil, over unhealthful sources, such as fatty meats and processed foods.

Favor water over sports drinks. As I said before, drinking liquids is important, no matter what your exercise program entails. But different liquids are better for different things. When it comes to training for strength, I suggest water over sports drinks and other sugar-laden liquids.

A weights-base workout usually uses less energy than a cardio workout and causes the body to lose fewer electrolytes. A strength-trainer's replenishment needs are therefore less dire than an endurance athlete's. In the end, water should be more than capable of keeping you hydrated during your workouts, allowing you to get your energy-stoking carbs from more nutritious sources, including grains, fruits, and vegetables. If you're a hardgainer, you might benefit from using a sports drink during your workouts. Go back to chapter 4 to find a meal plan for the hardgainer.

(*Note:* Athletes don't only abuse water by underdrinking it. Some, especially endurance athletes, overdrink. See page 202 for more on this.)

A Day in the Life of a Strength Eater

Here's how this all works out during a typical day.

Immediately before Training

Begin your workout well nourished but with your stomach pretty much empty. If you're undernour-

ished by having, let's say, skipped breakfast and lunch before an afternoon workout, your body will likely run out of fuel and crash before the workout ends. Conversely, if your stomach is full of food before you lift your first weight, too much blood will be drawn to your stomach rather than to your muscles, where you want it, and an insulin spike will have negative effects on growth-hormone release.

Ideally, you want to consume a high-energy meal 2 to 3 hours before your workout—one loaded with complex carbs, along with some protein. Then, an hour before training, get an added boost from a meal-replacement shake or a formulated energy drink with protein and some carbohydrates, plus 16 ounces of water. If you're an early-morning exerciser and just can't face breakfast before your workout, try to drink a cup of fat-free milk or eat a small carton of low-sugar yogurt. It will make a world of difference.

During Training

Fluid replacement should equal fluid loss. The recommended water intake per hour is 20 to 40 ounces. Drink cool or cold water (40 to 50 degrees) at a rate of 4 to 6 ounces every 15 to 20 minutes while training.

Remember, you probably won't need anything

FOODS THAT SHORT-CIRCUIT WORKOUTS

BECAUSE THESE FOODS SLOW DIGESTION AND ABSORPTION, avoid them before, during, and just after exercise.

High-fat foods
Baked goods

Dips

High-fat candies

Ice cream

Meats

Sauces

High-fiber foods
Dried fruit

High-fiber cereals

more than good old-fashioned water to rehydrate. If you want an extra dose of electrolytes, find a bottled water with them added.

Immediately after Training

This meal is really an extension of the workout because the results you get will depend directly on what you eat and drink after training. Secondarily, what you consume afterward will have a direct effect on your next workout, even if it's several days away.

The impact that post-workout nutrition can have on your body is profound. Along with hydration, a major priority is replenishing glycogen stores. (The average Joe stores 1,500 to 2,000 carbohydrate calories, equal to 375 to 500 grams, as glycogen in his muscles and liver.) You need to consume carbs to do that, and how many you take in is largely a function of your training goal. Because mass building and fat loss have dedicated chapters, for general training take a middle-of-the-road approach. In all situations, you need some carbs to help maximize increases in muscle mass and provide the fuel needed for your next workout.

Refill your muscles and liver with glycogen, in the form of carbohydrates, ASAP after exercising. Those carbs will raise your blood-sugar levels, and this is the one time of day when this is a good thing. In fact, now is when simple carbs that score up near 100 on the glycemic index are ideal. What this does postexercise is promote the release of insulin, the "master" hormone, which in turn will stimulate the transport of amino acids into muscle, promoting protein synthesis. What's more, it will blunt the rise of cortisol. Immediately after exercising, your body begins repairing damaged muscle proteins, so give your body all the help it needs.

Specifically, this is when you need a major slug of protein and carbohydrates—about 250 to 500 calories' worth, combined. Because it's often hard to eat a meal right after training, you might try bringing a premade smoothie with you to the gym for consumption after-

More Caffeine, More Muscle?

The research on caffeine and endurance dwarfs the research on caffeine and strength, and no evidence suggests that you'll lift more weight in a given workout if you take caffeine beforehand. However, some of the research does hint at the possibility that a reduced rate of muscle fatigue might allow you to lift the same weight longer.

Caffeine studies using animals have attributed enhanced muscle-force production to the supplement, but human studies have not. Still, the possibilities are intriguing.

One caveat: caffeine appears to negate the effects of another popular supplement, creatine, when they are taken together. Coffee drinkers who are taking creatine should probably limit themselves to no more than 2 cups a day.

ward. Depending on your size, the right mix for this drink is 20 to 40 grams of protein and 40 to 90 grams of carbs. By combining blended whole foods (bananas, berries, etc.) with some protein powder, fat-free milk, flaxseed oil and other essential fatty acids, and water or ice chips, you get a great combination that your body will soak up like a sponge.

2 Hours after Your Workout

Have a real meal. For example, combine protein and carbohydrates this time by eating 6 ounces of grilled salmon with an ear of corn, brown rice pilaf, and sliced tomatoes and mozzarella drizzled with extra virgin olive oil, all washed down with a big glass of water. For a different feel, go for ground sirloin with a slice of cheddar on a whole-grain bun with sautéed mushrooms and onions, bean soup, and a big salad with olives and balsamic vinaigrette dressing.

Rapid rehydration is also important here. As a rule of thumb, after exercising, you need to ingest at least 16 to 24 ounces, or 2 to 3 cups of water for every pound of body weight lost during that session.

Strength-Building Supplements

There's no substitute for consuming a muscle-friendly diet as outlined in this chapter and in the accompanying menu plans, but as you take your training to the next level, food alone often isn't enough. Consider adding some of the following supplements to the mix.

CREATINE. Your body relies on carbs and fats for most of its energy needs. But to fuel short bursts of energy, such as lifting a weight "X" number of times or sprinting "X" yards, it taps something called adenosine triphosphate (ATP). Through a series of biochemical reactions, creatine helps replenish ATP stores, providing more energy for your muscles. Creatine also pulls water into muscle cells, enhancing the "pumped" look that accompanies weight training.

In numerous studies, the supplemental form has been shown to improve the performance of high-intensity exercise performance and increase gains in both muscle mass and strength. What's more, it helps mitigate the lactic acid buildup that leads to the burning sensation in muscles near the end of a set.

Some people are still concerned that creatine may be dangerous if used long-term. But studies from the last 7 years have shown no adverse effects from the use of the supplement in healthy individuals. As always, it's your call, but to date there appears to be no cause for alarm.

Dosage: The typical recommendation calls for a 5-day loading phase of 5 grams, four times a day, followed by a maintenance dose of 2 grams a day. However, a study published recently in *Medicine and Science in Sports and Exercise* showed that a 2-day loading phase produces similar benefits to the 5-day one.

If you decide to use creatine, take 5 grams daily, mixed with at least 1 cup of grape juice, which will improve absorption. You'll need at least 35 grams of carbohydrates in your grape juice to do the job.

Adding in some protein may also help. (Citrus juices appear to interfere with the supplement's efficacy.) On workout days, take it immediately after your training with your recovery drink to improve absorption and recovery. Because creatine draws extra water into muscles, drink an extra 8 to 12 ounces of water for every 5 grams you take. A recent study showed that even though creatine enhances cell volumization and water transport into the cells, those subjects ingesting creatine had a lower risk of dehydration and cramping when compared with those not taking creatine.

GLUTAMINE. I'm not that excited about glutamine—it's in the "may help" category for me. Supposedly, it helps the body synthesize protein and prevent muscle-tissue breakdown, and it supports the immune system. Taking it as a supplement can spare glutamine in muscle tissue, blunting muscle-protein catabolism while improving nitrogen balance. If you train hard, glutamine may help to promote speedy muscle recovery.

Dosage: Depending upon your diet, health, and exercise regimen, take 8 to 20 grams per day. Taking a 2- to 5-gram dose two to four times a day is probably more effective than larger doses taken less frequently. On training days, try taking 2 to 5 grams before and after training. On off days, spread the same amount throughout the day.

CONJUGATED LINOLEIC ACID (CLA). A nonessential fatty acid, CLA taken as a supplement may help burn body fat while preserving muscle mass. The research is still equivocal, with different isomers of CLA showing either benefit or no effect.

Dosage: Take 3 to 6 grams daily.

PHOSPHATIDYLSERINE (PS). This supplement may reduce the production of cortisol. Secreted in response to long and heavy training sessions, "endogenous" phosphatidylserine has been shown to relieve overtraining symptoms such as muscle soreness. ("Endogenous" means this is stuff your body produces; its opposite is "exogenous," meaning it comes from outside sources. Supplements are exogenous versions of nutrients that may or may not also be produced endogenously.)

Dosage: 800 milligrams of PS taken 30 minutes before training has been shown in studies to reduce post-workout cortisol levels by 30 percent. Save it for hard training days.

MULTIVITAMIN/MINERAL. You won't always know if your diet is providing you with all the vitamins and minerals you need, especially because the roles many of them play are subtle, albeit crucial. The B vitamins, for example, help your body absorb food properly. A daily multivitamin/mineral is the cheapest insurance policy you'll ever buy.

Dosage: 100 percent of daily value.

HMB (BETA-HYDROXY BETA-METHYLBU-TYRATE). This is a metabolite produced by the breakdown of leucine. Because of its nitrogen-retaining effect, HMB is supplemented to prevent or lower muscle damage and blunt muscle breakdown associated with intense physical effort. It may also assist in the repair of muscle damage resulting from very strenuous training. When combined with intense training and adequate nutrition, HMB may enhance strength, increase muscle mass, and decrease body fat. It appears to be most effective when starting a training program, either for the first time or after a lapse, or when increasing the volume or intensity of training.

Dosage: Take 3 grams a day in three 1-gram doses. If you weigh more than 200 pounds, up that amount to 5 to 6 grams, equally divided. HMB is best taken with meals.

Fueling for Endurance

In 1974, Muhammad Ali and George Foreman fought their famed Rumble in the Jungle, an eight-round pummel fest that, blow for blow, is considered one of the greatest tactical boxing matches ever. The first seven rounds saw Ali take a heroic beating: Unable to stand up to a bigger, stronger Foreman, Ali seemed drawn to the ropes, where he faced one Foreman barrage after the next. By the eighth round, it appeared that Ali was doomed. Instead, Ali rose from his corner relaxed and poised, and proceeded to knock Foreman out.

The millions of stunned onlookers who couldn't believe what they saw learned later that Ali had spent those rounds letting Foreman wear himself out, using the ropes to absorb the power from most of Foreman's blows. Meanwhile, Foreman was throwing himself at Ali, assuming he was on the brink of a knockout. That knockout never came, and Ali left with the heavyweight title.

The Rumble in the Jungle is a prime example of the need for sports endurance, not so much on Ali's part (who, admittedly, had to endure a lot, ropes or no ropes), but on Foreman's. Foreman was easily the stronger, more vital man, having just won 41 straight bouts. In comparison, Ali, who was 32 years old at the time, was past his prime—a slower, less effective version of his former self. None of that matters when you are not tired and your opponent is. Foreman's body may have been a fantastic machine, but when the parts weren't working, he couldn't do a thing with it.

You probably don't consider boxing a traditional endurance sport. More often, people think of aerobic exercises, like marathon running or swimming. But endurance is a much more general idea. And it applies to nearly all sports. The entire range of athletes, from prototypical triathletes to football lineman, needs the physical endurance to avoid weariness and stay focused. That is the subject of this section.

All Roads Lead to Carbs

It is next to impossible to endure in sports if you haven't mastered the art of eating carbs. Your body hordes the stuff in its muscles, waiting until you need it—like when you are about to dive into the water to start a triathlon or explode from the starting blocks to begin a track meet. Without carbs, your personal best would be awfully similar to your worst performance. Carbohydrates make the difference.

Having enough carbs is especially important toward the end of a competition. Ideally, you'll have already prepared your body to take advantage of these carbs. With proper training, you can help your body reserve carbs longer in your muscles and revert to them only when your body has used a significant amount of another fuel source: fat.

Here's how that works: Your body will begin any athletic endeavor by burning carbs. If your body is well trained, it will soon stop burning carbs and move to your stores of body fat for energy. From about 10 to 20 minutes into exercise (depending on your training status) until just before you hit the wall with fatigue, you'll use that fat. After that, it's back to carbs again.

The logic here is simple. The faster you can access fats for fuel during exercise, the more glycogen (the stored form of carbohydrates in your muscles) you retain, and the more fuel you've got left for those last few moments of exertion at the end of a competition. Over time, the more well trained you are, the better your endurance.

None of this matters, though, if you don't have enough carbs in your system. The amount of carbohydrates stored (a.k.a. glycogen) in muscles is directly related to how many carbohydrates you eat and how well trained you are. In general, a diet with upward of 60 percent of calories from carbohydrates will allow for the greatest storage of glycogen in the muscles on a daily basis. In the meal plan I outline on page 218, that will come to just over 3 grams of carbohydrates per pound of body weight.

(*Note:* If you are training for more than 2 hours daily, you'll probably need more. I'd suggest increasing your carbs in that case to around 3.6 to 4.5 grams per pound. This high level of intake will re-duce the common risk of chronic fatigue and over-training syndrome. But beware of the trap in this diet strategy. You must still consume enough protein and fat. The body cannot perform on carbs alone! If you can't eat enough calories to consume adequate protein and fat and still maintain your body weight, then drop your carbs down a notch.)

Good Carbs, Bad Carbs

As you realize by now, not all carbs are created equal. If you don't know how certain carbs release in your body and how the nutrients they contain aid performance, you cannot effectively use your carbs. There's the right time for whole grains, vegetables, and fruits, and there's even a right time for sugar (especially if you are a long-distance runner). There's also the matter of how they all fit in with proteins and fats, and how carbs interplay with them. Knowing how to mix your macronutrients like a pharmacist mixes drugs will help you maximize certain effects.

Here's what you should concentrate on.

Consistency. The first rule of eating carbs for endurance is consistency. When you're fueling for endurance performance, you must include carbohydrates every time you eat throughout the day. Each meal and snack should have either some whole-grain bread, vegetable, fruit, legume, or milk product.

Variety. Notice how pasta is not listed as the only source of carbohydrates for the endurance athlete's diet? I'm certain that some of my clients used to think that the more pasta they ate, the faster and longer they'd run, until almost all they ate all day was pasta. Oh, and of course, potatoes.

This way of thinking couldn't be more wrong. Though pasta and potatoes are good carb sources, all the other foods listed above are so much fuller in vitamins, minerals, phytochemicals, and food factors, all incredibly important for supporting elite athletic performance. Athletes who focus solely on pasta and spuds consume a diet remarkably devoid of protein and fat. Ultimately, performance diminishes, and that's why they end up in my office looking for help.

Combination. Carbohydrate-rich foods should always be eaten in combination with protein and/or fat. The goal is to keep your body from absorbing the carbs too fast. The protein and fat act as gatekeepers, allowing carbs to enter the bloodstream at a time-released pace and avoiding a carbohydrate stampede. If carbs aren't controlled, you'll experience the super-elevated peaks and valleys of insulin secretion associated with high-carbohydrate diets. Your body will not rush to remove sugar from the bloodstream (which leads to fat storage) and instead will use that sugar as energy or put it into muscle storage. Also, you'll minimize the secretion of stress hormones, which will negatively impact muscle recovery and performance.

One Last Word on Carbs

With all the low-carb hype, you're probably wondering about the sanity of eating a moderately high-carb diet. A study at the University of Colorado showed that cyclists on a low-carb diet (100 grams per day) performed just as well on a 45-minute endurance test as those eating a high-carb diet (600 grams per day). But the high-carb group had much higher levels of muscle glycogen (carb storage) at the end of the test, and the low-carb group gained no fat-burning advantages, either. If this test had been performed on the same riders over the course of several days, I suspect the results would be different. If you're planning to do just one bout of exercise and no more, ever, then that low-carb diet is for you. If you plan to exercise day after day, then your exercise will become harder each day as your muscle fuel stores become depleted on a low-carb diet. If you exercise intensely more than 3 days per week, a low-carb diet is not for you.

Protein and Endurance

Even though you're not training to build muscle, you still need protein to repair your training muscles and help them recover and gain strength and endurance. You can't do any of this without adequate protein. You need protein to cover the jobs that only protein can perform throughout your whole body. An endurance athlete needs at least 0.54 to 0.64 grams of

VEGETA-FUEL

IF YOU ARE A VEGETARIAN, GETTING ALL THE VITAMINS and nutrients that build a resilient body can be tough. Here are some of your body's biggest needs and how to get them.

Nutrient	Sources
Protein	Soy and other legumes, grains, seeds, poultry, fish, and/or dairy if acceptable
Calcium	Dairy, dark leafy greens, fortified soy milk, legumes, peanuts, almonds, seeds, calcium-fortified fruit juice
Iron	Legumes, dark leafy greens, dried fruits, whole and enriched grains; combine sources of vitamin C with iron-rich food
Zinc	Whole-grain products, brewer's yeast, wheat germ, pumpkin seeds
Vitamin B_{12}	Dairy, eggs, nutritional yeast, fortified foods, fermented soy products
Riboflavin	Dairy, eggs, whole and enriched grains, brewer's yeast, dark leafy greens, legumes
Vitamin D	Fortified cow's milk and soy milk, fortified cereals, exposure of skin to sunshine

protein per pound of body weight per day. If you are a vegetarian, add another 10 percent. If you're eating fewer calories than you need in order to burn more fat, then you need at least 0.72 gram of protein per pound of body weight per day.

Speaking of vegetarians, you will benefit greatly from having a variety of sources of protein in your diet, just as I've been advocating variety in all the other food groups. Though poultry is high in tryptophan and pork is high in thiamine (vitamin B₁), red meat is highest in iron and zinc, two incredibly essential minerals supporting endurance performance.

If you avoid animal products, then you must supplement with fortified foods and dietary supplements to ensure adequate nutrition.

WHO CAN YOU TRUST?

Not Nutritionists

ANYTIME YOU READ OR HEAR ANYTHING FROM SO-CALLED NUTRITION EXPERTS, examine the credentials and qualifications of the specific voice you're reading or hearing. Every nutrition book has a disclaimer, and anybody can write anything—in fact, anyone can call him- or herself a nutritionist, as there isn't a universal or national licensure in the United States.

Standards vary widely from state to state. Two separate bona fide national certifications require stringent education, experience, testing, and continuing education in nutrition to be obtained and maintained. The certificates are for registered dietitian (RD) and certified nutrition specialist (CNS), but these are voluntary certifications and not required in many settings to practice nutrition counseling. In fact, close to half of the states don't require any licensure to do nutrition counseling. So if you're reading an unlicensed or uncertified person's content in print, buyer beware.

Although there are more than 70,000 registered dietitians in the country—which isn't very many—most are employed in hospitals and institutions, with only a handful of entrepreneurial private-practice dietitians. Few among them have specialized training in fitness and sports nutrition; for those who do, the system isn't really set up for them to do much because there's very little reimbursement for nutrition counseling (unless you're already sick). There's no system in place to allow for preventive nutrition counseling . I'm a registered dietitian and a certified nutrition specialist, and an insurance company would never pay me for what I do. I don't even bother taking insurance. They're not going to invest in prevention and health enhancement.

That's why it's too expensive for dietitians to spend much more time in school becoming more specialized, because they earn relatively little compared with physicians. Although dietitians with a busy consulting practice may be charging $70 to $100 an hour or more, I know dietitians in the country who are still being paid $20 an hour.

Good nutrition counseling, then, is scarce. That's why the Internet has become such a boon. But it is up to you to decide if you are reading bona fide information.

Fat Again

A healthy diet includes healthy dietary fats. Fat should make up between 20 and 25 percent of your calories. Stick with vegetable oils, avocados, nuts, and seeds. Choose lean meats and low-fat and fat-free dairy products. Just because you're active does not mean that you're protected from the health dangers of saturated fats.

When you are looking for great fatty snacks, choose nuts. They are dense in calories, healthy fats, protein, and fiber. They are also high in chromium and magnesium. Chromium, often found lacking in the diets of athletes, is essential for the transfer of glucose into cells for energy production. Magnesium helps relax muscles after contraction and plays a role in the conduction of nerve impulses.

Pay Even More Attention to Hydration

Getting dehydrated when you're working for strength is possible but not a given. But dehydrating when you're working toward endurance is almost guaranteed if you aren't replenishing your system regularly. Without fluid replenishment after exercise, your performance on successive days will decay, and your long-term health may be at risk. I suggest carrying water and fluids with you as a constant reminder to drink. Freeze fluids in water bottles to keep them cold during long-distance exercise. Don't forget that fruits and vegetables are great sources of water.

If you're working out for more than an hour (or even just working out intensely for less than an hour), you'll probably need more than water to stay appropriately charged. Carbohydrate-electrolyte sports drinks are an excellent choice to help you do this. By replacing carbs during exercise, you'll have more fuel available at the end of your training or competition, when you need it most. These drinks contain sodium to help drive your thirst mechanism, and they also enhance carbohydrate absorption by helping to usher glucose across the intestinal lining

into the bloodstream. During ultra and extreme events, you'll benefit from the electrolyte replacement, because your body will have lost significant amounts of electrolytes through sweat, and your performance could suffer without an external source.

If you want something even more cutting edge, new research suggests sports drinks that combine a little protein with carbs may be even better. A study done at James Madison University showed that a product with a 4:1 ratio of carbs to protein (Accelerade) enhanced endurance and reduced muscle damage after cycling to exhaustion in the lab. The jury is still out on these, but I think they're worth a try.

This is a story of trial and error. Try different products and see what works best for you. Find something you'll be willing to drink during your workouts and competition. No matter how scientifically based the product, if you don't like it, it won't keep you hydrated if you don't drink it.

Do the Goo

Long-distance, ultra-marathon, and extreme sport athletes sometimes need special products to keep their bodies from using up fuel. That means refueling on the fly, so to speak. There are many ways to do it, but among the most popular are gels and goos. Basically, these products provide concentrated sources of carbs in the form of sugar, allowing athletes to consume far more carbs than they would if they simply drank a bottle of Gatorade during competition. Also, many people's bodies cannot handle more-complex, dense foods (like bread and fruit) when they are in the middle of an event. Eating these can make an active body nauseous, which isn't a wonderful feeling when you're standing still, but it's even more burdensome when you're running 25 miles. Of course, some people get nauseous from goos and gels—it's all about figuring out what works for you.

Two words of advice on using gels and goos: First, try them out on training days before using them in competition. You never want to try a new product—especially not a goo or gel—on the day of a competition. Second, make sure you drink water with them. Although these products are designed to provide carbs without the extra liquid from a liter of sports drink, you'll still need a cup of water or two to regulate your body's fluid levels. Forget to drink, and your body will go looking for more liquid to dilute the carbs in your intestines. This will come from other cells, which will lead to dehydration.

Avoid Overhydration

On the flip side of dehydration, you must also worry about overhydration. Hydration is a delicate balance between fluids and minerals in your body. The concentration of sodium and other minerals (collectively known as electrolytes) in your bloodstream must fall within a very narrow range, or it can affect your muscle contractions. That includes the most important muscle: your heart.

When you take in too much water relative to the amount of electrolytes in your body, the result will eventually be a condition called "hyperhydration," or hyponatremia. The problem is that your blood has become too dilute, which is just as dangerous as dehydration, in which you have high levels of electrolytes without enough fluids.

Hyperhydration occurs more frequently than you might think, particularly in endurance and ultra-endurance sports like marathons. You can avoid hyponatremia with a few simple precautions.

- If you're training for your first marathon or triathlon, don't cut all the salt out of your diet (even though, as a general rule, most of us could

FOOD AS DEFENSE

FOOD CAN DO MORE THAN JUST IMPROVE the intensity and duration of your exercise sessions and then maximize the intended objectives, such as muscle growth and fat loss. It's also a way to protect your body against the potentially damaging side effects of training.

Although the benefits far, far outweigh the risks—and those risks can be mitigated with proper nutrition and rest—vigorous training can compromise your body's immune system, making you more susceptible to colds, infections, and other illnesses. It also subjects your muscles to serious trauma, which can produce something called delayed-onset muscle soreness 24 to 48 hours after a hard workout. That soreness is usually a natural response to doing new exercises or training at a higher level of intensity than before, or returning to the gym after a layoff. But another potential contributor to muscle soreness is the uncontrolled buildup during and after exercise of free radicals. That may sound like the latest punk group from London, but free radicals are molecules holding one or more unpaired electrons in their orbit. This makes them molecular loose cannons—highly reactive and potentially dangerous internal scavengers that can wreak havoc under your skin.

Free radicals aren't all bad. On the contrary: The immune system forms them to fight infections, and none of us would survive long without them. When you exercise, however, body temperature, lactic-acid production, and oxygen uptake all increase. In fact, oxygen

get away with a lot less than we currently take in).

■ If the day is cooler or less humid than you expected, compensate by drinking less than you'd planned during the event.

■ Go for sports drinks over pure water.

■ Don't think you have to match the more highly trained competitors drink for drink. Their sweat is literally different from yours, containing more water and fewer electrolytes. Your body is leaking sodium, while theirs are holding onto it.

■ If you find yourself slowing down toward the end of the race, don't take this as a sign that you should drink more. If you're running slower, you're also sweating less.

■ If you see pretzels being handed out along the course of a distance race, help yourself, assuming you're not sodium sensitive and you don't have high blood pressure.

Surprisingly, the symptoms of dehydration and hyperhydration are basically the same. If you collapse and require medical attention, that doctor or paramedic may not be able to tell if you've had too little or too much to drink. If you're in a condition to answer his questions, one of the first will concern your fluid intake.

A Day in the Life of an Athlete Who Endures

Here's how this all works out during a typical day.

Before Your Session

How you eat before your session will contribute greatly to your overall athletic development.

If you work out first thing in the morning: Replace the fluid and carbs lost during sleep by eating or drinking carbs in some form. Cereal and milk, a bagel

metabolism increases 10- to 20-fold during exercise. Along with the other changes, this inflicts oxidative damage on tissues and produces a lot of free radicals. Unchecked, free radicals produce chain reactions that can result in destructive biological fireworks. Throw in additional free-radical-producing factors like stress and the aging process itself, and it's easy to conceive of the body's own enzymatic defenses being overrun.

The key is to control free-radical generation beyond what the body needs to prevent tissue damage. Fortunately, the body produces enzymes that help control free radicals, and, paradoxically perhaps, these defense mechanisms also become stronger in response to exercise. More important, you can actively help your body control the production and accumulation of free radicals by making sure that your diet includes enough antioxidants, both from whole foods and from supplements. Antioxidants help neutralize free radicals and blunt their potential for causing damage.

Among whole foods, fruits and vegetables are chock-full of these free-radical fighters. Supplements can play a role as well. Most of the research has studied beta-carotene, vitamin C, vitamin E, selenium, coenzyme Q10, alpha lipoic acid, and proanthocyanins (grapeseed extract). Less well studied but also effective are melatonin, ginkgo biloba, green tea, garlic, quercitin, and lycopene.

and cheese, plain yogurt and fruit, even a cold slice of last night's pizza will all fit the bill. Going into your workout feeling good will enable you to work even harder and burn even more calories, and your ability to burn fat is going to be enhanced when you end a great workout still energetic. The food before exercise will improve endurance on a long-distance workout, decrease the muscle-damaging effects of exercise, and enhance your recovery afterward. Eat or drink just enough before your workout to feel good—but not so much that you feel sluggish and tired. What's more, leave the buckets of coffee and soft drinks for later in the day. A little caffeine is fine, but the last thing you want to do is ingest a potful of a diuretic before or immediately after your workout. That defeats the purpose of staying well hydrated.

If you do cardio at any other time of day: Consume your carbs long enough before exercise that they will have been assimilated into your body to some extent.

If you want to burn body fat, the best approach is to consume 60 calories of protein and 150 calories of low- to moderate-GI carbs 2 to 3 hours before exercise for nonathletes, and an hour to an hour and a half before exercise for athletes. Avoid an insulin response pre-workout. Manage insulin by keeping it within as narrow a range as possible. That way, the food you consume will be burned as fuel rather than stored.

Not only does combining protein and carbohydrates offer your body a good source of fuel before exercise, but it also appears to decrease the catabolic effects that naturally result from the exercise to come. As you exercise, you work your muscles, and that work inflicts damage. By repairing it, your body will build. It's just the natural way the body works. By minimizing that damage, you'll be less sore, allowing you to work out harder on successive days, but you'll still provide enough stimulus to produce an adaptive response.

During Your Session

Now that your session has started, your goal is to maximize your performance. That may not be possible, though, if you didn't take in carbohydrates beforehand. Fatigue will come sooner without those carbs.

That's why it's a good idea to sip liquid carbs from a sports drink throughout your session. Once you begin to fatigue, your body is less capable of making the enzymes available that are required to transport oxygen from your lungs to your working muscles. As your body is less and less able to get oxygen into the cells, fat will be less available as an energy source, and carbohydrates will come back into the picture with a vengeance as your primary fuel source. Remember, you've got to have oxygen around to burn fat but not to burn carbs. Even though your muscles are nearly out of carbs at this point, you'll get an extra burst of energy from that external fuel source toward the end of your session, and it will take you longer to reach fatigue.

After Your Session

Immediately after cardiovascular work, you have to replace the fuel stores you just tapped in your muscles. As soon as possible after your foot leaves the pedal or rubber, begin maximizing the muscle-recovery process by consuming a little over $\frac{1}{2}$ gram of carbohydrates per pound of body weight, along with about $\frac{1}{4}$ gram per pound of protein. The sooner, the better: This is the time when these nutrients are entering back into your cells the most rapidly. Repeat this strategy again within 2 hours of the workout. For the average 190-pounder, that would amount to 95 grams of carbohydrates and 47 grams of protein for the first meal immediately after exercise. If you are smaller, cut those numbers in half. You can eat slightly less for the meal 2 hours later. As you can see, a pretty big slug of your day's nutrition will come at these two times. Don't, however, neglect the rest of the day, because you will continue to recover all day long.

If your cardio session lasted for more than 1 hour—or much longer than 1 hour, if you're training for, say, a marathon—you really need to consume not only enough water but also electrolytes such as sodium, potassium, and magnesium. The best way to do that is by draining any one of the numerous sports drinks on the market formulated to include those electrolytes. They speed up the absorption of fluids and help your body retain them. Remember, if you are looking for an edge, try a sports drink with added protein.

Additional Endurance Supplements

Although most media discussions of pills, powders, and potions relate to those designed to spur muscle growth, elite endurance athletes have spent at least as much time exploring the frontier of performance-enhancing aids. So widespread is their use that the International Olympic Committee tests athletes for a laundry list of substances.

Most of these products aim to prolong the time it takes you to reach exhaustion. How quickly your body hits that wall depends largely on how much fuel it has and how efficiently it burns that fuel, which in this case comes primarily from carbohydrates and fat. Certain supplements that supposedly increase endurance, such as carb drinks and medium-chain triglycerides, attempt to boost endurance by increasing your body's stores of carbs and fat, respectively. Other supplements, such as pyruvate, attempt a metabolic shift from an emphasis on carb-burning to one that focuses on fat burning. Thus, your body would have more carbs for later, giving you the energy for a final kick.

Rest assured, the relationship between the human machine and its fuel is a bit more complicated than that. Even regarding supplemental carbohydrates, we're not sure that the only mechanism is the provision of a substrate (energy source). Yes, it seems to be useful, but in many studies we can't really distinguish between the energy that comes from blood glucose (the energy source in your bloodstream, which would have come from something you ate or drank recently) and the energy coming from muscle glycogen (the stored form of that sugar, which would have been created sometime before the test). So if you have a study in which one group gets supplemental carbs and one group doesn't, we can't necessarily tell from the results

of the study whether the supplemented group really used the additional carbs for energy during the event. The performance enhancement, if there is one, may come from something besides the carbs themselves.

Regardless of the mechanism, the key is to figure out which ones actually do what they purport to do, safely. For the times when you need one of those magic bullets, here's a rundown on what you should—and shouldn't—slide into the chamber.

Best Bet

CARB SUPPLEMENTS. The higher the energy demands you place on your body, the more carbs you need, so endurance athletes often resort to carb drinks to ensure that their body's reserves don't run dry in midstream. Supplementing with carbohydrates is very well documented way to improve performance in lots of types of prolonged exercise.

Whereas most endurance boosters are best taken before an event or workout, carbs are best "loaded" into your system after a workout, when muscle cells are most receptive to ushering them inside. I suggest going for liquid carbs over whole-food sources. Of course, if it's going to take you a while to eat after training, you can drain a carb drink ahead of time. Many such drinks are formulated with an optimal mix of moderate- and high-GI carbs for post-workout glycogen absorption and loading.

Dosage and timing: Variable. Endurance athletes should probably consume at least 1 gram of carbs for every 2 pounds of body weight immediately after training, or at least within a half-hour of training.

Take Your Chances?

PYCNOGENOL. The manufacturer of this supplement, which is an extract from the bark of a particular type of pine tree found in France, says it increased endurance by 21 percent in a recent California State University study. (It should be noted that the manufacturer funded the study.) The purported ergogenic effect is based on improved blood flow and pycnogenol's antioxidant properties, which the manufacturer claims mitigate damage to muscle tissue. These are early data and not conclusive, but with some positive possibilities and no apparent side effects, it may be worth a try.

Dosage and timing: 100 milligrams taken twice daily.

PYRUVATE. This is a naturally occurring substance that your body breaks down to form ATP, which is the molecule that provides the energy for your muscles to perform. The jury is still out on its synthetic form. Although some research suggests that pyruvate might be an effective fat burner, its benefits with respect to endurance are dubious.

Dose and timing: 5 to 10 grams taken an hour before event.

CIWUJIA. This Chinese herb is purported to delay lactic-acid buildup and increase the contribution of fat to energy during endurance exercise, thus prolonging time to exhaustion. Research in this area is sparse, with the majority of articles published in Chinese.

Dose and timing: The manufacturer of Endurox, a supplement derived from the herb, recommends taking 800 milligrams 60 to 90 minutes before a workout.

GINSENG. Endurance athletes typically experiment with the Asian version, known as panax ginseng. Termed an adaptogen because of its ability to "normalize" stress-induced abnormalities, ginseng has also been labeled an endurance booster by some. The research is inconclusive at this point.

Dosage and timing: 250 to 500 milligrams of extract per day.

MEDIUM-CHAIN TRIGLYCERIDES (MCTS). These occur naturally in some vegetable oils. The supplement is purported to provide an alternative fuel to carbohydrates, although the research is inconclusive.

Dosage and timing: 8 to 20 grams daily.

A VITAL LOAD

MOST ATHLETES WILL NOT NEED TO DEVIATE from the endurance meal plan on page 218. But those among you who compete in intense, long cardio sports (competitions lasting for 60 to 90 minutes or more, like a marathon) will need to change your methods a day before the race. The reason? Because, as effective as the endurance diet is, it won't give you enough stored carbs to make it through your event. For that, you'll need to carbo load.

There is no question that carbohydrate loading is a top effective performance aid if followed the week prior to competition, allowing athletes to push maximum amounts of glycogen into muscle storage. The basic strategy is twofold: Rest your muscles prior to the race, and eat as many carbohydrates as you can. Both parts are essential for success.

The one day you can relax and do whatever you want is race day. It may surprise you to hear that, but I have a story to explain why. I worked with a very successful female Olympic swimmer who, since the days of her earliest competitions, had shared a fast-food meal with her Dad just hours prior to the event. We're talking the big burger, the big fries, and a shake. Although it went against all the scientific advice that I knew, she was never willing to give up what had become an important ritual in her pre-event preparation routine. She was an incred-

RIBOSE. This naturally occurring five-carbon sugar is found in the body primarily as constituents of riboflavin, nucleic acids, nucleotides, and nucleosides. Some studies indicate that ribose supplementation (10 to 60 grams per day) can increase ATP availability in certain patient populations, among other medical uses. Whether it affects exercise capacity in trained athletes is still unknown.

Dosage and timing: Follow label instructions.

Long Shots

L-CARNITINE. This one looks great on paper: It chauffeurs fat into muscle cells for use as energy, thus sparing carbohydrates for later use. However, the literature suggests that L-carnitine ingested as a supplement doesn't necessarily end up in muscle cells.

LACTATE SALTS. As a precursor of blood glucose, lactate has been hyped in some circles as an endurance booster. Hype is right: A recent study in the *Journal of Sports Medicine and Physical Fitness* found that it produced no increase in time to exhaustion.

GLYCEROL. Some athletes take glycerol to attempt "prehydration." Getting more glycerol into the bloodstream, the theory goes, increases the volume of blood plasma by osmosis, which allows blood to hold more water. The research supports the theory of superhydration, but that hasn't been shown to improve performance. Unless you see yourself as a serious long-distance athlete, this is not worth trying.

Regardless of which of these supplements, if any, you take out for a test drive, keep in mind that the best way to improve endurance is to combine regular aerobic exercise with a balanced consistent diet and adequate sleep and recuperation. If you think you can abuse your body all week, only to pop a pill and set the world on fire come Saturday morning, think again. They haven't come up with a pill for delusions just yet.

ibly successful athlete, and the emotional attachment that she had to that meal was far more important than any possible negative nutritional impact it might have had.

In the same way, your personal likes and dislikes, and what feels good before a workout or a race, can be just as important as what you consume. If you are not emotionally attached to a routine and there may be something that could work better, then definitely try it. If you are willing to try to give up a practice you hold stock in, then do it months before the competition.

Here's the plan you should follow to carbo load.

Days Prior to Competition	Training Intensity	Diet
6	Flat out, hard—90 minutes	60 percent carbs; 2.7 grams per pound
5	Moderate—40 to 60 minutes	60 percent carbs; 2.7 grams per pound
4	Moderate—30 to 40 minutes	60 percent carbs; 2.7 grams per pound
3	Moderate—20 to 30 minutes	70 percent carbs; at least 4.5 grams per pound
2	Light—20 minutes	70 percent carbs; at least 4.5 grams per pound
1	Rest	70 percent carbs; at least 4.5 grams per pound
Race day	Go for it!	See above recommendations

THE EATING-FOR-STRENGTH MEAL PLAN

THIS IS THE DIET TO HELP YOU TONE UP, IMPROVE STRENGTH, and support all your sporting endeavors. It is the ideal program for a cross-trainer. There is enough carbohydrate to fuel your training but avoid fat gain. Proteins are carefully selected and timed for strength gain and muscle recovery. Use sports drinks for your high-intensity workouts and game days. If you're looking for bigger muscle gains, go to chapter 4 and follow the muscle-building diets.

Daily Assumptions*†

3,434 calories
489 grams carbohydrates
185 grams protein
82 grams fat

Daily Breakdown*†

14 bread
8 fruit
4 milk
23 teaspoons added sugar
6 vegetable
9 very lean protein
5 lean protein
1 medium-fat protein
7 fat

Note: Occasionally, a fat-free product, like mustard or cooking spray, is included on the menus. These do not count toward your daily breakdown but should not be overused.

*Use every day.

† Based on a 185-pound man.

THE MENU

DAY 1

Pre-Workout Snack

SMOOTHIE
Blend until smooth.

1 milk	1 cup fat-free milk
2 fruit	1 cup orange juice
2 very lean protein	14 grams whey protein powder
	Ice cubes

Workout

8 teaspoons added sugar	16-ounce sports drink
	Water

Breakfast

3 bread	3 slices whole-grain bread
1 milk	1 cup fat-free milk
2 fruit	1 cup cubed cantaloupe
	1 cup fresh raspberries
9 teaspoons added sugar	3 tablespoons 100% fruit spread
1 medium-fat protein	1 egg, scrambled in a nonstick pan
3 very lean protein	6 egg whites, scrambled with whole egg
2 fat	1/8 avocado, diced into egg
	1 1/2 tablespoons ground flaxseed
	Water
	Oil-free cooking spray (for eggs)

Snack

2 bread	8 whole-wheat crackers
1 vegetable	1 cup celery sticks
2 fat	2 tablespoons natural peanut butter

Lunch

5 bread	Foot-long Subway sandwich (choose from "6 grams fat or less" list)
2 vegetable	Lettuce, tomato, pepper, onion
2 fruit	1 small banana
	1 apple
1 milk	1 cup fat-free milk
4 very lean protein	Included (in sandwich)
1 fat	1 teaspoon olive oil or 1 tablespoon salad dressing

Snack

1 fruit	3/4 cup blueberries
1 bread	1/4 cup Grape Nuts cereal
1 milk	1 cup plain nonfat yogurt
3 teaspoons added sugar	1 tablespoon honey

Dinner

3 bread	1 sweet potato, baked
	1 small ear corn on the cob
1 fruit	1 slice watermelon
3 teaspoons added sugar	1/2 cup frozen yogurt
3 vegetable	Salad with 2 cups romaine lettuce, 1/2 cup tomato, 1/2 cup cucumber
	1/2 cup broccoli
5 lean protein	5 ounces salmon, grilled
2 fat	2 tablespoons olive oil (for dressing)
	Vinegar (for dressing)

DAY 2

Pre-Workout Snack

SMOOTHIE

Blend until smooth.

1 milk	1 cup fat-free milk
2 fruit	1 cup orange juice
2 very lean protein	14 grams whey protein powder
	Ice cubes

Workout

8 teaspoons added sugar	16-ounce sports drink
	Water

Breakfast

Combine yogurt, fruit, and honey. Combine muffin, avocado, and egg for sandwich.

3 bread	1½ whole-wheat English muffins
1 milk	1 cup fat-free unsweetened yogurt
2 fruit	2½ cups fresh strawberries
9 teaspoons added sugar	3 tablespoons honey
1 medium-fat protein	1 egg, hard-cooked
3 very lean protein	6 eggs, hard-cooked (discard yolks)
2 fat	1½ tablespoons ground flaxseed
	⅛ avocado, sliced
	Water

Snack

2 bread	4 rice cakes
1 vegetable	1 cup vegetable sticks
2 fat	2 tablespoons salad dressing (for dipping)

Lunch

5 bread	2 slices whole-grain bread
	1 ounce croutons
	1 cup brown rice
2 vegetable	Large salad with romaine lettuce, tomato, grilled eggplant, roasted red pepper
2 fruit	2 kiwis, sliced
1 milk	1 cup fat-free milk
4 very lean protein	4 ounces skinless white-meat chicken, grilled with lime juice
1 fat	2 tablespoons fat-free dressing
	1 teaspoon olive oil (for roasted vegetables)

Snack

1 fruit	8 dried apricot halves
1 bread	¾ ounce pretzels
1 milk	1 flavored latte, tall
3 teaspoons added sugar	1 tablespoons syrup (for latte)

Dinner

3 bread	1 cup cooked pasta
	1 slice garlic bread
1 fruit	1½ cups whole strawberries
3 teaspoons added sugar	½ cup flavored gelatin dessert
3 vegetable	2 cups ratatouille (over pasta)
	Salad with 1 cup lettuce, ¼ cup tomato, ¼ cup cucumber
5 lean protein	5 ounces lean ground beef (add to ratatouille)
2 fat	2 tablespoons fat-free dressing

DAY 3

Pre-Workout Snack

SMOOTHIE

Blend until smooth.

1 milk	1 cup fat-free milk
2 fruit	1 cup orange juice
2 very lean protein	14 grams whey protein powder
	Ice cubes

Workout

8 teaspoons added sugar	16-ounce sports drink
	Water

Breakfast

3 bread	3 slices whole-wheat bread
1 milk	1 cup fat-free cottage cheese (on bread; sprinkle with sugar and cinnamon)
2 fruit	4 ounces freshly squeezed orange juice (with pulp)
	1/2 cup sliced pineapple
9 teaspoons added sugar	3 tablespoons sugar
1 medium-fat protein	1 egg, cooked sunny-side up in a nonstick pan
3 very lean protein	6 egg whites, cooked with sunny-side up egg
2 fat	1 1/2 tablespoons ground flaxseed
	1 teaspoon oil (for egg)
	Water

Snack

2 bread	1 bagel
1 vegetable	Tomato, sprouts
2 fat	2 tablespoons cream cheese

Lunch

5 bread	2 1/2 cups rice
2 vegetable	1 cup Chinese vegetables, stir-fried with garlic, onion, fresh ginger
2 fruit	1 cup citrus sections
1 milk	1 cup fat-free milk
4 very lean protein	4 ounces scallops, stir-fried
1 fat	1 teaspoon oil (for stir-frying)

Snack

1 fruit	1¼ cups sliced strawberries
1 bread	1 slice 8-grain bread
1 milk	1 cup nonfat plain yogurt
3 teaspoons added sugar	1 tablespoon honey

Dinner

3 bread	2-inch square of corn bread
	1 cup kidney beans (for chili)
1 fruit	1 pear
3 teaspoons added sugar	½ cup frozen yogurt
3 vegetable	1 cup chopped cooked tomatoes with chili seasoning (for chili)
	½ onion, garlic (for seasoning)
	Salad with 1 cup lettuce, ¼ cup tomato, ¼ cup cucumber
5 lean protein	Included (in beans)
	3 ounces soy crumbles (for chili)
2 fat	2 slices bacon, cooked very crisp (crumble into chili)
	Included (in corn bread)

DAY 4

Pre-Workout Snack

SMOOTHIE

Blend until smooth.

1 milk	1 cup fat-free milk
2 fruit	1 cup orange juice
2 very lean protein	14 grams whey protein powder
	Ice cubes

Workout

8 teaspoons added sugar	16-ounce sports drink
	Water

Breakfast

2 fruit	2 cups raspberries
1 milk	1 cup fat-free milk (½ cup for French toast)

FRENCH TOAST *(See recipe directions on page 44.)*

3 bread	3 slices whole-wheat bread
9 teaspoons added sugar	3 tablespoons maple syrup
1 medium-fat protein	1 egg
3 very lean protein	6 egg whites
1 fat	1½ tablespoons ground flaxseed
	1 teaspoon oil (for frying)
	Water

Snack

2 bread	24 Wheat Thins
1 vegetable	1 cup sliced bell pepper
2 fat	4 tablespoon reduced-fat salad dressing (for dipping)

Lunch

2 fruit	1½ cups blueberries
1 milk	1 cup fat-free milk

FAJITAS

Combine ingredients.

5 bread	1½ cups Spanish rice
	2 tortillas
2 vegetable	1 cup sautéed onions, peppers
	2 tablespoons salsa
4 very lean protein	4 ounces skinless white-meat chicken, grilled with lime juice
1 fat	1 teaspoon olive oil (for cooking)

Snack

1 bread	¾ ounce pretzels

SMOOTHIE

Blend until smooth.

1 fruit	½ large frozen banana
1 milk	1 cup fat-free milk
3 teaspoons added sugar	1 tablespoon chocolate syrup
	Ice cubes

Dinner

3 bread	1 ounce croutons (for salad)
	1 cup chicken noodle soup
	4 crackers
1 fruit	1 nectarine
3 teaspoons added sugar	1 cup reduced-calorie cranberry juice cocktail
3 vegetable	3 cups salad with lettuce, tomato, cucumber, pepper
5 lean protein	5 ounces swordfish, grilled with ginger and scallions
2 fat	4 tablespoons reduced-fat salad dressing

DAY 5

Pre-Workout Snack

SMOOTHIE

Blend until smooth.

1 milk	1 cup fat-free milk
2 fruit	1 cup orange juice
2 very lean protein	14 grams whey protein powder
	Ice cubes

Workout

8 teaspoons added sugar	16-ounce sports drink
	Water

Breakfast

3 bread	1$\frac{1}{2}$ cups quick oats (not instant)
1 milk	1 cup fat-free milk
2 fruit	1 apple, diced
	1$\frac{1}{4}$ cups sliced strawberries
9 teaspoons added sugar	3 tablespoons brown sugar
1 medium-fat protein	1 egg, hard-cooked
3 very lean protein	6 eggs, hard-cooked (discard yolks)
2 fat	1$\frac{1}{2}$ tablespoons ground flaxseed
	6 slivered almonds (for oatmeal)
	Water

Snack

2 bread	1$\frac{1}{2}$ ounces baked tortilla chips
1 vegetable	$\frac{1}{2}$ cup salsa
2 fat	8 black olives
	$\frac{1}{8}$ avocado, cubed

Lunch

5 bread	1$\frac{1}{2}$ cups minestrone soup
	1$\frac{1}{2}$ cups cooked linguini
2 vegetable	1 cup marinara sauce
2 fruit	1 whole grapefruit, sectioned
1 milk	1 cup fat-free milk
4 very lean protein	4 ounces shrimp, grilled
1 fat	1 teaspoon olive oil (for cooking)

Snack

1 fruit	$\frac{1}{2}$ cup canned pineapple
1 bread	$\frac{1}{4}$ cup Grape Nuts cereal
1 milk	1 cup plain nonfat yogurt
3 teaspoons added sugar	1 tablespoon honey

Dinner

3 bread	1 large pita
	1 ounce croutons
1 fruit	2 large figs
3 teaspoons added sugar	10 ounces apricot nectar
3 vegetable	3 cups salad with lettuce, tomato, cucumber, pepper
5 lean protein	5 ounces lean lamb, grilled with lime juice
2 fat	2 tablespoons vinaigrette

DAY 6

Pre-Workout Snack

SMOOTHIE

Blend until smooth.

1 milk	1 cup fat-free milk
2 fruit	1 cup orange juice
2 very lean protein	14 grams whey protein powder
	Ice cubes

Workout

8 teaspoons added sugar	16-ounce sports drink
	Water

Breakfast

3 bread	3 slices multigrain toast
1 medium-fat protein	1 egg, scrambled in a nonstick pan
3 very lean protein	6 egg whites, scrambled with whole egg
	Oil-free cooking spray (for eggs)

SMOOTHIE

Blend until smooth.

1 milk	1 cup fat-free milk
2 fruit	½ cup orange juice
	1 fresh peach
9 teaspoons added sugar	3 tablespoons honey
2 fat	2 teaspoons flaxseed oil
	Water

Snack

2 bread	2 slices whole-wheat bread
1 vegetable	Tomato, lettuce
2 fat	2 slices bacon
	Fat-free mayonnaise

Lunch

5 bread	1 whole-wheat bagel
	1 cup potato salad (made with reduced-fat mayonnaise)
	3/4 cup vegetable noodle soup
2 vegetable	1 cup carrot sticks
	Onion, tomato
2 fruit	2 cups honeydew melon
1 milk	1 cup fat-free milk
4 very lean protein	4 ounces smoked salmon
1 fat	1 tablespoons reduced-fat cream cheese

Snack

1 bread	5 reduced-fat Triscuits

SMOOTHIE

Blend until smooth.

1 fruit	1 cup frozen raspberries
1 milk	1 cup fat-free milk
3 teaspoons added sugar	1 tablespoon vanilla syrup

Dinner

3 bread	2 slices rye bread
	1/2 cup pasta salad
1 fruit	17 grapes
3 teaspoons added sugar	1/2 cup frozen yogurt
3 vegetable	1 cup coleslaw
	1/2 cup chopped vegetables (cucumbers, carrots, onions; mix into tuna)
5 lean protein	5 ounces tuna in olive oil, drained
2 fat	2 tablespoons reduced-fat mayonnaise

DAY 7

Pre-Workout Snack

SMOOTHIE

Blend until smooth.

1 milk	1 cup fat-free milk
2 fruit	1 cup orange juice
2 very lean protein	14 grams whey protein powder
	Ice cubes

Workout

8 teaspoons added sugar	16-ounce sports drink
	Water

Breakfast

3 bread	1 1/2 cups Shredded Wheat
1 milk	1 cup fat-free milk
2 fruit	2 cups raspberries
9 teaspoons added sugar	3 tablespoons sugar
1 medium-fat protein	1 egg, hard-cooked
3 very lean protein	6 eggs, hard-cooked (discard yolks)
2 fat	1 1/2 tablespoons ground flaxseed
	6 almonds
	Water

Snack

2 bread	2 tortillas
1 vegetable	1/2 cup sliced vegetables
	1/2 cup salsa
2 fat	8 black olives, chopped
	1/8 avocado, diced

Lunch

5 bread	1 large multigrain roll
	6 ounces baked yam
2 vegetable	Sliced tomato, lettuce (for sandwich)
	1 cup radishes, celery, carrots
2 fruit	2 nectarines
1 milk	1 cup fat-free milk
4 very lean protein	4 ounces skinless white-meat chicken, grilled with lime juice
1 fat	2 tablespoons low-fat ranch dressing (for dipping)

Snack

1 fruit	2 tablespoons dried sweetened cranberries
1 bread	3/4 ounce pretzels
1 milk	1 nonfat latte, tall
3 teaspoons added sugar	Included (in cranberries)

Dinner

3 bread	3-inch square of corn bread
	1 ounce croutons
1 fruit	1 large tangerine
3 teaspoons added sugar	1/2 cup flavored gelatin dessert
3 vegetable	3 cups salad with lettuce, tomato, cucumber, pepper
5 lean protein	4 ounces salmon, poached
	1 ounce shredded cheese
2 fat	2 tablespoons low-fat Caesar dressing
	Included (in corn bread)

THE EATING-FOR-ENDURANCE MEAL PLAN

THE GOAL FOR THIS DIET IS TO KEEP YOU WELL-FUELED to go the distance. It's got the right carbs at the right times to power your body and your mind. The combinations of protein and fat with carbohydrates are timed to maximize performance, minimize muscle damage, and allow for maximum recovery so that you can go long and strong at your next training session. The plan is packed with vitamins, minerals, antioxidants, and phytochemicals to catalyze energy production and keep you healthy throughout your training and competitive seasons.

Daily Assumptions*†

3,500 calories
550 grams carbohydrates
141 grams protein
80 grams fat

Daily Breakdown*†

14 bread
10 fruit
3 milk
31 teaspoons added sugar
6 vegetable
4 very lean protein
4 lean protein
1 medium-fat protein
9 fat

Note: Occasionally, a fat-free product, like mustard or cooking spray, is included on the menus. These do not count toward your daily breakdown but should not be overused.

*Use every day.

† Based on a 185-pound man.

THE MENU

DAY 1

Breakfast

3 bread	3 slices whole-grain bread
1 milk	1 cup fat-free milk
2 fruit	1 cup cubed cantaloupe
	1 cup fresh raspberries
9 teaspoons added sugar	3 tablespoons 100% fruit spread
1 medium-fat protein	1 egg, scrambled in a nonstick pan
2 fat	$^1/_8$ avocado (dice into egg)
	$1^1/_2$ tablespoons ground flaxseed
	Water

Snack

2 bread	$1^1/_2$ ounces whole-wheat pretzels
1 vegetable	1 cup celery sticks
3 fat	30 peanuts

Lunch

5 bread	Foot-long Subway sandwich, with extra meat (choose from "6 grams of fat or less" list)
2 vegetable	Lettuce, tomato
2 fruit	1 small banana
	1 apple
4 very lean protein	Included (in sandwich)
2 fat	2 teaspoons olive oil or 2 tablespoons salad dressing

Snack

1 bread	$^1/_2$ cup Grape Nuts cereal
1 milk	1 cup nonfat plain yogurt
3 teaspoons added sugar	1 tablespoon honey
1 fruit	$^3/_4$ cup blueberries

Dinner

3 bread	1 large sweet potato, baked
1 fruit	1 slice watermelon
3 teaspoons added sugar	$^1/_2$ cup frozen yogurt
3 vegetable	Salad with 2 cups romaine lettuce, $^1/_2$ cup tomato, $^1/_2$ cup cucumber
	$^1/_2$ cup broccoli
4 lean protein	4 ounces salmon, grilled
2 fat	2 tablespoons olive oil (for dressing)
	Vinegar (for dressing)

Pre-Workout Snack

SMOOTHIE

Blend until smooth.

1 milk	1 cup fat-free milk
4 fruit	1 cup orange juice
	1 large banana
	Ice cubes

Workout

16 teaspoons added sugar	32-ounce sports drink
	Water

DAY 2

Breakfast

Combine yogurt, fruit, and honey. Combine muffin and egg for sandwich.

3 bread	1 whole-wheat English muffin
	$^1/_2$ cup graham cereal (for yogurt)
1 milk	1 cup fat-free, unsweetened yogurt
2 fruit	$1^1/_2$ cups fresh strawberries
9 teaspoons added sugar	3 tablespoons honey
1 medium-fat protein	1 egg, hard-cooked
2 fat	$1^1/_2$ tablespoons ground flaxseed
	6 almonds, sliced
	Water

Snack

2 bread	2 rice cakes
1 vegetable	1 cup vegetable sticks
3 fat	3 tablespoons salad dressing (for dipping)

Lunch

5 bread	2 slices whole-grain bread
	1 ounce croutons
	1 cup brown rice
2 vegetable	Large salad with romaine lettuce, tomato, grilled eggplant, roasted red pepper
2 fruit	2 kiwis, sliced
4 very lean protein	4 ounces skinless white-meat chicken, grilled with lime juice
2 fat	2 tablespoons fat-free dressing
	2 teaspoons olive oil (for roasted vegetables)

Snack

1 bread	$^3/_4$ ounce pretzels
1 milk	1 cup fat-free milk
3 teaspoons added sugar	1 tablespoon chocolate syrup
1 fruit	15 grapes

Dinner

3 bread	1 cup cooked pasta
	1 slice garlic bread
1 fruit	1 cup strawberries
3 teaspoons added sugar	$^1/_2$ cup flavored gelatin dessert
3 vegetable	2 cups ratatouille (over pasta)
	Salad with 1 cup lettuce, $^1/_4$ cup tomato, $^1/_4$ cup cucumber
4 lean protein	4 ounces lean ground beef (add to ratatouille)
2 fat	2 tablespoons reduced-fat dressing
	1 teaspoon butter (for garlic bread)

Pre-Workout Snack

SMOOTHIE

Blend until smooth.

1 milk	1 cup fat-free milk
4 fruit	1 cup orange juice
	1 large banana
	Ice cubes

Workout

16 teaspoons added sugar	32-ounce sports drink
	Water

DAY 3

Breakfast

3 bread	3 slices whole-wheat bread
1 milk	1 cup low-fat cottage cheese (on bread; sprinkle with brown sugar and cinnamon)
2 fruit	4 ounces freshly squeezed orange juice (with pulp)
	1/2 cup sliced pineapple
9 teaspoons added sugar	3 tablespoons brown sugar
1 medium-fat protein	1 egg, cooked sunny-side up in a nonstick pan
2 fat	3 tablespoons ground flaxseed
	Water
	Oil-free cooking spray (for egg)

Snack

2 bread	1 bagel
1 vegetable	Tomato, sprouts
3 fat	3 tablespoons cream cheese

Lunch

5 bread	2 1/2 cups rice
2 vegetable	1 cup Chinese vegetables, stir-fried with garlic, onion, fresh ginger
2 fruit	1 cup citrus sections
4 very lean protein	4 ounces scallops, stir-fried
2 fat	2 teaspoons oil (for stir-frying)

Snack

1 bread	1/2 cup puffed rice cereal
1 milk	1 cup fat-free milk
3 teaspoons added sugar	1 tablespoon honey (drizzle on berries)
1 fruit	1 cup strawberries

Dinner

3 bread	2-inch square of corn bread
	1 cup kidney beans (add to chili)
1 fruit	1 pear
3 teaspoons added sugar	1/2 cup frozen yogurt
3 vegetable	1 cup chopped cooked tomatoes with chili seasoning
	1/2 onion, garlic for seasoning
	Salad with 1 cup lettuce, 1/4 cup tomato, 1/4 cup cucumber
4 lean protein	Included (in beans)
	2 ounces soy crumbles (for chili)
2 fat	2 slices bacon, cooked very crisp (crumble into chili)
	Included (in corn bread)

Pre-Workout Snack

SMOOTHIE

Blend until smooth.

1 milk	1 cup fat-free milk
4 fruit	1 cup orange juice
	1 large banana
	Ice cubes

Workout

16 teaspoons added sugar	32-ounce sports drink
	Water

DAY 4

Breakfast

2 fruit	1 cup raspberries
	1/2 cup orange juice
1 milk	1 cup fat-free milk (1/2 cup for French toast)

FRENCH TOAST *(See recipe directions on page 44.)*

3 bread	3 slices whole-wheat bread
9 teaspoons added sugar	3 tablespoons maple syrup
1 medium-fat protein	1 egg
2 fat	3 tablespoons ground flaxseed
	4 walnut halves, chopped
	Water

Snack

2 bread	24 Wheat Thins
1 vegetable	1 cup sliced bell pepper
3 fat	3 tablespoons salad dressing (for dipping)

Lunch

2 fruit	1 1/2 cups blueberries

FAJITAS

Combine ingredients.

5 bread	1 cup Spanish rice
	2 tortillas
2 vegetable	1 cup sautéed onions, peppers
	2 tablespoons salsa
4 very lean protein	4 ounces skinless white-meat chicken, grilled with lime juice
2 fat	1 teaspoon olive oil (for cooking)

Snack

1 bread	2 rice cakes
1 milk	1 cup fat-free milk
3 teaspoons added sugar	1 tablespoon 100% fruit spread (for rice cakes)
1 fruit	½ large banana

Dinner

3 bread	1 ounce croutons for salad
	1 cup chicken noodle soup
	4 crackers
1 fruit	1 nectarine
3 teaspoons added sugar	1 cup reduced-calorie cranberry juice cocktail
3 vegetable	3 cups salad with lettuce, tomato, cucumber, pepper
4 lean protein	4 ounces swordfish, grilled with ginger and scallions
2 fat	2 tablespoons dressing

Pre-Workout Snack

SMOOTHIE

Blend until smooth.

1 milk	1 cup fat-free milk
4 fruit	1 cup orange juice
	1 large banana
	Ice cubes

Workout

16 teaspoons added sugar	32-ounce sports drink
	Water

DAY 5

Breakfast

3 bread	1½ cups quick oats (not instant)
1 milk	1 cup fat-free milk
2 fruit	½ cup diced apples
	1 cup sliced strawberries
9 teaspoons added sugar	3 tablespoons maple syrup
1 medium-fat protein	1 egg, hard-cooked
2 fat	1½ tablespoons ground flaxseed
	6 almonds, sliced (for oats)
	Water

Snack

2 bread	1¹/₂ ounces baked tortilla chips
1 vegetable	¹/₂ cup salsa
3 fat	8 black olives
	¹/₄ avocado, cubed

Lunch

5 bread	1¹/₂ cups minestrone soup
	1¹/₂ cups cooked linguini
2 vegetable	1 cup marinara sauce
2 fruit	1 whole grapefruit, sectioned
4 very lean protein	4 ounces shrimp, grilled
2 fat	1 teaspoon olive oil (for cooking)

Snack

1 bread	10 melba toast rounds
1 fruit	1 cup pineapple tidbits in natural juice
1 milk	¹/₂ cup fat-free cottage cheese
3 teaspoons added sugar	Included (in pineapple)

Dinner

3 bread	1 large pita
	1 ounce croutons
1 fruit	2 figs, large
3 teaspoons added sugar	¹/₂ cup apricot nectar
3 vegetable	3 cups salad with lettuce, tomato, cucumber, pepper
4 lean protein	4 ounces lean lamb, grilled with lime juice
2 fat	2 tablespoons vinaigrette

Pre-Workout Snack

SMOOTHIE

Blend until smooth.

1 milk	1 cup fat-free milk
4 fruit	1 cup orange juice
	1 large banana
	Ice cubes

Workout

16 teaspoons added sugar	32-ounce sports drink
	Water

DAY 6

Breakfast

3 bread	3 slices multigrain toast
1 medium-fat protein	1 egg, scrambled in a nonstick pan
	Oil-free cooking spray (for egg)

SMOOTHIE

Blend until smooth.

1 milk	1 cup fat-free milk
2 fruit	1/2 cup orange juice
	1 fresh peach
9 teaspoons added sugar	3 tablespoons honey
2 fat	2 teaspoons flaxseed oil
	Water

Snack

2 bread	2 slices whole-wheat bread
1 vegetable	Tomato, lettuce
3 fat	2 slices bacon
	1 tablespoon reduced-fat mayonnaise

Lunch

5 bread	1 whole-wheat bagel
	1 cup potato salad, made with reduced-fat mayonnaise
	1/2 cup vegetable noodle soup
2 vegetable	1/2 cup carrot sticks
	Onion, tomato
2 fruit	1/4 honeydew
4 very lean protein	4 ounces smoked salmon
2 fat	2 tablespoons low-fat cream cheese

Snack

1 bread	4 crispy rye crackers
1 milk	1 cup fat-free milk
3 teaspoons added sugar	1 tablespoon 100% fruit spread
1 fruit	2 tablespoon raisins

Dinner

3 bread	2 slices rye bread
	½ cup pasta salad
1 fruit	24 grapes
3 teaspoons added sugar	1 tablespoon 100% sugar (sprinkled on fruit)
3 vegetable	1 cup coleslaw
	½ cup chopped vegetables (cucumber, carrots, onion; mix into tuna)
4 lean protein	4 ounces tuna in olive oil, drained
2 fat	2 tablespoons reduced-fat mayonnaise
	Tea

Pre-Workout Snack

SMOOTHIE

Blend until smooth.

1 milk	1 cup fat-free milk
4 fruit	1 cup orange juice
	1 large banana
	Ice cubes

Workout

16 teaspoons added sugar	32-ounce sports drink
	Water

DAY 7

Breakfast

3 bread	1½ cups Shredded Wheat
1 milk	1 cup fat-free milk
2 fruit	1 cup raspberries
	½ cup grapefruit juice
9 teaspoons added sugar	3 tablespoons sugar
1 medium-fat protein	1 egg, hard-cooked
2 fat	1½ tablespoons ground flaxseed
	10 peanuts
	Water

Snack

2 bread	2 tortillas
1 vegetable	½ cup sliced vegetables
	½ cup salsa
3 fat	8 black olives, chopped
	¼ avocado, diced

Lunch

5 bread	1 large multigrain roll
	6 ounces baked yam
2 vegetable	Sliced tomato, lettuce (for sandwich)
	½ cup radishes, celery, carrots
2 fruit	2 nectarines
4 very lean protein	4 ounces skinless white-meat chicken, grilled with lime juice
2 fat	4 tablespoons low-fat ranch dressing (for dipping)

Snack

1 bread	3 cups popcorn (air-popped)
1 milk	1 cup fat-free milk
3 teaspoons added sugar	¼ cup chopped dried fruit
1 fruit	Included (in dried fruit)

Dinner

3 bread	3-inch square of corn bread
	1 ounce croutons
1 fruit	2 large tangerines
3 teaspoons added sugar	Sprinkle on fruit
3 vegetable	3 cups salad with lettuce, tomato, cucumber, pepper
4 lean protein	4 ounces salmon, poached
2 fat	2 tablespoons low-fat Caesar dressing
	Included (in corn bread)

Pre-Workout Snack

SMOOTHIE

Blend until smooth.

1 milk	1 cup fat-free milk
4 fruit	1 cup orange juice
	1 large banana
	Ice cubes

Workout

16 teaspoons added sugar	32-ounce sports drink
	Water

CHAPTER SIX

Food and Daily Health

FEELING TIRED? SICK? NURSING AN INJURY? FOOD MAY BE THE ANSWER TO YOUR PROBLEMS

A recent cover of a popular magazine portrayed a still life of pills. What a fitting record of this, The Medicated Age. From each pill, a line extended outward to the margin, identifying the target of that prescription medicine, from anxiety and depression to erections that aren't quite so erect anymore. . . . About the only thing missing was a pill to make you taller. Researchers are no doubt working on that, too.

A cover filled with a bunch of fruits, vegetables, fresh fish, and whole grains wouldn't have sold as many copies, but it would have painted a better picture of what really makes you healthy: food. As it turns out, Mom was right. You *should* eat your vegetables, as well as other healthy foods (although perhaps not for the reasons she thought). Hot peppers can reduce your risk of heart disease. Grapefruit can make blood flow more easily through your arteries, if they've begun to accumulate plaque. Green tea can combat those viral infections that seemingly wipe out a few weeks of your life most winters. Oranges can help reduce the length and intensity of cold symptoms. Yogurt can kill bacteria that contribute to colorectal cancer, and celery can prevent constipation.

This is just a sampling of the overall effect that eating a balanced diet can have on the health of your body. Imagine going a whole year or more without getting sick. Imagine needing fewer over-the-counter medicines and remedies, like antacids and laxatives. If you have the misfortune of undergoing surgery for an injury, imagine amazing even your expert therapists by recovering faster than they have ever seen.

It's all possible, thanks to better eating. In chapter 7, we'll look at how food can help you live longer. For now, let's focus on how food can help you today—this hour, even this minute.

The Side-Effect Cure

Although the use of food as a day-to-day cure for minor problems has been all but forgotten over the past, say, 50 years, the tradition actually goes back millennia. Garlic was used in ancient Egypt to ward off disease. Hippocrates, known as "The Father of

Medicine," prescribed myriad foods for healing and is famous for saying "Let food be thy medicine." Herbs like rosemary were the health aids of choice in Medieval Europe, and 17th-century Englishmen believed that bird meat had the ability to heal, as well as improve the voice, help the appetite, and even aid breathing.

Of course, most of us don't roast a turkey when we feel a flu coming on. Over the past century, we've increasingly turned to drugs to treat our illnesses and our infirmities. But although drug manufacturers have introduced some miraculous products—let's all clap for penicillin—they haven't found a way to fix a big problem with drugs: side effects. Drugs aren't discriminating and can't target just one thing. Many of their unintended effects are bad, and many of them affect the gut. Because the pharmaceutical industry is predicated upon risk-to-benefit ratios, there's no guarantee a drug will come free of dangerous side effects.

Sometimes the risk is worth taking. Metoprolol, for instance (known as Lopressor or Toprol XL by patients), is used to lower high blood pressure. Patients with blood-pressure problems get to choose: Take it, and possibly feel dizzy or experience diarrhea or even develop a rash; don't take it, and possibly die. Not a hard choice to make. But frustration over side effects from drugs that aren't saving our lives—for instance, a drug for irritable bowel syndrome that's also habit-forming—has started to create a backlash. We're learning that our magic pills aren't always worth a headache, an upset stomach, or a rash, especially when the right vegetable or protein can do the job without side effects.

Water: The Fountain of Youth

Before I even get to the wonder foods for daily recovery, we need to look at water and hydration again. There are going to be times when you just generally don't feel good but aren't sure why. Allow me to make a suggestion: Drink a glass of water or two and see if the feeling passes. About 50 percent of the time, that's probably all you'll need.

Dehydration is a common problem, although not one that most people take too seriously. Most of us will never experience acute and severe dehydration—the kind that causes disorientation, coma, and sometimes death—and therefore don't think about it much. It's something that nags us after a hard workout, something that sneaks up on us after a long day at the beach.

But mild dehydration is a problem, and a common one at that. Too many of us make poor hydration a way of life. Day to day, this can be a bigger problem than you realize. It's a simple equation: Water is the body's most important nutrient. It is critical to our bodies in so many ways: controlling our blood volume, distributing nutrients to the body, and aiding in digestion, joint lubrication, and reproduction. Even if you're only mildly dehydrated most of the time—the equivalent of being down 1 to 2 percent of body weight in fluid loss—you could suffer cardiovascular and thermoregulatory responses that have real health consequences.

Preventing Kidney Stones

There's a major link between the development of urinary tract stones and mild dehydration. These excruciatingly painful ailments are more common than you probably think. Anywhere from 12 to 15 percent of the general population will form a kidney stone at some time, and men are at a higher risk than women are.

The link between water and kidney stones comes down to urine. The less water you drink, the lower your urinary volume, and the less fluid you pass. The more concentrated your urine, the greater the chance that solids, like minerals, will precipitate out and form stones. Studies show that stone patients who increased their urine output to 2 liters daily had a significantly lower level of recurrence than patients who didn't increase their water intake. If you think about it, that's incredible: You don't have to take any medicine. You don't have to have any kind of treatment. Just drink more water. There's probably no other health problem we know of that's affected so dramatically by drinking more water.

How much more? The researchers recommended that people at risk for urinary stone formation consume at least 250 milliliters (roughly 1 cup) of fluid with each meal, between meals, before bedtime, and if and when they get up at night to go to the bathroom. That's about 8 cups a day.

Another weapon in the arsenal against stone formation is something called black-currant juice.

SMART THINKING ABOUT DRINKING

SEDENTARY PEOPLE LOSE ABOUT 8 CUPS of fluid daily just through required metabolic processes like energy metabolism, respiration, digestion, and, of course, going to the bathroom. But if you exercise, travel (the dry air on planes is notorious for sucking the moisture out of you), are dieting, have been sick, or are recovering from an injury or surgery, you'll need more fluids.

Fluid losses occur naturally during the day, but the exact rate has really not been documented. Much more work has been done with people exercising, and we know that you can lose about 4 cups of fluid for every hour of exercise, depending on your size and perspiration rate. Working out moderately in a mild climate, you are probably losing 1 to 2 quarts of fluid each hour. That means a 150-pound person can easily lose 2 percent of his body weight in fluid (3 pounds, or 6 cups) within an hour. With more-intense exercise or in a more extreme environment, fluid losses are greater.

We recommend drinking small amounts regularly throughout the day, not a quart all at one time. The stomach and intestines can't absorb huge loads. Here's a good target drinking schedule to prepare for and sustain your exercise regimen.

- Drink 2 cups of fluid 2 to 3 hours before you exercise.
- Drink another cup just before exercise.
- Drink 4 to 6 ounces every 15 to 20 minutes during exercise.
- Drink at least 2 to 3 cups after exercise.

Stress of all sorts increases your need for fluids. If you are traveling, sick or injured, dieting, or living in an extreme environment, add at least another 2 cups for each factor to the 8-cup basic need every day.

Both men and women need fluid for reproduction, as the whole process occurs bathed in fluids. However, I can't tell you exactly how much difference hydration makes in fertility. On the other hand, a guy who is dehydrated by 2 percent or more won't have much endurance or stamina, that's for sure.

German researchers found that it can increase the pH level of your urine, making it less likely that you'll develop kidney stones.

Preventing Short-Term Heart Problems

As I'll discuss later, increased water consumption is linked with a decreased risk of heart attack and stroke. The short-term effects of dehydration hint at this: As a general rule, the greater your fluid volume, the lower your blood pressure. For example, researchers have found that mild dehydration can induce mitral valve prolapse (a.k.a. a heart murmur). When cells aren't fully hydrated, they lack something called turgor: enough fluid pushing against the cell wall. The same thing keeps plants erect, and when it's lacking they fall over. Assuming the plant isn't dead, once it's watered the cells are again volumized, and the plant stands up. The effect is similar to that of a balloon, which can be blown up or deflated, making it very tight or flaccid. That's exactly what happens to the cells in your body. Think of the heart as a muscle with valves that open and close; when you're dehydrated, they don't close tightly but become wobbly.

If a guy isn't predisposed to this condition, dehydration probably won't trigger it; then again, if he is, it might. I've spoken with cardiologists who say that many men who come to see them in a dehydrated state—whether it's from a gastrointestinal flu, nausea, vomiting, or diarrhea—have a heart murmur. If you test them a month later, after they're rehydrated, the heart murmur is gone. It's really important for guys to know this in advance because you could be misdiagnosed just because you're dehydrated. It doesn't mean it happens in everybody, but it can happen.

Aiding Digestion

If you have gut problems, water alone may not do the trick (see page 240). Then again, dehydration may be the one thing keeping you from regularity. Not only does fluid keep everything lubricated and moving through the gut, but it also combines with dietary fiber to make your solid waste bulkier. This may not sound terribly desirable, but I assure you it is. Imagine for a moment the gut during *peristalsis,* the alternating contracting and releasing of the smooth muscle that surrounds the gut. If there's nothing there for it to squeeze and work on, that smooth muscle gets flaccid and out of shape—sort of how your abs would look if you never exercised: flabby, detrained, and unhealthy. Then you're not totally healthy. When you've got a larger stool, your gut has something to work against, which keeps it much healthier. You don't have to strain as much, and things get pushed through much more efficiently. That's also how you'll avoid hemorrhoids and other abnormal features that develop in the walls of your intestine that not only are uncomfortable, but can potentially become precursors to life-threatening ailments.

Aiding Oral Hygiene

I'm amazed by how many people brush their teeth three or four times a day but never think to drink extra water to keep their teeth clean. Water has a big effect on oral health and hygiene, specifically because you need it to create saliva. Having saliva wash over your teeth is part of the natural process of keeping your teeth cleansed. If you get dehydrated and produce less saliva, you'll be at higher risk for dental problems ranging from cavities to periodontal disease. This is especially important at meals, so try to drink some water at each one. If you don't like drinking water with food, simply drink some soon after.

Curing Headaches

If you are suffering from a headache, you might want to reach for a glass and the tap before you reach for Advil. A few years back, a study was done with a group of chronic-headache sufferers. Half the people took water and aspirin; the other half, water and a placebo. Those taking water and a placebo showed the same improvement as those taking water and aspirin. Logically, the researchers concluded that the headache sufferers lacked water, not aspirin. They were dehydrated.

Wondering how long it takes to find out? Next time you get a headache, drink a glass or two of water and wait 30 minutes. If your headache hasn't begun to subside, *then* reach for the aspirin.

A Replacement for Caffeine

Burning eyes, dry mouth, fatigue, and, in some cases, a burning sensation in the stomach are signs of dehydration. Ask the average guy, and he probably gets these symptoms most every afternoon. To compensate, he drinks a cup of coffee.

He should hit the water bottle first. Granted, coffee is not the diuretic people once thought it to be. Fewer than three cups of coffee won't flush water from most well-hydrated people, research has shown. However, a German study done a few years ago found that six cups of coffee had a definite dehydrating effect on the drinker. If you are already dehydrated, caffeine can only make things worse. Bottom line: When you are feeling that mid-afternoon slump, reach for a glass of water or two instead of the coffee. If you still need a pick-me-up, *then* go ahead and have some Joe.

Recovering from a Hangover

On the flip side of caffeine is alcohol. No guy who has ever pounded a 12-pack by his lonesome needs to be told he'll be in pain the next day, and most of us know that the pain—commonly called a hangover—is directly related to dehydration. How exactly does he come to be a few pints short after downing beer all night?

It helps to know a little more about how the kid-

neys work. These smallish organs contain tubules through which fluids and then minerals and electrolytes are filtered. As fluids pass through these filters, balance is maintained in other parts of the body through the secretion of enzymes and hormones. They come to the kidneys for their marching orders, basically. Do we need more salt, or less? Do we need more potassium, or less? Do we need more calcium, or less? Do we need more fluid, or less?

One of the key players in this dance is called the anti-diuretic hormone (ADH), which turns off or on, depending on whether the body needs more or less fluid. If the body is becoming dehydrated, ADH turns on, telling the kidneys to absorb more fluid back into the body, rather than letting it flush out into the bladder and exit as urine.

Add alcohol, however, and suddenly your ADH turns off, regardless of your body's needs. Virtually all of the fluid passing through the kidneys will get excreted rather than reabsorbed, resulting in dehydration.

How much fluid you lose depends on how much alcohol you drink and how long the potency stays in your bloodstream. Assuming that you have normal liver function and body fat levels, alcohol is cleared from the bloodstream at a rate of one drink per hour. At that pace, the effect of one glass of wine will be fairly insignificant, but draining a six-pack of beer will take a toll.

Hangover Helpers

To help work the alcohol out of your system and replace your fluid losses, choose a beverage (or even a food) that contains some of the minerals you're losing. Here's a quick rundown of some of your options.

■ **Flavored water.** Consumer research has shown that given a choice, guys will take a flavored beverage over old-fashioned water. Flavor usually means sugar, though, and sugar means added calories. A new breed of "fitness" waters may provide the answer: They contain vitamins and minerals, taste pretty good, and have 10 to 30 calories per 8 ounces. Propel, Aqua-Lean by Pinnacle, Reebok Fitness Water, and Dasani Nutriwater are among my favorites.

- **Sports drinks.** Sports drinks are a great option for your big night out because they contain minerals and electrolytes, which can help replace what your body loses. Try slipping a bottle of Powerade or Accelerade in between the Jack-and-Cokes, and you won't feel quite so trashed in the morning.
- **Watermelon.** This may not always be available, especially at times other than summer, but watermelon is more than 90 percent water, making it great for rehydration purposes. As an added health bonus, it's loaded with the antioxidant lycopene, which has been shown in studies to help prevent prostate cancer.
- **Iced tea.** A little of this can help, but don't go crazy with it—too much caffeine and you'll get that secondary diuretic effect. Opt for unsweetened teas rather than sugary alternatives.
- **Cucumbers.** If the place where you're drinking has a salad bar or serves appetizers, munch on cucumbers between or with drinks. They're almost all water—96 percent.
- **Tap water or bottled water with added minerals.** There are no data regarding what type of water is best for rehydrating after drinking alcohol. In principle, you will always rehydrate better when there is sodium in the fluid. Avoid purified water, and head for the tap water or a bottle of mineral water.

The Immune System

There are some problems that hydration alone can't fix. When it comes to boosting your immune system, food is the way to go.

We're used to thinking of the immune system in mysterious terms—your body somehow "builds re-sistance" to a disease or "fights off" the flu. In reality, the immune system is a very real network of cells and molecules whose job is to maintain the well-being of our bodies and kill (or at least isolate) foreign particles, like bacteria, that find their way in. It's become standard practice today to bolster our immune systems with a barrage of antibiotics and other drugs, a practice that some argue will hurt our immune systems in the long run. One thing is for certain, though: Eat right, and you'll need antibiotics a whole lot less.

Plenty of foods can kick bacteria's butt and jump-start your immune system, and I'll give you the best of them later in this section. But I can't go any further without making this point:

The number-one way to protect your immune system through food is to just eat.

If you aren't getting enough calories, your body switches to starvation-adaptation mode. That means it effectively decides to channel calories to body parts that need them most, like your heart and your brain. The flip side is that your body slowly begins to stop feeding the systems that aren't critical to staying alive at the moment. Your immune system is toward the top of that list. If you have only so much energy to go around, and you have to keep your heart beating and your blood pumping, the immune system is secondary. It's not critical to staying alive at the moment. That's why immune function diminishes in people who starve themselves thin. Test their immune function and you won't get much response.

This doesn't mean that you can't be on a weight-loss diet. It means there's a point at which you won't have enough critical calories to go around. To help you understand how many calories your body needs, do a simple test.

1. Figure out your Resting Energy Expenditure (REE—the number of calories you would need for survival if your daily routine consisted of

nothing more than watching television and sleeping) by multiplying your weight times 11.

2. Use the chart below to pick your Activity Factor (AF—a number that scientists use to represent the amount of activity you do in a day).

3. Multiply your REE times your AF. That is your base number of calories per day, known as your Total Energy Expenditure (TEE).

To maintain your health, I'd recommend straying no more than 300 calories from your daily TEE and definitely no more than 500 calories. For example, a 180-pound guy with an activity factor of 1.7 has a TEE of 3,397. To lose weight, he should eat around 3,097 calories, and he must eat at least 2,897 per day. On the other hand, if he wants to gain muscle, he should eat between 3,697 and 3,897 calories. (If you

ACTIVITY FACTORS (AF) FOR DIFFERENT LEVELS OF ACTIVITY

USE THIS CHART TO DETERMINE YOUR ACTIVITY FACTOR. Use that number to help determine your Total Energy Expenditure.

Activity Level	Male	Female
RESTING		
Sleeping, reclining	1.0	1.0
SEDENTARY		
Minimal movement, largely bedridden		
Activities include watching television, reading	1.3	1.3
LIGHT		
Office work, sitting, day consists of sleeping 8 hours with 16 hours of walking or standing		
Activities include walking, laundry, golf, ping-pong, walking on level ground at 2.5 to 3 mph, restaurant trades; usually includes 1 hour of moderate activity	1.6	1.5
MODERATE		
Light manual labor		
Activities include walking 3.5 to 4 mph, carrying a load, cycling, tennis, dancing, weeding, and hoeing	1.7	1.6
VERY ACTIVE		
Full-time athletes, agricultural laborers, active military duty, hard laborers (mine and steel workers)		
Activities include walking with a load uphill, team sports, climbing	2.1	1.9
EXTREMELY ACTIVE		
Lumberjacks, construction workers, coal miners, some full-time athletes with daily strenuous training	2.4	2.2

TOTAL DAILY CALORIE NEEDS

_____ × _____ = _____ (the daily number you need for maintaining weight)

Your REE   Your AF   Your TEE calories

are truly inactive and have no plans to exercise, make sure you never consume fewer calories than your REE, unless a doctor tells you otherwise. *Note:* I would *never* recommend this kind of lifestyle.)

Proteins

All three macronutrients (and most micronutrients as well) are important for immune function, but let's forget the carbs and fats for a minute. Next to generic calories, nothing is more important for defending your body than proteins. These are the building blocks of the cells, enzymes, cytokines, hormones, growth factors, and antibodies that make up and control the immune system. Without enough protein, the critical cells of the immune system can't function. An extreme example of this can be seen in patients with HIV, whose damaged immune systems have difficulty creating antioxidants to fight decay in their bodies. In a recent study, scientists gave whey protein supplements with key amino acids to HIV patients and found that their immune systems were strengthened.

FEED A COLD, STARVE A . . . HUH?

OR IS IT THE OTHER WAY AROUND? Most guys have a hard time keeping the sequence of that crusty aphorism straight, let alone figuring out if it's true or is an old wives' tale.

The saying goes, "Feed a cold, starve a fever," and let's debunk it once and forever, shall we? It's hokum. When a guy runs a fever, he needs *more* calories, not the same amount or fewer. Granted, you might not feel like eating anything, but keep the nourishment coming anyway. Especially the fluids. In fact, at any time, the more well nourished you are, the better.

Years ago, some researchers studied starving cancer patients to see which would starve first: the cancer or the patient. Undeniably, the fewer nutrients that were made available, the slower the cancer grew. At the same time, the body's immune functions diminished down to almost nothing. So the body had nothing, basically, with which to battle this diminished foe. So it was a wash.

On the flip side, there seems to be little reason, medically and nutritionally speaking, to gorge yourself when you've got the sniffles. When you get sick, you lose your appetite, and it becomes difficult to eat. One of the reasons is functional: When you're eating, you're digesting, and that takes energy away from the site where you're trying to ward off an intrusion.

What you *do* want to consume in either case is plenty of fluids, which are essential for the transport of nutrients into the body and to the site where an illness is occurring, as well as for transporting toxins away and out of the body. You also need fluids to keep cells volumized, so that protein metabolism can move forward as rapidly as possible, with everything functioning at peak levels. So fluids are absolutely essential when you're sick.

As for Mom's cure-all, chicken soup, several studies have shown that it does have an anti-inflammatory effect. Whether it's strong enough to replace your over-the-counter cold medicines is another matter. But it sure tastes better than any other medicine you'll take.

The average sedentary man needs about 0.36 grams of protein for every pound he weighs. That's about 65 grams of protein per day for a 180-pound man. As I've said before, men who want to build muscle will need much more, but 0.36 gram per pound will keep you in basic health.

Additional Immuno-Defenders

Once you've got the basics down—eat, and eat protein especially—there are still plenty of ways to boost your immune system. Below, you'll find some of the more reliable foods, vitamins, and minerals.

Get to zincing. Study after study has shown that zinc is vital for nearly every aspect of your immune system, from fighting off disease to healing wounds. Without it, your body works slower and loses effectiveness when fighting illness; in extreme cases, zinc deficiency has been shown to stunt growth and significantly delay healing. Ideally, you should consume around 11 milligrams (mg) of zinc a day, and no more than 40 mg; take too much and your body will act as if you are zinc deficient. Foods rich in zinc include meat, liver, eggs, and seafood (especially oysters). Whole-grain products also contain zinc. Vegetarians may need more zinc than meat eaters do.

Mind your magnesium. Your body's need for magnesium resembles its need for zinc. According to some nutrition scientists, it is one of the most important micronutrients and is intimately involved in the immune system, from fighting inflammation to breeding new cells and prolonging the life of older cells. Men ages 19 to 30 should try to get 400 mg each day, and men over 30 should get 420 mg. For best results, try to get no more than 350 mg from supplements daily. The best food sources of magnesium are green leafy vegetables, legumes, whole grains, nuts, meat, seafood, and milk.

Bet on beta-carotene. Beta-carotene and the other carotenes are potent antioxidants your body needs to fight free radicals (potentially dangerous substances in your cells that I'll talk about soon). There are no established recommendations or limits for beta-carotene; 2,500 international units (IU) from supplements are safe, although daily intakes of 20,000 IU from either food or supplements over several months may cause skin yellowing. There are hundreds of carotenoids in nature, found mostly in orange and yellow fruits and vegetables, and in dark green vegetables. You should include these with abundance in your diet, and depend on food and not supplements to meet your needs.

Don't go easy on the green. Green tea, that is. The catechins in green tea wage war against viral infections by enhancing the immune system and acting as an antioxidant. Research on mice has shown that catechins decrease the risk of certain types of cancers. It is difficult to say how much green tea you should drink each day, because the research has been done almost exclusively with extracts, and potency varies. But if you are drinking a cup or two each day, you are probably helping the cause.

Load up on yogurt. Though this area is still somewhat controversial, it appears that several bacteria in yogurt, known collectively as probiotics, have a beneficial effect on the health of the intestinal lining by decreasing the inflammatory processes in the gut. Among their benefits, probiotics appear to reduce the diarrheal symptoms of gut infections and irritable bowel syndrome, and even reduce the risk of colon cancer. Eating a daily yogurt labeled as containing "Live active cultures" or using a probiotic supplement appear to be equally effective.

Selenium, copper, and manganese. Your body contains certain disease-fighting enzymes, called metalloenzymes, that can't function without these three minerals. You can easily get enough of all three if you eat whole grains, egg yolks, green leafy vegetables, and seafood regularly.

Inflammation

Inflammation is a tricky subject. Maybe you associate it with the zit on your nose that appeared miraculously as you headed out the door for a hot date last week, or with a painful ingrown nail. My coauthor, Jeff, associates it with the color his grapefruit-size ankle turned the last time he went up for a rebound and landed funny.

Red, puffy, and sore to the touch—that's how most of us experience inflammation. In fact, beneath the skin's surface, it is one of the body's most constant underlying phenomena. Your body is filled with tissues, and anytime they become irritated or damaged, they also become inflamed. The sources of this irritation are nearly endless—an injury, a hard workout, lack of sleep, a fat-laden meal, and pretty much everything in between.

When this happens, your body reacts fast. The inflammatory response kicks in, and blood flows with haste to the damaged tissue, permeating it with nutrients and immune cells, whose job it is to clean up the microscopic materials that are causing the inflammation. This is all part and parcel of the healing process.

GOOD FOOD TO GO

YOUR IMMUNE SYSTEM IS ESPECIALLY SUSCEPTIBLE DURING TRAVEL. It's bad enough that going somewhere usually means picking up a bug on a flight, after breathing air that has been circulated continuously for several hours. (Although the airline industry vehemently refutes this.) There's also the havoc travel can wreak with your diet. Room service, meals out, business dinners. . . . By the time you get home, it often takes a month to undo a week's worth of dietary damage.

When I travel on business, I bring breakfast with me, and I eat it in my room. Part of it is principle: I just have a hard time accepting the costs for ridiculously expensive room-service breakfasts. I also want to control what I eat, so along with plastic bowls and plastic spoons, I bring Shredded Wheat, ground flaxseed, wheat bran, and raisins in separate zip-top bags. All I have to do then is go to the gift shop, get a few cartons of milk, and refrigerate them in my room—voilà! Breakfast when I want it.

If you do order from room service, eat your usual meal. Don't get trapped into the whole pancakes-and-eggs-and-bacon thing. This is one of the critical factors to successful travel. Sometimes I'll order scrambled eggs to go along with my cereal, but skip the heavy, fat-laden stuff.

Nail breakfast, and the rest of the day will usually work out, assuming you plan ahead. I carry nuts with me, always. I carry a protein-energy bar or two as a last resort in case I get stuck somewhere. I'm not a big fan of the energy bars, but they're a better choice than a bag of chips or a candy bar from a vending machine. And they will help you ward off panic eating episodes where you eat whatever isn't nailed down just because you're so famished.

Many of the offending materials that immune cells clean up are free radicals. To understand free radicals, think back to high school chemistry. Your cells are full of atoms and molecules. Sometimes, these atoms become unstable—caused by any number of things, from cigarette smoke and UV rays to damage, stress, or simply breathing—and let off an errant electron. That electron will bounce around until it can latch onto another atom, which becomes a temperamental, highly reactive structure: a free radical. At the same time, the new free radical lets off an electron of its own, sparking a chain reaction of new free radicals. We're not talking about a bad apple here and there, either. Every breath you take, for example, produces some 10,000 of these molecules within each of your body's cells. When you exercise, you create even more (see "The Exercise/Free Radical Connection" on this page).

Over time, the effects of free radicals on your body are far-ranging and can be quite dangerous. We'll get to that later. For now, all you need to know is that anytime you experience inflammation, be it a swollen knee, a bee sting, or a sore throat, free radicals are playing a part.

Antioxidants

To combat free radicals, turn to foods rich in antioxidants, which work in several different ways to fight free radicals and reduce lipid peroxidation (a.k.a. oxidation of fats in your cells.) For instance, beta-carotene can actually destroy free radicals after they are formed. Vitamin C keeps free radicals from destroying the outermost layers of cells. Vitamin E scavenges free radicals, saving tissues from damage.

The best-known antioxidants come at the end of a fork or in pill form: vitamins C and E; beta-carotene, a precursor to vitamin A; and minerals such as copper, zinc, manganese, and selenium. Getting most of your antioxidants from whole foods has major advantages—you get not only the antioxidants but also a whole host of other nutrients. Although the science of antioxidants is still unraveling, researchers suspect that your body may best absorb and use antioxidants when these other nutrients are present. When isolated and placed in a pill, they don't seem to have the same effect on the body.

Spotting the Antioxidants

The easiest way to point you toward foods packed with antioxidants is to show you the U.S. Department of Agriculture's Oxygen Radical Absorbance Capacity (ORAC) chart (see next page). The title is confusing, but the idea is simple: The chart ranks the top antioxidant-rich foods, starting with the very best and working down to the very good. We're not going to bore you with a dissertation on every food on the list, but I would like to hand out a few "Antioxidant Awards."

The Exercise/Free Radical Connection

A lot of guys scratch their heads with this seeming contradiction: "So, on the one hand you're telling me to exercise, and on the other you're telling me that exercise creates millions of free radicals that could harm me in the long run?"

Actually, no. In reality, it's exactly the opposite: Because of exercise, your body is better equipped to fight harmful free radicals, even when there are more than usual to deal with. Over time, your body adapts to oxidative stress by boosting its internal antioxidant production. That's why you don't see world-class athletes, who train constantly, contracting cancer left and right, or succumbing to heart disease prematurely. That's also why sedentary people, whose sloth has minimized free radical production, don't live to a ripe old age.

Best overall. It's hard to find a better snack than raisins, dried plums, or any of the dark-colored fruits, especially when it comes to antioxidants. Prunes (now officially called dried plums) are the king of the hill. Yes, those shriveled purple blobs are the butt of more jokes than any other food (except possibly baked beans), but they have twice the anti-oxidants of raisins, which are ranked second. Both foods are nearly devoid of water, making their anti-oxidants heavily concentrated. Incidentally, the antioxidant content of red grapes helps explain why red wine reduces the risk of heart disease better than white wine, liquor, or beer.

Best for fighting pain. Cherries are another amazing inflammation fighter. They rank among the top 10 in terms of antioxidant content, making them a powerful anti-inflammatory. A study at Michigan State University found that eating tart cherries could relieve inflammatory pain as capably as aspirin or ibuprofen but with less potential stomach irritation. And because there are only 51 calories per cup, you can forget about getting heavy and concentrate on getting healthy.

Runners-up. One antidote for a sprained ankle or a broken tibia might be eating beef, chicken, seafood, and other foods high in B vitamins. In animal trials, vitamins B_1, B_6, and B_{12} seemed to disrupt the transmission of pain signals between the rest of the body and the brain. Olive oil and nuts also have anti-inflammatory action that can help minimize sprains and tendinitis. In contrast, the saturated fat in meats can aggravate such problems.

Most underrated antioxidant. The award here goes to herbs. The U.S. Department of Agriculture recently tested dozens of culinary herbs and spices for antioxidant content and found that many of them outpace fruits and vegetables in this department. For example, Mexican, Italian, and Greek

OXYGEN RADICAL ABSORBANCE CAPACITY (ORAC)

HERE ARE THE FOODS THAT BEST PROTECT YOUR CELLS from free radicals and oxidation. Although scientists are still studying these foods, initial results show that eating fruits and vegetables high in ORAC levels may be highly beneficial.

Top Antioxidant Foods (ORAC units per 100 grams)

FOOD	VALUE	FOOD	VALUE
Prunes	5,770	Alfalfa sprouts	930
Raisins	2,830	Broccoli florets	890
Blueberries	2,400	Red bell peppers	840
Blackberries	2,036	Oranges	750
Kale	1,770	Red grapes	739
Strawberries	1,540	Beets	710
Brussels sprouts	1,260	Cherries	670
Spinach	1,260	Onions	450
Raspberries	1,220	Corn	400
Plums	949	Eggplant	390

Pill Power

Supplements can help fill in some of the holes in your diet, particularly when it comes to vitamin E. The current recommended daily allowance for men is 30 international units (IU) daily, but studies published in *The New England Journal of Medicine* found that 200 to 400 IU reduces the risk of heart disease significantly. Because vitamin E comes primarily from nuts and oils, that's perhaps 10 times more than the average guy will get from even a healthy diet.

oregano all outscored vitamin E when measured for antioxidant activity. Bay, dill, coriander, thyme, and rosemary scored nearly as well. Keep in mind that because herbs and spices tend to be sprinkled lightly on whatever you happen to be eating, they're not a substitute for the quantities found in fruits and vegetables. But it's an easy way to amp up your overall antioxidant consumption, with the added bonus of making your food tastier.

Best for stopping muscle cramps. There may be a number of different causes of muscle cramps, but one that you can easily eliminate is dehydration and loss of salts, especially sodium, potassium, and magnesium. Slathering a banana with some salted natural peanut butter and drinking a huge gulp of water is a great antidote for your muscle cramps. If the cramps persist, seek medical advice.

Best for curing headaches. Ginger may help relieve standard headaches, as well as migraines. It may work as an analgesic and halt the headache prophylactically by inhibiting the release of serotonin into the brain. For migraines, enjoy some nuts, beans, whole grains, and even spinach. All contain magnesium, which a recent study on children suggests can ease the length and severity of migraine pain.

Most likely to beat arthritis. Here's yet another malady whose sufferers may benefit from a Mediterranean-style diet. Norwegian researchers recently found that when arthritis patients switched from a standard American diet to one emphasizing fruits, vegetables, and fish, their joint pain decreased by half.

That would be consistent with the anti-inflammatory effects attributed to those Mediterranean foods. The omega-3 fats in fatty fish, for example, have been shown to help people with autoimmune diseases like rheumatoid arthritis.

Most likely to prevent cavities. Again, green tea is great here. Its catechins combat the bacteria that cause tooth decay. Primarily, catechins inhibit the bacteria's ability to attach to the tooth, along with a number of other factors that diminish the risk of tooth decay.

Runner-up. Another way to support the integrity of your teeth is by strengthening your gums with calcium. So grab a quart of milk and drink up. Researchers at the State University of New York found that guys who take in 800 milligrams of calcium or more per day have half the risk of periodontal disease as compared with men consuming 500 milligrams a day or less. However, most men consume only half the recommended three servings a day of dairy.

Gastrointestinal Problems

Next time you're strolling around a drugstore, discreetly looking for the condoms or the Rogaine, notice the far more visible section jammed full of purported remedies for heartburn. The shelves are lined with these products from one end to the other, and no wonder: As the years pass, I hear about so many people taking antacids and related products that I wonder if maybe I'm in the wrong business. In meetings, people literally break into a sweat and excuse themselves from the table because they're so horribly uncomfortable.

I firmly believe that a lot this discomfort can be fixed if guys would just pay better attention to what they are eating. Almost all stomach upset, heartburn, and gas (and even things like chronic constipation and some irritable bowel syndrome) can be traced back to food and, specifically, a guy's food intolerances and food allergies. Recognizing these can help relieve unnecessary pain and discomfort in the short run. In the longer run, some of these nagging problems can be a prelude to life-threatening conditions like cancers of the gut, which I'll discuss in the next chapter.

The logical questions here: What is the difference between a food intolerance and a food allergy,

and how do I know if I have one? To answer these questions, you have to understand how intestines work. Think of your intestines as a long, porous hose. As your digestive system breaks food into nutrients, the intestinal wall allows those nutrients to pass through and enter your bloodstream, which in turn takes the nutrients to your organs. Conversely, your intestinal lining is also an incredibly important barrier, keeping foreign particles from invading the inside of your body where your organs are housed.

The size of the particles that can get through the lining of your intestines varies depending on your age. When you were born, your gastrointestinal sys-

COMMON TRUE FOOD ALLERGIES IN ADULTS

HERE ARE THE MOST COMMON FOODS THAT CAUSE actual allergic reactions in adults.

Crustaceans
(shrimp, crab, lobster, crawfish)

Eggs

Fish

Milk

Peanuts

Soy

Tree nuts

Wheat

Symptoms of Food Allergies and Intolerances

True food allergy symptoms*

Cutaneous (skin): swelling, hives, skin rashes

Gastrointestinal: abdominal cramps, diarrhea, nausea, vomiting

Oral allergy syndrome: mouth, palate, and tongue itching and swelling; hives

Respiratory: runny nose, asthma, constriction of the throat

Systemic: anaphylactic shock (severe generalized shock)

Food intolerance symptoms†

Gastrointestinal: abdominal cramps, diarrhea, nausea

Metabolic: hemolytic anemia (in severe cases, jaundice and kidney failure)

*Usually people experience only a few of these symptoms, not all of them. Onset of symptoms may occur immediately or within an hour of ingesting the food.
† These may be mild and transient and do not involve the immune system. Onset is 30 minutes to several hours after ingesting the food or beverage.

tem was not quite fully developed, allowing bigger molecules to pass through. This is why infants are fed mainly a protective diet of breast milk or formula and water. Their bodies cannot handle the huge protein molecules in cow's milk. The proteins in breast milk and processed formula are smaller and are more easily digested and broken down.

One of the theories behind the development of food allergies relates to this early stage of gastrointestinal development. Scientists theorize that exposure to certain complicated proteins in infancy or early childhood may startle the immune system. Recognizing these large molecules as foreign bodies, the immune system develops antibodies and immunoglobulins to fight them off. Even after the gut lining is fully developed, the immune system still recognizes these food proteins as intruders and creates an immune reaction, or a true allergic reaction, to the food.

These reactions can range from annoying disturbances like hives and eczema to life-threatening reactions like anaphylactic shock. The most common foods that cause allergies are peanuts, tree nuts, wheat, eggs, shellfish, milk, and soy.

More common than food allergies are food intolerances. These are not caused by your immune system. Instead, they are usually either metabolically based (as in lactose intolerance, when an ingredient cannot be fully digested or absorbed), or they are abnormal, almost inexplicable responses to food (as in sulfite-induced asthma, where exposure to sulfites results in severe difficulty breathing). Food intolerances are generally not as severe as true food allergies, but the symptoms can resemble those of an allergy, ranging from abdominal cramps and diarrhea to anemia (low iron and red blood cells).

Adults with true food allergies usually know their trigger foods and avoid them. On the other hand, symptoms of food intolerance can often go unnoticed or ignored. Many people live a lifetime with gut problems and think it's a normal thing. Others realize that certain foods make them uncomfortable but won't stop eating them.

I'm here to suggest paying more attention to these problems. The constant barrage of foods that cause disturbances in the gut may ultimately lead to inflammation of the gut lining and discomfort that can no longer be ignored. The same holds true for any kind of viral or bacterial infection that you may have encountered, like a bout with intestinal flu. You need to heal any damage that occurred. Luckily, both disturbances can be handled naturally: the first by learning what to include in your diet to promote better gastrointestinal (GI) health, and the second by learning what might need to go.

Fiber

There's little fiber in the typical American diet, another reason that you should try extra-hard to get more of it down your throat. There are two primary types of fiber: water-soluble and water-insoluble. It's the water-insoluble fiber that really helps you stay regular. We mentioned before that fiber makes for a bulky stool, a very good thing. Now let's get more specific.

Unless you're actively tracking it, it's hard to know how much fiber you're consuming. The general recommendation from organizations such as the American Heart Association is 25 to 35 grams a day, but they usually base that on a diet of 2,000 calories. We want you to eat more than that, so your fiber intake should be higher, too. The diets I design tend to be very high in fruits and vegetables, and those foods alone can contribute 50 grams or so of fiber a day.

Adding fiber to your diet if you didn't consume much before is best done in short steps. If you add 35 or 40 grams of fiber to your diet, when you were consuming only 5 or 10 grams total before that, you'll blow up like a balloon. The body will adapt and adjust to the extra fiber, but it's going to take some time. Start by trying to add about 10 grams a day.

You might have to live through some intestinal discomfort—gas—for a week or two, but thankfully for you (and anyone who knows you) that should subside. Then you can add more.

In the real world, a hearty slice of whole-grain bread contains 3 grams of fiber, and two oblong biscuits of Shredded Wheat contain 5½ grams. When you're reading the side of a food box or package, something that's a good fiber source should have at least 2 to 3 grams.

There's no downside to being a little bit higher than normal on your fiber intake. Being very, very high will eventually interfere with your ability to eat enough food—you'll be too full to continue. Adding fiber supplements can also be tricky—at a minimum, you have to drink enough fluid to avoid getting an obstruction, which does happen. Some guys get carried away and add a ridiculous amount of wheat bran to their daily diet, or double-fist fiber tablets all day. Do that without drinking enough and you'll get an obstruction. Painful? Let's put it this way: It's probably the closest a guy will ever come to experiencing childbirth. I add 2 to 3 tablespoons of wheat bran to my cereal in the morning. That's enough for most people.

The irony is that guys who have irritable bowel syndrome often have been eating a low-fiber diet because they're afraid of all these foods. They think fiber is going to make their gut hurt, so they avoid it, and things gets worse. This is true only if your gut has become so inflamed that you're approaching an ulcer. Then you need to cut fiber out of your diet and just let everything quiet down. It would be like having a wound on your knee, only you keep bending it and reopening it—the wound never heals. If you keep your knee straight for a while, it can mend. The same goes for your stomach. Usually, the easiest thing for guys to do at that point is to follow a liquid or soft diet for a little bit and then slowly begin adding bulkier foods back in. If you think that this describes your problem, you should definitely get a referral to a registered dietitian, who can help you design a nutritionally sound liquid or soft diet, and then work you back onto whole foods.

Foods That Heal Your Gut

Certain foods can help improve the odds that your stomach contents will move through your intestines without a hitch. Here are some tips for your daily diet.

Buy more broccoli. Perhaps no food presents a better introduction to the health intersection of nutrition and the GI tract as broccoli. It has long been

PASS ON GAS

ADDING FIBER INTO YOUR DIET IS ONE OF THE HEALTHIEST moves you can make. But you don't want your social life to suffer while your health is improving. That's why you have to look out for the fibrous foods that will give you gas and learn to manage them.

Among the biggest culprits are onions and cruciferous vegetables—broccoli, cauliflower, Brussels sprouts, etc. Our suggestion: Find the ones you like, or eat smaller portions of the ones you can tolerate. You can also try boiling the veggies, which will help cut down on their sulfur content. Broccoli or cauliflower, for instance, should be boiled for 10 minutes in an uncovered pot without a lid. Your house may stink, but the acids will escape from the food.

known that many compounds found in vegetables inhibit the growth of pathogens, but as it turns out, perhaps none is as powerful as broccoli. The stomach contains bacteria, called *Helicobacter pylori,* that have been implicated in stomach ulcers and stomach cancers. Broccoli contains the chemical sulforaphane, which kills these potentially deadly bacteria. It's so strong, in fact, that it even kills helicobacter that are resistant to antibiotics. What's more, lab tests have revealed that there's probably enough sulforaphane in the broccoli we eat to do the job. Try to eat several servings (1 cup raw or ½ cup cooked) each week.

Eat more strawberries and oranges. Since high levels of vitamin C have been linked to a reduced risk of developing an ulcer, a handful of strawberries or some orange slices also help fight ulcers. Researchers at the San Francisco VA Medical Center found that individuals with the highest levels of vitamin C in their blood are one-fourth less likely to be infected with *H. pylori.* Try to have at least one serving of vitamin C–rich foods every day.

Try turmeric. Those suffering from inflammatory intestinal diseases might try turmeric, a spice used in curry. Researchers at the Hamamatsu University School of Medicine in Japan found that the spice contains an anti-inflammatory agent called curcumin, which appears to help colitis sufferers, as well as sufferers of certain neurological diseases. Along with traditional foods like Indian and Thai, add it to squash soups, stews, roasted vegetables, and even mashed potatoes. A couple times a week would be a huge increase from what most people eat now. If you are heading to the hospital for elective surgery, add it to your menu before and after surgery.

Make friends with pectin. If you've got diarrhea, make pectin your pal. This water-soluble fiber helps absorb the extra water in your large intestines that, for some reason (infection, food intolerance) has appeared in higher abundance than usual. As pectin moves through your intestines, it dissolves in water and turns into a gel-like structure. This helps

reduce that flushing process, just as it turns runny cooked strawberries into strawberry jam. Apple skins are high in pectin.

Eat more celery. The insoluble fiber found in celery helps prevent constipation and gallstones. In truth, any fiber will do, but celery is particularly high in fiber for the calories it contains. And three-quarters of the total fiber content is insoluble. An 8-inch stalk of celery is only 6 calories and gives you about 1 gram of fiber. If you went all-out and ate five stalks of celery, you'd have eaten 5 grams of fiber and a measly 30 calories! To get the same amount of fiber in broccoli, you'd have to eat 50 calories worth, and only one-half of the total fiber would be insoluble.

Get your peppermint. Peppermint oil is a spasmolytic, meaning that it relaxes the smooth muscle lining of the stomach and intestines. Drink some peppermint tea, and you'll reduce bloating and cramping by avoiding gas buildup. (*Note:* If the reason for your upset stomach is esophageal reflux, stay clear of peppermint. It won't help, and it may injure the esophageal lining.)

Know your calcium alternatives. For anyone with lactose intolerance, yogurt is a great way to get calcium. Many people who can't drink milk or eat ice cream can still tolerate 6 to 8 ounces of yogurt because the bacterial culture actually consumes much of the lactose for its own nutrition. The same goes for other cultured dairy products, like kefir and ripened cheeses.

What You Need to Watch Out For

A classic case of food intolerance goes something like this: The offending particle (let's say it's the lactose from a piece of American cheese) enters the stomach and proceeds through digestion. In most cases, guys aren't actually allergic to lactose (a.k.a. milk sugar), but they don't produce enough of the enzyme lactase, which is what it takes to break down the lactose molecule into the monosaccharides glucose and galactose, allowing them to be absorbed across the intestinal barrier and metabolized. Lactose-intolerant guys don't metabolize those molecules normally, so they get down lower into the gut.

Once there, lactose becomes a feast for bacteria living in that part of the body. Normally, these bacteria never see lactose molecules. As a result of their newfound food, the bacteria reproduce at a much faster rate than normal, and the by-product of that metabolism is a lot of gas and digestive acids. Also, all that sugar low down in the gut changes the concentration of the solids dissolved in the fluid passing through the gut. The body tries to improve digestion by adding more fluids to the mix, but that ends up causing diarrhea. The end result is an inflammation—there's that word again—of the gut.

Your best bet is to figure out which foods are hurting you—and stop using them. The gut is a moist setting, and once you get rid of the offending element, it heals incredibly rapidly, just as your mouth recovers comparatively quickly from oral surgery. You should see marked improvement over 1 week, and total healing by the end of 3 weeks.

Some guys think they can just tough it out, but here's something to think about: If you constantly abuse that lining, you're always going to have impaired nutritional absorption, like a wound never being allowed to heal. It'll be constantly inflamed, and this ongoing hyperimmune response will result in so much cellular damage that you'll increase the risk of some kind of mutation happening in that area. In a worst-case scenario, that kind of cell damage can increase the risk of something catastrophic occurring, like the formation of cancer cells. Here are some major culprits:

Fructose

When it comes to intestinal turmoil, fructose is Public Enemy No. 1 these days. It sounds harmless enough. After all, isn't it basically just fruit sugar? Yep, fruit sugar is the largest natural source of fruc-

tose, and it's also found in vegetables and the saps of some trees—honey and maple syrup, to be precise.

But today we have high-fructose corn syrup, a highly engineered sugar that has hijacked the average American diet. (If you've skipped to this chapter and haven't read about the dangers of high-fructose corn syrup already, please see page 92 before you continue.)

At the same time, the incidence of irritable bowel syndrome (IBS) in the country is exploding (no pun intended). As the name implies, IBS is a constellation of symptoms affecting the large intestine, including cramping, bloating, gas, diarrhea, and constipation. In reality, labeling someone with IBS is a diagnosis of exclusion. It isn't like cancer, where your doctor takes a biopsy and says, "Okay, you've got a malignant tumor." He or she will diagnose you with IBS, in all likelihood, only after exhausting all of the other options that could conceivably affect the bowel.

Nobody really knows with any certainty what causes IBS. Is it stress? Lactose intolerance? If it were well understood, a portion of IBS sufferers could be categorized and "cured" thusly—but not others. Is it an allergy to, say, wheat? People who suffer from something called gluten allergies do so because of an inflammatory process in the bowel that produces horrible discomfort: diarrhea, gas, pain—the whole nine yards. Again, when the offending food or foods are subtracted from the diet, the bowel irritation disappears with them.

Yet there is a whole other group of men for whom elimination diets don't work. Until recently, doctors hadn't been able to tease out what causes IBS in them. Some researchers set their sights on high-fructose corn syrup as a stealth culprit in IBS, however, and the results of a handful of studies suggest that they may be on to something. In fact, it now appears that at least 40 percent of the people who "present" with irritable bowel syndrome are actually fructose intolerant. Eliminate all sources of fructose, including high-fructose corn syrup from their diet, and in short order their guts settle down and heal. Then, when fruit is reintroduced into their diet, they can handle a natural amount. The real problem—which should be avoided—is the soda, fruit-ades, and highly sweetened cereals loaded with high-fructose corn syrup. Even soup and pasta sauce contain the stuff now. It's everywhere.

There's no reason guys need to feel like they have to avoid fruit. What they do need to avoid is sitting down and eating two pints of strawberries, or drinking a quart of orange juice or apple juice. (The latter is particularly high in fructose.) That may disturb them. In fact, when a client tells me he can't drink apple juice without diarrhea, I know immediately that he's fructose intolerant.

When it comes to gut health, a huge bell should be ringing about this issue.

Dairy products

If you are lactose intolerant, you have plenty of company, as the condition affects a significant portion of the world's adult male population. The severity of the condition varies widely, according to the body's ability to secrete lactase. Some guys can drink one glass of milk with no problem, but they can't drink two or three glasses without feeling queasy. Others can drink a glass in the morning and another at night and feel okay but get sick when they have more. Still others can't handle so much as a pat of butter on a slice of bread or they risk becoming deathly ill. Those people who have no tolerance at all are lactase deficient.

The more that food scientists learn about lactose intolerance, the better the solutions they offer. In fact, the lactase-replacement enzyme found on grocery store shelves allows most people who are lactose intolerant to consume dairy products in normal amounts. You might have to take more than the amount suggested on the side of the box— perhaps even double or triple that amount—to get the amount of the enzyme you need. (Every guy secretes lactase at different rates and in different amounts, so while one guy might do just fine with the dosage in the instructions, another guy might need considerably more. Taking more is fine; it can't hurt you.)

Alcohol

Booze also affects the lining of the gut, impairing its ability to absorb nutrients, which is one reason alcoholics are often deficient in B vitamins. For some guys, alcohol carves into the gut lining, making it really, really inflamed, and perhaps even causing an ulcer if the abuse persists long enough. A bleeding ulcer can lead to iron deficiency, and at a certain point the gut can even rupture. Suddenly your insides are full of all kinds of bacteria that otherwise never get into the rest of the body, and in worst-case scenarios, can result in death.

How much alcohol is too much? There's a question for the ages, huh? We don't know a one-size-fits-all answer to that question, but two drinks a day is a good limit for almost every guy. None of the data showing health benefits from alcohol refer to any more booze than that. Moreover, drink beyond that cutoff point and the alcohol starts to have a significant influence on your body's physiology—most of it negative. There's some play here depending on a guy's size and even his background.

But men who drink three alcoholic beverages on weekdays are probably drinking more than that on weekends. There's no good reason to drink regularly like that unless you're looking to ruin your body (not to mention your mind).

Heart Health

Most of the discussion about the relationship between fats and your arteries arguably applies more to longevity than to short-term health. After all, it usually takes a while to clog an artery. (To learn more, turn to the next chapter.) Increasingly, however, researchers think that high-fat meals can present an immediate danger.

The potential problem comes when you consume a meal containing more than 50 grams of fat. (This may seem like a high threshold. After all, when people enter a hospital to see if they have a problem with fat absorption, they receive a loading dose of approximately 100 grams of fat, which is supposed to be extraordinarily high, but gourmet and fast food meals alike frequently exceed 50 grams of fat. And people who eat junk all day spend much of their day above that level.) All of that fat enters your body, driving up the level of triglycerides in your bloodstream while simultaneously driving down HDL, the good cholesterol that ushers fat out of the body. Regarding the triglycerides, we're not talking about a little bump in the night, either, but a surge that can persist for up to 8 hours. That's assuming you don't take in even more fat, pushing triglyceride levels into the stratosphere.

The short of it is, if you are on the threshold of a heart attack, one 50-fat-gram meal could cause your ticker to stop ticking—on the spot.

Provocative new research has found that post-meal surges in blood fats increase the "coaguability" of blood by making blood platelets stickier. The smooth muscle cells lining the arteries suddenly lose some of their ability to contract, and if those arteries are already somewhat hardened, the odds rise that a blockage will form, which could lead to a stroke or a heart attack.

Keep in mind that alcohol can play a role in this scenario. People who drink a lot of alcohol tend to have high triglyceride levels. The medical community used to be more preoccupied with cholesterol, with triglycerides considered a secondary concern, but the latter is now also seen as key, specifically be-cause of their platelet-aggregation effect, which can lead to clotting.

Food for Your Heart

The best thing you can do to make sure that your arteries remain open thoroughfares, free from bottle-necks, is to reduce the amount of saturated fat in your diet. In the shorter term, though, these foods can help blood flow more freely.

Eat fatty fish. Your heart's best friend is fatty fish like herring, mackerel, salmon, and tuna. A study in the journal *Circulation* found that fatalities from heart attacks or heart disease were cut in half among those who ate tuna or other fish three times or more each week.

Granted, fish eaters tend to have healthier lifestyles in general. They tend to be better educated, less inclined toward saturated fat and more toward fruits and vegetables, and much less likely to smoke. Still, even after researchers statistically adjusted these factors, fish stood out as a major heart helper.

Chomp on celery. A substance inside these stalks, called 3-butylphthalide, helps prevent blood vessels from constricting, as they do after high-fat meals.

Get garlic and onions. Nothing stinks about these where cardiac health is concerned. The adenosine contained in garlic can lower blood pressure, as can the ajoene in garlic and onions.

Up your ginger. This root will protect you from the blood clots that eventually cause heart attacks and strokes. It works in a similar manner to aspirin, thinning the blood by making your blood platelets less sticky. Because ginger is also an effective anti-inflammatory, reducing the body's inflammatory-response chemicals helps to decrease risk of cardiovascular disease.

Buy more bananas. Potassium, found in large quantities in bananas (about 500 milligrams per fruit), is well known for helping lower blood pressure and is getting noticed for its ability to protect against stroke as well. In a study of men and women over age 50, those who took in more than 3,500 milligrams of potassium daily were less likely to die from stroke than those who consumed less than 1,950 milligrams daily.

Switch to whole grains. The magnesium they contain helps regulate your heartbeat and, studies show, may restore damaged blood vessels' ability to open up when the body needs more blood.

Eat licorice. The coumarone it contains also lowers blood pressure.

Postoperative Nutrition

Food cannot only help keep you from getting sick, it can assist in the recovery process from illness, even after something as invasive as surgery.

The best postoperative nutrition strategy begins well before you ever enter a hospital. First, stockpile nutrients ahead of time. This can have a huge impact on the outcome. Surgery isn't always predictable and foreseeable, but if it is, ask your doctor for a day or two to prepare for it nutritionally. If it's an elective surgery, you've got weeks to plan ahead. Eating well ahead of time makes an enormous difference.

One goal should be to consume plenty of foods that have an anti-inflammatory effect, that break down the materials that cause inflammation in the body's tissues. After all, usually after some kind of treatment, surgery, illness, or soreness, a doctor will give you a nonsteroidal anti-inflammatory drug. Everyone reacts differently to these drugs. Some people take them and have no problems, and some people take them and have horrible gut problems as a result. (For example, if I take a nonsteroidal anti-inflammatory for more than a day or two, I get terrible mouth ulcers.)

For those who do have problems with these drugs, an alternative is food that naturally produces an anti-inflammatory effect. So if you're getting ready to go into the hospital for some kind of surgery, consume those foods for several weeks ahead of time to build up levels of those nutrients. That will help you build up effective levels of anti-inflammatory in the blood. (Drugs, in contrast, require less preparation and work faster—in some cases, almost immediately. Unfortunately, so do many of the negative side effects.)

The first place you should turn is to foods rich in bioflavonoids. If you want to keep inflammation to a minimum, these are the guys that do it. Every day, bioflavanoids help protect your cells by fixing and strengthening the cell membrane. They really get to do their stuff when inflammation hits, though. Think of inflammation as an invading army and your cells as a fort under attack: You need soldiers to protect the fort internally and soldiers to abate the enemy outside. Here, the soldiers are your bioflavonoids. While maintaining the integrity of your cells, they go out to stop pro-inflammatory enzymes. The more you've got, the less damage you incur and the more healing that occurs.

You may ask, "Doesn't the inflammatory response serve an important function, though?" Yes, but sometimes the inflammatory response itself can inhibit the healing process by causing more cell damage. The free-radical-fighting qualities of bioflavanoids are so desirable because they decrease cell damage while maintaining the integrity of the cell membrane.

Soy, onions, kale, green beans, apples, citrus foods and juices, and prunes are all good sources of bioflavanoids. You may also want to turn to herbal remedies, like China's wogonin. In a study where researchers used wogonin as a topical treatment for skin inflammation, it was shown to have a powerful anti-inflammatory effect on inflamed skin.

Another nutrient that's great before and after

surgery is bromelain. Found in pineapple, bromelain is an enzyme that breaks down protein. It also increases the anti-inflammatory chemicals in the body, decreasing clotting, walling off injured areas, improving drainage, and diminishing swelling. It also decreases pro-inflammatory mediators, so it offers benefits on both sides of the inflammatory process.

Other foods and nutrients with anti-inflammatory properties are the omega-3s found in fatty fish, the antioxidant vitamins, algae, wheat germ, and the minerals iron and zinc. The latter two present a good reason to eat red meat and the dark meat of poultry, which are the most efficient sources of those minerals. That doesn't mean you have to have something fat-laden like brisket. Instead, go for lean sources and, in the case of chicken, remove the skin.

So if you know you have surgery coming up, there are some very specific things you can do with your diet to enhance the outcome. Eat lots of fruits and vegetables, including pineapple every day. The new "gold" varieties of pineapple from Hawaii are lower in acid than the common varieties, and they are incredibly sweet. Sprinkle some wheat germ or ground flaxseed on your cereal. Have fatty fish as often as possible, and eat lean beef and chicken occasionally.

All of your dietary choices before and after surgery should be made in consultation with a medical professional. Ask to meet with one of the hospital dietitians before you go under the knife, and set up a plan. Some meal-replacement products, like various formulations of Ensure, have been formulated specifically with ill populations in mind. Go with whatever the hospital dietitian recommends—he or she will know best if you need low fiber or specific medium-chain fatty acids for some reason, as well as what diet or supplement is formulated specifically for the type of procedure you are undergoing.

Here's one final word about nutrition and surgery:

creatine. This muscle-building supplement has received a bad rap in the past for being ineffective and possibly even dangerous. That's all unscientific mumbo-jumbo. Data from a 2001 study show that using this supplement before an operation and then continuing to use it postoperatively can speed up your recovery.

If you're going to have surgery for any kind of injury, the smartest strategy you can employ is something called "prehab," where you see a physical therapist prior to surgery. The idea is that by exercising that area beforehand, you'll be able to maintain as much muscle as possible there after the surgery, when function will be limited and the body part in question will be subject to atrophy. When they do actually get you moving again—which they'll want to do as soon as possible—your rehab will progress relatively quickly, and you'll have the best outcome.

Now researchers are finding that, by supplementing with creatine during your prehab and then continuing to use the supplement during your rehab, you get an improved outcome in the form of less muscle lost.

My personal experience is only anecdotal, of course, but I took creatine during the two weeks preceding surgery for an ACL (for the uninitiated, that's the anterior cruciate ligament in the knee) that I tore skiing. (Doctors often don't want to do the surgery immediately after the injury occurs. They want to wait for the inflammation to go down a little bit after your injury.) I didn't do a loading phase; I took the standard daily dose of 5 grams of creatine daily. I continued taking it into my rehab, and I had the sort of accelerated recovery shown in the study. Several of my therapists said, "Oh, my! I've never seen anyone rehab so quickly." There is no question in my mind that I had a faster recovery than I would have had without taking creatine.

If you're interested in pursuing that strategy

yourself, always ask your physician before taking creatine or any supplement you may take before or after surgery. For example, vitamin E is a fantastic supplement, but you don't want to take extra before or immediately after surgery because it's a blood thinner. Too much bleeding is not a good thing around surgery.

Healthy Eating: It's Up to You

We said this earlier in another context, but if you really want to eat healthy, you have to get your act together. What I mean by that is that at some point, the responsibility is squarely on your shoulders. Nobody can do this for you. All we can do is prescribe. You have to do it.

That brings us to the subject of obesity. In this era of political correctness, in some circles you can't even talk about the reality of being fat. Not horizontally challenged, not large-size, and not pleasantly plump. *Fat.* Well, here's the deal: If you're fat, you're almost certainly going to get sick, both in the short term and the long term. A researcher at the Cooper Institute looked into the whole notion of being fit and fat, meaning someone who's overweight but who exercises and has chronic-disease risks that are low, and can thus be deemed healthy. After studying the phenomenon, he estimated that it applies to a very small percentage of the overweight population. Those rare individuals probably are genetically predisposed to carry high amounts of muscle tissue to begin with, and they probably exercise a lot on top of that. Why they're obese, we don't really know.

Other researchers have also found that fitness and fatness are in fact separate risk factors for heart disease. Even if you are fit, if you are fat you have a great risk of succumbing to the illnesses associated with heart disease. If you're seriously overweight and you're reading this now, let's just assume you're not among the miniscule percent of the population that may be fit and fat. That means you're too fat right now. It's not *sizism* or anything else other than medical fact. Telling people that they're okay at any size isn't okay. They may be good people, but that's not the issue; people who are obese are going to get sick and contribute to the huge strain on the whole medical system, which has become a huge strain on the country's economy. Ultimately, overweight people die before their time. Is that really how you want your epitaph to read?

We can't overemphasize this enough. You have to do it yourself. If your diet is unhealthy and you've been putting off fixing it till "tomorrow" for 10 years now, wake up. You don't have to change everything at once—and, in fact, trying to do it that way is probably setting yourself up for failure. But you have to start somewhere.

Special note: If you've been reading the other chapters and meal plans, you'll find that they have been fairly consistent in labeling proteins, fruits, nuts, vegetables, and so forth. For instance, a garbanzo bean was labeled as a "very lean protein plus one bread." But in this chapter, you'll be using foods a little more precisely. Instead of a very lean protein, for example, we might indicate that you need a specific number of bean or soy servings or certain types of vegetables daily. This will help you to use those foods to treat and prevent illnesses, much like a prescribed drug. Once you get the hang of it, you'll find it's not terribly difficult—just a few more details to remember.

THE DEHYDRATED-GUY FLUID PLAN

THE KEY HERE IS TO HAVE A FLUID PLAN, just as you have a food plan. You need a minimum of 9 to 11 cups of fluid each day, with at least 5 of those cups being water. Additional fluids, at least a couple of cups, will be needed if you travel or get sick. Eat foods that are high in fluid, specifically fruits, soups, and vegetables, and you can cut out several cups of fluid. And remember: stay away from alcohol.

The diet for the hypertensive guy (page 308) is a good one to follow for the dehydrated guy.

FLUID PLAN

Wake Up

1 cup water

Breakfast

2 cups fluid — 1 cup fat-free milk and 1 cup orange juice; or 1 cup fat-free milk and 1 cup coffee* or tea*

Snack

2 cups water — Sparkling water, or any bottled, filtered, or tap water

Lunch

1 to 2 cups fluid — Water, fat-free milk, tea*, coffee*, soda*, or fruit juice; 1 cup soup may be included here

Pre-Workout Snack

2 cups water

Workout

7 to 10 ounces every 10 to 20 minutes, more in extreme temperatures

Post-Workout

At least 2 cups fluid — A better guideline: Weigh yourself before and after exercise; drink 2 to 3 cups fluid within 2 hours after exercise for every pound of body weight you've lost

Dinner

1 to 2 cups fluid

*2 to 3 caffeinated beverages per day can be included as part of your total fluid intake. If you drink more than 3 caffeinated beverages per day, those above the first 3, as well as any alcoholic beverages, should not be counted toward your total daily fluid intake.

THE PRE- AND POST-OP MEAL PLAN

THE FOUNDATION OF THIS DIET IS ADEQUATE FLUIDS, protein, and calories; enough carbs to spare protein; an array of fruits and vegetables; and a healthy assortment of fats to get all the vitamins, minerals, phytochemicals, and antioxidants associated with keeping the immune system operating at peak levels. Then there are some special added attractions to enhance healing, decrease oxidative damage, diminish inflammation, and boost your natural anti-inflammatory processes. Last but not least, daily moderate exercise will also boost your immune function. So even if you're in the healing phase, as long as your doc says its okay, get out and move.

Daily Assumptions*†

2,500 calories
305 grams carbohydrates
163 grams protein
73 grams fat

Daily Breakdown*†

4 bread
6 fruit (2 citrus, 2 berry, 2 other)
4 milk
1 yogurt
8 teaspoons added sugar
6 vegetable (3 carotenoid,
   2 brassica, 1 allium)
6 poultry
4 fish
1 medium-fat protein
4 fat
1 bean
2 nut
2 soy

Note: Occasionally, a fat-free product, like mustard or cooking spray, is included on the menus. These do not count toward your daily breakdown but should not be overused.

*Use every day.

† Based on a 185-pound man.

THE MENU

DAY 1

Breakfast

2 bread	1 cup Shredded Wheat
1 milk	1 cup fat-free milk
1 citrus	1/2 cup orange juice
1 berry	3/4 cup fresh blueberries
1 medium-fat protein	1 egg, scrambled in a nonstick pan
1 fat	1 1/2 tablespoons ground flaxseed
	Water
	Oil-free cooking spray (for egg)

Snack

2 soy	1 cup edamame
1 carotenoid	1 cup carrot sticks
	Tea

Lunch

1 milk	1 cup fat-free milk
2 carotenoid	Salad with 1 1/2 cups romaine lettuce, 1/2 cup tomato, 1/2 cup cucumber
6 poultry	6 ounces turkey
1 bean	1/2 cup garbanzo beans
1 fat	1 tablespoon oil and vinegar

Pre-Workout Snack

1 other fruit	Peach
2 nut	20 peanuts
1 yogurt	1 cup fat-free yogurt

Post-Workout

SMOOTHIE

Blend until smooth.

1 milk	1 cup fat-free milk
1 citrus	1/2 cup orange juice with calcium
1 berry	1 1/4 cups frozen whole strawberries
6 teaspoons added sugar	2 tablespoons honey

Dinner

2 bread	Small ear corn on the cob
	Small whole-wheat roll
1 other fruit	Apple
2 brassica	1 cup steamed broccoli and cauliflower
1 allium	1/2 cup grilled onions
4 fish	4 ounces salmon, grilled
2 fat	8 Kalamata olives
	1 teaspoon olive oil
2 teaspoons added sugar	2 teaspoons sugar or honey
	Tea

DAY 2

Breakfast

Combine yogurt, fruit, and honey. Combine muffin and egg for sandwich.

2 bread	1 whole-wheat English muffin
1 milk	1 cup fat-free unsweetened yogurt
2 fruit	1/2 cup grapefruit juice
	1 1/4 cups fresh whole strawberries
1 medium-fat protein	1 egg, hard-cooked
1 fat	1 1/2 tablespoons ground flaxseed
	Water

Snack

2 nut	1 tablespoon peanut butter
1 carotenoid	1 cup carrot sticks
	Tea

Lunch

1 milk	1 cup fat-free milk
2 carotenoid	1 cup lettuce, $^1/_2$ cup tomato, $^1/_2$ cup roasted red pepper
6 poultry	6 ounces skinless white-meat chicken, grilled with lime juice
	1 teaspoon olive oil (for roasted vegetables)
1 fat	2 tablespoons fat-free dressing

Pre-Workout Snack

1 other fruit	Plum
2 soy	2 ounces soy nuts
1 yogurt	1 cup plain nonfat yogurt

Post-Workout

SMOOTHIE

Blend until smooth.

1 milk	1 cup fat-free milk
1 citrus	$^1/_2$ cup orange juice with calcium
1 berry	$^3/_4$ cup frozen blueberries
6 teaspoons added sugar	2 tablespoons honey

Dinner

2 bread	$1^1/_2$ cups cooked pasta
1 other fruit	Pear
2 brassica	1 cup Brussels sprouts, cooked
1 allium	$^1/_2$ cup shallots and garlic, grilled (with shrimp)
1 bean	$^1/_2$ cup kidney beans
4 fish	4 ounces shrimp, grilled
	2 teaspoons olive oil
2 fat	2 tablespoons fat-free dressing (for Brussels sprouts)
2 teaspoons added sugar	2 teaspoons sugar or honey
	Tea

DAY 3

Breakfast

2 bread	2 slices whole-wheat bread
1 milk	1 cup fat-free cottage cheese (on bread)
1 citrus	4 ounces freshly squeezed orange juice (with pulp)
1 berry	$^{3}/_{4}$ cup blueberries
1 medium-fat protein	1 egg, cooked sunny-side up in a nonstick pan
1 fat	$1^{1}/_{2}$ tablespoons ground flaxseed
	Water
	Oil-free cooking spray (for egg)

Snack

2 soy	2 ounces soy nuts
1 carotenoid	$^{1}/_{2}$ cup V8 juice
	Tea

Lunch

1 milk	1 cup fat-free milk
2 carotenoid	2 cups spinach and bok choy, stir-fried
6 poultry	6 ounces chicken, stir-fried with ginger and garlic
1 bean	$^{1}/_{2}$ cup black beans
1 fat	1 teaspoon oil (for stir-frying)

Pre-Workout Snack

1 other fruit	Nectarine
2 nut	10 cashews
1 yogurt	1 cup plain nonfat yogurt

Post-Workout

SMOOTHIE

Blend until smooth.

1 milk	1 cup fat-free milk
1 citrus	$^{1}/_{2}$ cup orange juice with calcium
1 berry	1 cup frozen raspberries
6 teaspoons added sugar	2 tablespoons honey

Dinner

2 bread	1 ounce croutons (for salad)
	1 cup chicken noodle soup
1 other fruit	1 slice watermelon
2 brassica	1 cup steamed cauliflower and broccoli
1 allium	$\frac{1}{2}$ cup onion (for salad)
4 fish	4 ounces swordfish, grilled with ginger and scallions
2 fat	2 teaspoons olive oil (for fish)
2 teaspoons added sugar	2 teaspoons sugar or honey
	Tea

DAY 4

Breakfast

1 milk	1 cup fat-free milk ($\frac{1}{2}$ cup for French toast)
1 citrus	$\frac{1}{2}$ cup orange juice
1 berry	1 cup raspberries

FRENCH TOAST (*See recipe directions on page 44.*)

2 bread	2 slices whole-wheat bread
1 medium-fat protein	1 egg
1 fat	$1\frac{1}{2}$ tablespoons ground flaxseed
	Water
	Oil-free cooking spray

Snack

2 nut	1 tablespoon almond butter
1 carotenoid	1 cup carrot sticks
	Tea

Lunch

1 milk	1 ounce skim milk mozzarella
2 carotenoid	2 cups tomatoes with balsamic vinegar
6 poultry	6 ounces turkey
1 fat	$\frac{1}{8}$ avocado
	Tea

Pre-Workout Snack

1 other fruit	1 apple
2 soy	1 cup edamame
1 yogurt	1 cup fat-free yogurt

Post-Workout

SMOOTHIE

Blend until smooth.

1 milk	1 cup fat-free milk
1 citrus	$\frac{1}{2}$ cup orange juice with calcium
1 berry	$1\frac{1}{4}$ cups frozen strawberries
6 teaspoons added sugar	2 tablespoons honey

Dinner

2 bread	1 hamburger bun
1 other fruit	17 grapes
2 brassica	1 cup coleslaw
1 allium	$\frac{1}{2}$ cup onion, garlic (for seasoning)
1 bean	$\frac{1}{2}$ cup baked beans
4 fish	4 ounces salmon burger
2 fat	8 Kalamata olives
	Included (in coleslaw)
2 teaspoons added sugar	Included (in baked beans)
	Tea

DAY 5

Breakfast

2 bread	1 cup quick oats (not instant)
1 milk	1 cup fat-free milk
1 citrus	$\frac{1}{2}$ cup orange juice
1 berry	$1\frac{1}{4}$ cups whole strawberries
1 medium-fat protein	1 egg, hard-cooked
1 fat	$1\frac{1}{2}$ tablespoons ground flaxseed
	Water

Snack

2 soy	1 cup edemame
1 carotenoid	$\frac{1}{2}$ cup V8 juice
	Tea

Lunch

1 milk — 1 cup fat-free milk

FAJITAS

Combine ingredients.

2 carotenoid — 1 cup sautéed peppers

2 tablespoons salsa

6 poultry — 6 ounces skinless white-meat chicken, grilled with lime juice

1 bean — 1/2 cup fat-free refried beans

1 fat — 1 teaspoon olive oil (for cooking)

Pre-Workout Snack

1 other fruit — 1 pear

2 nut — 2 tablespoons almond butter

1 yogurt — 1 cup plain nonfat yogurt

Post-Workout

SMOOTHIE

Blend until smooth.

1 milk — 1 cup fat-free milk

1 citrus — 1/2 cup orange juice with calcium

1 berry — 1 cup frozen blackberries

6 teaspoons added sugar — 2 tablespoons honey

Dinner

2 bread — 1 small pita

1/2 cup couscous

1 other fruit — 1 cup honeydew melon

2 brassica — 2 cups broccoli slaw

1 allium — 1/2 cup combined onion, shallot, garlic (in couscous)

4 fish — 4 ounces fresh trout (stuff with couscous)

2 fat — 2 tablespoons vinaigrette

2 teaspoons added sugar — 2 teaspoons sugar or honey

Tea

DAY 6

Breakfast

| 2 bread | 2 slices multigrain toast |
| 1 medium-fat protein | 1 egg, hard-cooked |

SMOOTHIE

Blend until smooth.

1 milk	1 cup fat-free milk
1 citrus	1/2 cup orange juice
1 berry	1 cup raspberries
1 fat	1 1/2 tablespoons ground flaxseed
	Water

Snack

2 nut	1 tablespoon peanut butter
1 carotenoid	1 cup carrots
	Tea

Lunch

1 milk	1 cup fat-free milk
2 carotenoid	1 cup tomato, 1 cup spinach
6 poultry	6 ounces turkey
1 fat	2 tablespoon reduced-fat ranch dressing

Pre-Workout Snack

1 other fruit	1 small banana
2 soy	2 ounces soy nuts
1 yogurt	1 cup fat-free yogurt

Post-Workout

SMOOTHIE

Blend until smooth.

1 milk	1 cup fat-free milk
1 citrus	1/2 cup orange juice with calcium
1 berry	1 cup frozen raspberries
6 teaspoons added sugar	2 tablespoons honey

Dinner

2 bread	2 slices rye bread
1 other fruit	1 cup cantaloupe
2 brassica	1 cup coleslaw
1 allium	$^1/_2$ cup chopped onion (mix into tuna)
1 bean	$^1/_2$ cup fava beans
4 fish	4 ounces tuna in olive oil, drained
2 fat	2 tablespoons mayonnaise (mix into tuna)
2 teaspoons added sugar	2 teaspoons sugar or honey
	Tea

DAY 7

Breakfast

2 bread	2 cups Kashi
1 milk	1 cup fat-free milk
1 citrus	$^1/_2$ cup grapefruit juice
1 berry	1 cup blackberries
1 medium-fat protein	1 egg, hard-cooked (for egg salad)
1 fat	$1^1/_2$ tablespoons ground flaxseed
	Water

Snack

2 soy	1 cup edamame
1 carotenoid	1 cup red pepper sticks
	Tea

Lunch

1 milk	1 cup fat-free milk
2 carotenoid	1 cup romaine lettuce, 1 cup tomato
6 poultry	6 ounces skinless white-meat chicken, grilled with lime juice
1 bean	$^1/_2$ cup pinto beans
1 fat	2 tablespoons reduced-fat ranch dressing
	1 teaspoon oil (to cook chicken)

Pre-Workout Snack

1 other fruit	17 grapes
2 nut	10 walnuts
1 yogurt	1 cup plain nonfat yogurt

Post-Workout

SMOOTHIE

Blend until smooth.

1 milk	1 cup fat-free milk
1 citrus	1/2 cup orange juice with calcium
1 berry	3/4 cup frozen blueberries
6 teaspoons added sugar	2 tablespoons honey

Dinner

2 bread	3-inch square of corn bread
1 other fruit	1 pear
2 brassica	1 cup broccoli, steamed
1 allium	1/2 cup leeks (for salmon)
4 fish	4 ounces salmon, poached
2 fat	1 teaspoon olive oil
	Included (in corn bread)
2 teaspoons added sugar	2 teaspoons sugar or honey
	Tea

CHAPTER SEVEN

Food and Longevity

FIGHT DISEASE WITH THE BEST ALLIES YOUR MONEY CAN BUY—FOOD

The human race has put a man on the moon, mapped its own genome, and developed a computer architecture that can link a guy in the heart of Manhattan with someone on Pitcairn Island in the South Pacific with a few keyboard clicks. Yet we've only scratched the surface of understanding the impact of food on longevity.

Your body is infinitely complex—a walking, talking collection of chemicals. Foods, too, are a complicated mishmash of chemical ingredients. Bring them together and you've got a science experiment whose intricacies rival anything the world's best physicists and engineers have ever devised. You probably don't think of yourself as a human test tube, but every time you bite into an apple or drink a beer, you're essentially performing a chemistry experiment. Each piece of food that enters your mouth is broken down into its smallest fractions—atoms and molecules—which ultimately interact with your genes. That turkey sandwich you scarf down at lunch may cause a chemical reaction in your cells that helps you get through your afternoon workout; that charcoal-grilled burger you inhale each night may spark the chemical change in your cells that eventually metastasizes into full-blown cancer.

Such are the mysteries of food, longevity, and life spans.

It wasn't long ago that mankind didn't need to worry about how food affected life spans. In earlier centuries and millennia—in fact, for most of human history—human life expectancy was 25 to 30, give or take a few years. Those short life spans had little, if anything, to do with the makeup of the human body. Genetically speaking, men have been the same for the past 40,000 years. If time travel were possible and you brought a caveman to the 21st century, there's no reason he couldn't live into his 70s and beyond.

Instead, we can blame early man's short life span on environmental factors like famine, pestilence, and flood (not to mention causes that were decidedly less biblical). Back then, guys usually were killed or otherwise perished long before their body had a chance to reach its natural expiration date. They had to worry about being devoured by predators, frozen to death by a sudden blizzard, or done in by something that today could be cured through a routine medical procedure, like an appendectomy. Think back to the worst toothache you've ever had. If dentists and painkillers didn't exist, what would you have done? Something that mundane could have killed you.

In a way, that's what makes the past 50 years so amazing: In a single half-century, we've advanced human control of our environment light years beyond the generations before. In the developed world, we can avoid environmental factors, or at least manage them with great success. Paramount among our advances is how we've learned to fight disease and treat injuries. We sanitize our food. We can transplant organs from one body to another. We can unblock blocked arteries, repair collapsed lungs, and even operate effectively on damaged brains.

In the process, we've redefined the idea of a "natural life span." Today, most men expect to live into their 70s and 80s, with some pressing well into their 100s and beyond. How long will we ultimately be able to live? Only the future can answer that, but it's not unreasonable to think that men will someday celebrate 100-year birthdays with regularity. The question that faces us today is: What is keeping us from getting there?

Our diets, for one thing. As medicine has advanced, our diets have gone rapidly downhill. The percentage of men and women over 50 with a chronic disease has skyrocketed. In one example from the American Diabetes Association, 18.2 million people in the United States alone have diabetes, a disease in which the body does not produce or properly use insulin. Another 20.1 million have "prediabetes"—blood glucose levels that are higher than normal but not yet high enough to be diagnosed as diabetes. In both cases, the number of patients for these diseases has jumped by the millions over the past three decades. Diabetes is the fifth leading cause of death by disease in the United States, and it contributes to higher overall rates of morbidity. People with diabetes are at higher risk for heart disease, blindness, kidney failure, extremity amputations, and other chronic conditions. The major cause? A diet loaded with calories, refined carbohydrates, and unhealthy fats—the diet that causes obesity.

The economic costs of such diseases are staggering, and diabetes alone cost the American public an estimated $132 billion in 2002. The social costs are also enormous, as a swelling population of individuals who can no longer support themselves must depend on others. When you see debates about Medicare and Social Security in the context of the ballooning federal budget deficit, one of the underlying truths is that supporting a nation of old, fat, unhealthy eaters is expensive.

The following review of the various ways nutrition can contribute to your ultimate demise is intended as a wake-up call, so it might be a little alarming at times. Looked at as a glass half-full, however, this information will show what an extraordinary positive impact food can have on your life.

Just to preface what follows with one example, Harvard researchers recently studied 3,000 subjects and found that eating breakfast daily resulted in a 35 to 50 percent reduction in the risk of getting diabetes, cancer, and heart disease.

On that note, here we go.

Inflammation

We mentioned free radicals in the last chapter, but they are far more dangerous over the long term than the short. To get an idea of what they do to your body over the long haul, picture a golf club that's been left outside for a few days and is beginning to rust. Or an apple that turns brown less than an hour after you bite into it. In both cases, you're witnessing oxygen's corrosive effects on a solid, known as oxidation.

If oxygen can do that to your nine-iron, imagine what it can do to your body's delicate tissues over the course of 80 years. Free radicals form from oxygen and can actually oxidize many of the structural components of your body's cells, zapping everything from the membrane down to receptors and enzymes, and, ultimately, DNA, your body's genetic software. When too many cells begin to mutate or die from this molecular onslaught, this program gets corrupted, and some very bad stuff can begin to happen—like cancer, heart disease, Alzheimer's, and arthritis. Somewhere at the root of all these diseases of lifestyle and aging is oxidative damage.

(Keep in mind, however, that you do need free radicals to some amount and degree. In fact, you'd

THE ORGANIC TRUTH

DOES ORGANIC FOOD MAKE A HEALTH DIFFERENCE? It depends on whom you ask. Yes, if you listen to the Organic Trade Association.

After a 1995 meeting, the trade association's standards board defined "organic agriculture" as "an ecological production management system that promotes and enhances biodiversity, biological cycles, and soil biological activity. It is based on minimal use of off-farm inputs and on management practices that restore, maintain, and enhance ecological harmony."

The board goes on to define "organic" as "a labeling term that denotes products produced under the authority of the Organic Foods Production Act." The principal guidelines for organic production are to use materials and practices that enhance the ecological balance of natural systems and that integrate the parts of the farming system into an ecological whole.

The association and other proponents say organic foods contain fewer pesticides and other harmful chemicals than nonorganic foods do. It's not just what organic foods lack, though. Advocates say they also have more of nature's good stuff, whether it's vitamin C, minerals like iron and magnesium, or phytonutrients like polyphenols—naturally occurring antioxidants that may help bolster the body's immune system.

Some scattered, fairly small-scale research has offered intriguing indications that this may well be the case. For example, one study found that frozen organic corn contained 52 percent more vitamin C than conventional corn did.

For others, though, the answer to the organic-foods question is a resounding . . . maybe. Though intriguing, the results from the studies that have been done to date in this area are inconclusive overall. Some research, like the aforementioned study, suggests that organic foods have enhanced nutritional value; other studies indicate that any differences may be insignificant. We have good data showing that populations with low intakes of fruits and vegetables have high levels of disease morbidity and mortality, but we have zero data showing that people who eat lots of traditionally grown fruits and vegetables are ill, and that people who eat organic fruits and vegetables are not.

die quickly without free radicals. Just to cite a few examples, they're employed by white blood cells to eradicate any foreign bodies that invade our cells, and the body also needs them to produce essential materials like prostaglandins, a group of hormone-like substances that help along numerous important processes that are underway inside the body.)

Our bodies take a free-radical beating every day. An increasingly compromised ozone layer, the heavy metals found in the environment, secondhand cigarette smoke—40,000 years ago, the human body had other things to worry about, but it didn't have to deal with those things, all of which produce a lot of free radicals. In an evolutionary sense, we haven't had time to adapt to them yet. The best we can do, probably, is to fortify our bodies with large amounts

I think organic produce does offer several obvious benefits. For one, farming methods employed by organic-foods manufacturers are much kinder to the earth than those of agribusiness conglomerates. As a result, farm workers harvesting organic produce aren't exposed to harmful chemicals.

Although that may not affect you directly, the higher levels of chemicals found in foods that haven't been produced organically almost certainly does. A small pilot study done recently at the University of Washington found that pesticide levels are much lower in children who eat organic fruits and vegetables than in those who eat traditionally farmed produce. So it looks like at least some of the chemicals used in farming do enter your body in measurable amounts.

Do I know for a fact that this makes a health difference? No. But it's not a huge stretch to think that chemicals formulated to kill molds, spores, pests, and fungi probably aren't great for human cells, either.

Without question, many conventional food producers adhere to strict government standards for pesticide use, intent on doing the right thing. But large quantities of food enter the United States from abroad, and you probably won't know if the produce on your table comes from Brazil, Chile, Mexico, or the Central Valley in California. Agricultural standards around the world vary greatly, with standards far more lax in some countries than others. FDA inspectors can't be everywhere all the time.

So why not just err on the side of fewer chemicals? Because organic foods can be significantly more expensive than standard produce, although this depends to some extent on where you live. Here's the bottom line, from my perspective: Buy organic produce if you want it, if it's available, and if you can afford it, but don't buy simply because you're afraid you're going to get sick from standard produce.

One footnote: Regardless of whether your produce is grown organically or through traditional means, always wash it before eating.

of the antioxidants that whole foods provide. It's a matter of self-defense, really.

Free radicals are also produced in abundance by modern methods of preparing food, like frying foods in fats and oils. It's yet another reason to avoid fast food, although heavy processing elevates the free-radical potential of even mundane foods. The body is designed to manage free radicals below a certain threshold, but when that threshold was hardwired 40,000 years or so ago, men were scavenging for berries and hunting game with rocks, not having their dinner dipped into a vat of scorching fat by a fast-food employee.

All this is compounded when you look at the stresses our bodies encounter every day. I'm not talking about a small cut that gets infected, swollen, and sore. A joint can also become inflamed and sore from a one-time event, like a vigorous workout, or from something more chronic, like arthritis. Regardless, free radicals are proliferating, and your body is basically sending out chemical sentries to deal with the damage. When you see the redness and the swelling, you're looking at an army of cells that have come to repair the damage. It's a battlefield.

Targeting Hidden Inflammation

The inflammation we're aware of is one thing; what we see or feel is just the smaller pockets of inflammation occurring in our bodies. There are other inflamed areas in our body that we aren't even aware of and that spell trouble.

Progressive gum disease is a perfect example of inflammation that can go largely undetected for years—it doesn't produce any acute pain, even though you might see some redness if you look closely enough. To make things worse, these stealth inflammation processes send chemicals out into the body that can cause further disease unrelated to the inflammation's place of origin. For example, science has shown that the aforementioned gum disease can actually increase the risk of developing heart disease. A study published recently in the *Journal of Periodontology* reported that effects from periodontal disease, a chronic bacterial infection of the gums, causes the waste from oral bacteria to enter the bloodstream and encourage your body to manufacture C-reactive protein. That protein inflames arteries and promotes blood-clot formation, increasing your risk of heart disease over time.

Gum disease, not surprisingly, could have a lot to do with what you're eating. If your diet is heavily dependent on things like fruits and vegetables, especially those high in fiber, you'll probably develop less plaque than someone eating a diet of highly processed foods, especially sugar. Left to accumulate, plaque becomes tartar, and tartar can produce the symptoms of gingivitis—more inflammation. (Look for more on food and dental care in chapter 9.)

Digestion

Although it can hit anywhere, the source point for much of the body's internal inflammation is concentrated in the digestive system. Constant distress in this region increases the risk of developing cancer in the colon or other parts of the gastrointestinal (GI) tract. Just imagine how much inflammation is caused by constipation, one of the most common ailments in the United States. Characterized by an infrequent passing of stools, constipation can lead quickly to hemorrhoids—pretty much the inflammation poster child—and, left untreated, can eventually increase your risk of getting bowel cancer.

The point here is that one of the best nutritional strategies for life extension is to eat foods that counter inflammation. Think of the doctor who prescribes an anti-inflammatory for you after surgery. He wants to control your postoperative pain, but by bringing inflammation down, he moves the entire healing process forward much more rapidly. Like that doctor, you want to decrease the level of inflammatory chemicals; in this case, though, they are circulating throughout your body. Do that and you can decrease your risk of developing a disease down the line. And by accomplishing this with whole foods, you avoid the side effects that these potent pharmaceuticals can produce, including more GI irritation (which kind of takes you back to square one).

Antioxidants Redux

The best antidote to swelling and free-radical damage is to try and prevent it with antioxidants, or at least let those antioxidants bolster the immune system once the damage has been done. Antioxidants are a quadruple threat to free radicals. They can scavenge and destroy them, or turn them into safe and useful molecules. They can protect tissues against the damage that free radicals inflict, or boost chemicals essential to the immune system's front line of defense. There is no escaping them; they can save your life. And, when it comes to jamming as many antioxidants as you can into your diet, there are only two rules:

1. Get as many as you can, as often as you can.
2. Look for bright and deeply colored food: orange, yellow, green, and red.

A note on number 2 there: We're not talking about M&Ms. We're talking vegetables and fruit, from leafy green spinach to sweet, bright oranges. It won't surprise you that Americans don't eat enough fruits and vegetables. But you may be surprised that, every day, half of us don't eat a single piece of fruit all day long. The American diet is decidedly brown and beige, the colors of meats and starches.

Invariably, diets like these don't fight free radicals efficiently. Without fruit, guys don't get enough phytonutrients or phytochemicals, which your body needs to fight disease, including cancer. You can get some of these and other nutrients from other sources, including dairy products, eggs, and fish (be-

lieve it or not, they are now referred to as zoochemicals), but you don't get as much variety from them, and what you do get can be accompanied by high calories and unhealthy fats.

The Foods to Choose

We covered the specific foods that fight inflammation in the last chapter, but we didn't discuss which ones are best for fighting long-term problems. Here's a rundown of those.

Citrus. If I die trying, I'm going to convince you to get more citrus in your diet. Citrus fruits are especially important disease-protectors. The high content of vitamin C, a natural antioxidant, may protect cell membranes and DNA from oxidative damage that can lead to cancerous changes. Citrus also contains about 20 carotenoids, all antioxidants associated with reducing macular degeneration, the leading cause of blindness in the United States after age 65. Pink grapefruit contains a high level of lycopene, the red pigment popularized in tomatoes that has a significant antitumor property. Berries, which are great sources of vitamin C, are also excellent sources of the antioxidants anthocyanins, which protect against heart disease.

Broccoli. Again, a food that is high in vitamin C, as are all leafy green vegetables. For anyone who bristles at the idea of munching on the leafy heads of broccoli, here's a thought: Just eat the stalks. Though some nutrients, like vitamin A, are concentrated in broccoli's leafy florets, you'll find rich amounts of vitamin C in both the stalks and the florets. Again, I'd prefer that you eat the entire veggie. But if it means the difference between broccoli or no broccoli at all, then by all means, off with their heads.

Tomatoes. Tomatoes contain as many as 10,000 phytochemicals. One of the most important is lycopene, an antioxidant that may help prevent not only cancer but heart disease as well. One study indicates that men who eat tomato-based meals at least six times per week reduced their chances of getting prostate cancer by more than 60 percent.

Carrots. Carrots, of course, contain one of the best-known and best-studied phytochemicals, beta-carotene. Responsible for making carrots orange, beta-carotene is an antioxidant nutrient known to dampen oxidation, keeping that normal metabolic process from becoming dangerous. These antioxidant properties have been demonstrated in laboratory studies.

One important thing to note here: Beta-carotene can, depending on the environment and quantity in which it occurs, act as a pro-oxidant. In other words, it can hurt you by promoting oxidation rather than fighting it. Before you go questioning everything you've read in this book, understand that

RIPE FOR THE PICKING

MOST GUYS EQUATE FRUIT WITH APPLES, ORANGES, AND BANANAS, maybe with a pineapple thrown in on occasion for good measure, but the choices are legion. Virtually all fruits are jam-packed with phytonutrients that can protect you from disease, prolonging your life. Add some or all of these lesser-known fruits to your repertoire.

- **Star fruit (carambola).** Why: More antioxidants than in big-name fruits like avocados and pineapples. And antioxidants are a great weapon against age-related illnesses such as cancer, cardiovascular disease, and diabetes. Tastes: Sweet and tangy. Look for: Firm and shiny ones with few blemishes.

- **Papaya.** Why: It's over-the-counter stroke medicine, with vitamin E and folate. Tastes: Like nothing else; light and somewhat tart. Look for: The yellowest ones.

- **Kiwifruit.** Why: All the vitamin C of an orange, about half the potassium of a banana, and a cache of potentially cancer-preventing chlorophyll. Tastes: Vaguely strawberryish. Look for: Firmness, no shriveling.

- **Blood orange.** Why: The antioxidants called anthocyanins, which make these oranges red, protect you from cancer and help improve blood flow. Tastes: Like a really sweet orange. Look for: Firm, heavy ones.

- **Passionfruit.** Why: Contains more phytosterols, compounds similar to cholesterol, than any other fruit. USDA research shows that phytosterols crowd LDL cholesterol out of arteries, lowering levels by as much as 17 percent. Tastes: Like tart watermelon. Look for: Bigger ones with slightly wrinkled skin.

- **Mango.** Why: Just one provides almost 90 percent of your daily allowance of vitamin A, more than any other fruit. That'll protect your skin and maybe even fend off liver cancer caused by alcohol abuse. Tastes: Like a collision between an apricot and a peach. Look for: One that has a strong, sweet smell.

- **Prickly pear.** Why: More magnesium than in any other fruit, which helps control blood pressure, relieve migraines, regulate blood sugar, and fight fatigue in people who are magnesium deficient. Tastes: Like a melon, only milder. Look for: Deep, uniform color. Spots signal decay.

the beta-carotene in food has never shown negative effects. Only when given as a supplement in research studies have scientists seen negative consequences of beta-carotene. The moral? Get your beta-carotene from food.

Others. There are other plant foods of utmost importance, including a variety of beans, especially soybeans, cereals, nuts and olives, avocados, and vegetable oils. It's all about variety. Not just having variety among food groups, like a fruit, a vegetable, and a grain, but great variety *within* each food group as well. And you'll soon see that the food groups in *Power Food* only vaguely resemble those you learned about in fourth grade. Ours are separated by much finer detail and health needs of the body. We leave much less room for error.

Your Heart

My coauthor, Jeff, once interviewed an extraordinary guy named Christopher Michael Langan. His IQ is 196, well above Einstein's. Some people think he's the smartest man on earth today, and what ultimately convinced Jeff of that assertion is that he finds a way to live on $6,000 a year—in New York, no less. He works occasionally as a bar bouncer on Long Island, earning just enough to rent his living space and eat, so that he can dedicate himself to his true passion: figuring out how the universe came to be, how it works now, and how it will all end. Hoping to catch a glimpse into such weighty intellectual explorations, Jeff drew up a list of profound questions to ask, including the big one: What happens to us when we die?

Drum roll, please.

"Your heart stops beating," he said.

That pretty much sums it up: If you want to live a long, healthy life, you have to keep that sucker pumping.

Sadly, I know plenty of guys in their 30s and 40s who think they still have a few years until they need to think about heart health seriously. That's a common mode of thinking, albeit a significantly outdated one. Back during the Korean War, many autopsies were performed on American GIs killed in battle. Most were 18- to 20-year-olds—boys, basically. Much to the amazement of doctors and medical examiners, many of these young men already showed signs of arterial damage. It was the first time medicine documented that arteries could be affected at such a young age.

In the spirit of those autopsies, I send a message to anyone out there in their 20s and 30s: The time to eat better is *now*. Ignore me and by the time you hit 40, your ticker could be a ticking time bomb.

Saturated and Trans Fats

The biggest culprit when it comes to arteries hardening is saturated fat, featured prominently in fatty red meat and high-fat dairy products. Solid at room temperature, saturated fat has been shown in study after study to raise harmful cholesterol—LDL—which is a major risk factor for heart disease, not to mention cancer and a host of other diseases. One Finnish study puts this issue in plainer terms. In the study, scientists followed a group of children from age 7 months until 7 years. Some of the children received nutritional counseling to help steer their saturated-fat consumption, but others had no counseling. By 7 years old, the boys from the intervention (counseling) group had lower total cholesterol and LDL cholesterol levels, as well as smaller LDL particle sizes—all factors that help prevent heart disease.

Saturated fats aren't a problem in moderation; in fact, your body needs some to store for last-resort energy and to keep warm. But as those roles suggest, saturated fat isn't dynamic—it basically just sits in your body. If too much is sitting around, you are in trouble.

Possibly far worse for you are saturated fat's

Fat-Fighting Tips

If you are looking to cut out fat, here are some of your safest plays.

- Meat is a major source of saturated fats. When you eat meat, go for lean cuts of round, sirloin, or flank in portions sized no bigger than your palm. Or have chicken, turkey, or fish instead.
- If you can actually see fat on the meat, trim if off before you eat or cook it.
- To avoid melting fat back into the meat, bake, broil, grill, or steam it using cooking racks.
- Eschew, don't chew, bologna and salami sandwiches. Choose low-fat chicken or turkey breast instead.
- Especially because you should be eating or drinking dairy two to four times a day, choose low-fat or fat-free alternatives to products like whole milk.
- If you eat eggs, a potentially major source of cholesterol, substitute three egg whites and one yolk for two whole eggs, or use egg substitutes.

partners in crime, the trans fats. These pop up most frequently in fried foods, commercial baked goods, microwave popcorn, and margarines. Some experts think they're even worse for your heart than saturated fats. After all, that Finnish study showed that saturated fat is associated with heart disease. But studies have shown that trans fatty acids, gram for gram, put people at a $2^1/_2$- to 10-fold higher risk of developing heart disease than saturated fat does. Bottom line: If you want to live a long, healthy life, you should minimize these fats in your diet.

Among foods loaded with saturated and trans fats, some of the worst foods are butter, choco-late, American cheese, piecrust, pork sausage, and bacon.

The Good Fat

Notice we didn't say that the biggest issue regarding food and your heart was fat. That's because the un-saturated plant and fish oil fats—such as those in fish, olive oil, and nuts—actually protect your heart. Unsaturated fats are far more biologically active than saturated fats, and much of what they're doing inside the body is beneficial. Studies show that people who eat fatty fish at least once a week dramatically lower their risk for a heart attack. The reason is that the fatty acids in these fish carry LDL (bad) cholesterol out of the bloodstream, before it can attach to fat molecules and stick to the walls of your arteries.

The fatty acids in these fish, called polyunsaturated fats, are considered "virtually essential," meaning that although your body may manufacture a small amount, you need to consume them to acquire enough of them. That means you need to know what you're looking for. Omega-3 fatty acids, for example, are found in high-fat, cold-water fish such as salmon, sardines, tuna, halibut, mackerel, and trout. Flaxseed is the best plant source of the essential fats linoleic and linolenic acid, precursors of omega 3s. Pumpkin seeds and walnuts also contain them.

Monounsaturated fats can help your heart, too. Like polyunsaturates, they're liquid at room temperature but sometimes get mushy and almost solidify when cooled. These fats are abundant in several oils—olive, peanut, and canola—as well as in nuts, olives, and avocados.

For decades, monounsaturated fats were sort of the ignored middle child of fats, stuck between the big, bad saturated fats on one side and the revered polyunsaturated fats on the other. Increasingly, however, food researchers think monounsaturated fats rank right up with polyunsaturated when it comes to heart health. In some cases, mono may even be better.

Not only do they appear to lower LDL, as the polyunsaturated fats do, but they also elevate HDL, which has a beneficial effect. This potent double-whammy helps explain why the Mediterranean diet, with its heavy reliance on olive oil, is so heart healthy.

Get a Heart-y Helping

As with all long-term disease, heart problems can be counteracted and prevented by focusing on phytochemicals—not coincidentally, the same high-antioxidant, high-phytochemical foods that we keep talking about. Eat your fatty fish and omega-3 fats. Get your water-soluble fiber from fruits, vegetables, oats, and beans, and you'll keep cholesterol levels lower. Target vitamin E—rich vegetable oils, olives, and nuts for their antioxidant powers. And drink your red grape juice and wine for the resveratrol it contains, an antioxidant that is important and may even be antiaging.

One thing I want to emphasize: The disease-preventing power of fruit, a recurring theme in this book, is felt acutely in the heart. Anthocyanins are the water-soluble, reddish pigments found in many fruits, such as strawberries, cherries, cranberries, raspberries, blueberries, grapes, and black currants. They inhibit cholesterol synthesis and provide protection against heart disease. The carotenoids are powerful antioxidants that also stimulate the immune system, and guys with high levels of them in their blood have a reduced risk of both heart disease and cancer, not to mention macular degeneration. Carotenoids are the pigments found in yellow-orange fruits, and yellow-orange, red, and green vegetables.

Several studies have shown that the risk of heart disease drops with increasing consumption of vitamin C, carotenoids, and citrus fruits. One of those studies showed that men with low levels of vitamin C and carotene were two to four times as likely to develop heart disease and stroke as those whose

Good Taste, Bad Choice

One common denominator of foods high in saturated fats and trans fats is that they taste really good. That may seem like a cruel joke from on high, or perhaps an invisible test of willpower, but the truth is that American consumers have conditioned themselves (and allowed themselves to be conditioned) to enjoy the taste of these foods. Your parents' parents probably ate that stuff and fed it to your parents, who in turn fed it to you.

Maybe you still eat it. After all, it's classically American to eat a high-fat diet—as American as Mom, baseball, and apple pie.

You can recondition your taste buds, however. Eat "clean" for a few months, and then see how appealing three greasy strips of bacon seem. With a cleaner palate, you'll also start to enjoy the amazing flavor of fresh fruits and vegetables, whole grains, and fish.

antioxidant consumption from fruits and vegetables was adequate. In the United States, men with low vitamin C intakes have a significantly higher risk of cardiovascular disease and death compared with men eating the highest levels of vitamin C. Heart disease risks appear to be the lowest in people eating an average of at least 11 pounds of citrus fruit per year.

High Blood Pressure

At day's end, the best measure of whether you're winning the battle for heart health is blood pressure. Except for your body temperature, arguably no single number or set of numbers offers a more accurate quick read on the state of a man's health. Blood pressure measures how easily your life force is flowing throughout your body, which in turn gives a good indication, albeit not a complete or infallible one, of the exertion level of your heart.

High blood pressure is a warning that something is wrong and possibly getting worse. The greater the pressure, the harder your ticker has to work—and, more often than not, the sooner your circulatory system will break down. At best, you'll likely need a lifestyle change or some medication to fix it. At worst, you'll suffer a stroke or heart attack that no doctor can save you from.

What's happening is that the pressure against the artery walls is too high. Think about a fire hose, where you leave the water on but the sprayer on the end is turned off or very restricted. There's only so much pressure that fire hose can handle. If the pressure is too high, a bubble forms in the hose. Eventually, it bursts.

You don't want that to happen in your brain or anywhere else in your body.

The problem of high blood pressure, a.k.a. hypertension, has slowly grown into an epidemic in the United States over the past three decades, thanks largely to the prevalence of saturated fats in the American diet. But the problem got a lot worse overnight on May 14, 2003—or at least some new information cast a clearer light on just how insidious the problem had become. On that day, federal health officials changed their blood pressure guidelines, having decided the old guidelines misled people about the severity of their problems. The new guidelines were far more strict, moving 45 million Americans away from borderline status and placing them squarely in a category called "prehypertension," which describes individuals with a systolic reading (measuring when the heart contracts) of 120 to 139, and a diastolic reading (measuring between heartbeats) of 80 to 89.

One in four Americans—roughly 50 million adults—are even worse off: They *have* hypertension, meaning they score above the high end of the ranges for prehypertension. The most commonly treated ailment in the United States, hypertension is called a silent killer because many or all of the symptoms often don't become manifest until extensive damage has already been done. It's also a particularly lethal problem because it precedes so many pathologies, like kidney disease, and some catastrophic health events, including heart disease and stroke.

Unfortunately, only one out of three people with hypertension succeed in lowering it to safe levels. Particularly because genetics play a role in high blood pressure, lowering it isn't easy. Drugs are the quickest and easiest way to manage high blood pressure, but they have side effects. No drug targets one problem and that problem only.

Introducing the DASH Diet

Your diet is a more natural and extremely effective way to manage hypertension. First, a high correlation exists between having high blood pressure and being overweight, so weight loss alone can make a huge difference. There's also a diet specifically for lowering hypertension, recommended by the National Heart, Lung, and Blood Institute. It's called the DASH diet, which stands for Dietary Approaches to Stop Hypertension. This approach mirrors much of what is emphasized throughout *Power Food:* going heavy on the fruits, vegetables, low-fat dairy products, and whole grains while lowering intake of saturated fats. My diet for high blood pressure will be similar to DASH, albeit with a *Power Food* twist. For example, I like you to have more protein than it allows for—specifically, more fish.

Those minor differences aside, the DASH diet's creators have a lot of research behind their work, and they've come up with a beautiful dietary model to treat and prevent hypertension. If a guy doesn't eat that way already, switching to a DASH-based diet often can lower his blood pressure within a month.

In the original 454-subject study, those who followed DASH compliance had average decreases of

11.4 points in systolic blood pressure and 5.5 points diastolic blood pressure. That's significant, and that's without any weight change, without any reduction of sodium intake, and without medication. The effects of the latter shouldn't be underestimated. If you're taking a beta-blocker, which is the most common hypertensive medication, you can't exercise as well as you did before because it slows your heart rate, making it harder to train at higher intensities. Walking uphill becomes a challenge, and chasing after your dog can become practically impossible. So even as a guy's blood pressure falls, he doesn't necessarily feel better. When the choice is between lowering your blood pressure and feeling rotten, or lowering it and feeling fine, is the decision really that hard?

Losing weight on top of that makes a huge additional impact, but one thing the DASH diet designers discovered is that hypertension isn't just about body weight. A variety of blood-related factors also affect hypertension. For example, having the right levels of electrolytes in your blood is key. So the DASH diet not only is calorie-controlled but also prescribes specific levels of consumption for potassium, magnesium, and calcium. Too much or too little of these can negatively affect hypertension. The designers of DASH recommend that you get these minerals in ample supply as part of whole foods, by and large. For example, the 2,100-calorie-version DASH diet contains 4,700 milligrams of potassium, 500 milligrams of magnesium, and 1,240 milligrams of calcium. That's two to three times higher than what's found in the average American diet. You'll get your magnesium from grains and nuts, your potassium from fruit, and your calcium from dairy. Sweets are restricted to control the added sugar in your diet.

One thing I hear from guys is how much they hate vegetables. As you've probably guessed by now, it's pretty difficult to improve anything in your body

So What about Sodium?

Notice I haven't mentioned the negative effects of sodium in the discussion of high blood pressure. After all, isn't excessive salt consumption synonymous with high blood pressure?

Not necessarily. Some people are sodium sensitive, but most of the population isn't. For them, playing with sodium levels isn't going to help much. In fact, most people are more sensitive to minerals like potassium, magnesium, and calcium. These are actually more important in controlling hypertension than sodium is. (That said, buckets of sodium can be harmful. Try to use in moderation.)

if you aren't eating enough of them. The same goes for lowering blood pressure. But if you think about it, there are a lot of guy-friendly ways to get color into your diet.

■ Cut veggies up and hide them in your food. Zucchini, squash, and carrots work well this way.
■ Mix 'em with meat. Glutamate dulls bitterness.
■ Load them onto a pizza.
■ Dull their bite by steaming, microwaving, or stir-frying them.
■ Throw some salt on there; it interferes with bitterness somehow. (But avoid this step if you've already got hypertension.)
■ Sauté them in olive oil, sesame oil, or peanut oil.
■ Smother things like chicken or ground turkey in tomato paste—it's a vegetable.
■ Dip them in salsa or low-fat dressing.

The more you do this, the faster your body will get used to eating veggies, and the quicker your taste for them will grow. If you're looking to see your blood pressure drop, few things are more important.

Cancer

Two facts to start:

- Your risk of developing cancer increases dramatically with age. One in five men older than 60 are diagnosed with it.
- Other than smoking or maybe living across the street from a toxic waste dump, nothing puts you at greater risk of getting cancer—and dying from it—than obesity.

We've known for years that being overweight—or worse, obese—is a major risk factor for all kinds of bad things, including hyperinsulinemia, insulin-resistance, Type 2 diabetes mellitus, hypertension, high cholesterol, and heart disease. Now, thanks to a recent study sponsored by the American Cancer Society and published in the *New England Journal of Medicine,* we can add virtually all types of cancer to that list as well.

Obesity and Cancer

In the study, scientists tracked a large group of men and women for over 16 years. Starting out, the height and weight of the men and women were recorded. Subsequently, their illnesses and causes of death were also tallied and recorded. Comparing those two

HERE'S TO YOUR . . . HEALTH?

DEPENDING ON WHOM YOU LISTEN TO, alcohol is either a fountain of youth or the first thing that will kill you. Not surprisingly, our opinion falls somewhere in between.

As long as you drink in moderation, alcohol isn't going to kill you (unless you get behind the wheel of a car while drunk, but that's another story). Drink too much, though, and it's pretty clear that alcohol isn't good for you. Alcohol is a toxin. The more you drink, the worse it is for you.

Usually, two drinks is considered the limit. They could come in the form of wine, beer, or both.

Here are some of the key considerations regarding alcohol and longevity. As you'll see, it's a bit of a mixed bag:

- The antioxidant properties of red wine are intriguing. Red wine (red grape juice and grapes) contain a heart-protecting phytochemical called resveratrol, which has antioxidant properties. That would also allow red wine to fight free radicals, the molecular motors of the aging process. Whether you get enough resveratrol from one or two glasses of red wine with dinner is uncertain.
- Dark beers also have antioxidants that protect the heart. In studies at the University of Wisconsin–Madison Medical School, dark beer showed an ability to inhibit blood platelets from clotting. Israeli researchers found a link between lager and a lower risk of blocked blood vessels.
- Wine belly? Because obesity is a leading cause of diabetes, that belly hanging over your belt from too much drinking is a longevity issue. Regarding that fat fold around your

data sets through statistical analysis, researchers found that their obese subjects—people with a body mass index (BMI) over 29.9—showed a dramatically increased risk of dying from all types of cancer. (See page 100 to calculate your BMI.)

Some questioned the design of the study, saying that having subjects report their own body weight and height, rather than measuring them, was a suspect methodology, as people have a tendency to underestimate the actual figures or willfully misstate them. Critics also said that basing a research study on a height and weight reported only once doesn't necessarily give a real picture of how their body weight might have changed over the 16 years. The researchers themselves raised this point: Obese patients are often underdiagnosed and undertreated for disease. If that's true, even if obesity was a risk factor in the development of the cancer, substandard medical care might have actually caused death.

But the study's overall implications cannot be ignored: If these BMI levels were in fact *below* the actual values, and the risk of dying from cancer *increases* as BMI values rise, it's possible that the risk of dying from cancer when you're obese may be even higher than reported. And, yes, multiple measures of BMI done over the course of 16 years would have been more representative of subjects' body weight evolution, but research into the body-weight patterns of

waist, is it more likely to come from wine, beer, or liquor? The studies are varied, sometimes even contradictory. The most relevant experiment for you in this case is probably the one you do on yourself.

▪ Alcohol and the liver. Alcoholics are more likely to get hepatitis and liver cancer than non-alcoholics are. (The liver processes and detoxifies alcohol.) Alcohol intake is also positively associated with colon cancer: The more you drink, the greater your risk. Needless to say, that's a longevity issue.

▪ Alcohol as a cholesterol fighter. A recent French study found that alcohol raised levels of HDL, the good cholesterol.

▪ Alcohol as a diuretic. Throughout this book, we've hammered home the importance of hydration, so it should be noted that alcohol is a natural diuretic, meaning it causes you to lose more fluid. Alcohol does this by turning off the hormones that help the body reabsorb fluids.

▪ Wine as a blood thinner. A little vino may be similar to aspirin in this respect. By keeping platelets from getting sticky, it appears to lower the risk for heart attacks and strokes.

The bottom line here goes to the prestigious *New England Journal of Medicine,* which recently published a study showing that moderate daily alcohol consumption lowers a man's risk of heart disease, but regularly having more than a couple of stiff ones at a time increases your risk for a variety of ailments, including high blood pressure and various cancers.

I'll drink to that.

adult Americans shows that they tend to get fatter, not leaner, as they age. The odds are slim that most subjects grew skinnier over the duration of the study.

What the study appears to show is that a guy's risk of dying of cancer rises dramatically if he's obese even once as an adult. It reinforces what many of us in the health and nutrition fields already suspected: The more overweight you are, the better the chances are that you'll die from cancer, regardless of the underlying factors. And if you're obese—really, really fat—the risk you'll die from cancer probably doubles.

What this study doesn't tell us is why being overweight causes cancer, or whether your risk of cancer death decreases if you become overweight and then lose some of the excess baggage. But other studies have shown that increased adipose tissue— a.k.a. body fat—disturbs hormone control and cell chemistry. A study in Poland in 2002 investigated the influence of body fat levels on the secretion of the hormones leptin and cortisol. The author found that increased body fat alters secretion of leptin, cortisol, or both, leading to abnormal levels of the hormones and disturbed metabolic states. Consider that one carcinogen alone can make a healthy cell cancerous, and you begin to understand the danger such a change can bring.

In contrast to the bad news linking obesity with cancer are studies examining the link between energy intake, metabolic syndrome, and cancer. A study investigating calorie restriction and rates of illness and death in rhesus monkeys has been ongoing for more than 15 years. One group of monkeys has been fed a slightly calorie-reduced diet; a group of their peers has been allowed to eat at will. The restricted monkeys seem to maintain a healthy body-fat range between 10 and 22 percent. At those body-fat levels, they seem to avoid the age-related changes that lead to abnormal blood-sugar control, obesity, and diabetes in the unrestricted monkeys. The data suggest that calorie restriction is allowing the monkeys to live longer.

So what can you do with this information? If you're already fit, keep up the good work. Continue eating well and getting to the gym. If you're overweight, losing weight will decrease your risk of developing cancer. The status quo puts you at above-average risk for this devastating illness. Undoubtedly, you'll be healthier if you eat a more balanced diet and exercise consistently. And if you control your calorie intake, you'll ultimately lose weight.

If you're intent on losing weight with an eye toward lowering your cancer risk, you'll need to establish an action plan, including good eating (see the meal plans in this chapter and in chapter 3), good exercise (see chapter 5), regular physical exams (see your doctor), and stress reduction (see a therapist, if necessary.) A carefully planned, well-thought-out program of exercise and nutrition almost always precedes success. Flying by the seat of one's pants inevitably leads to disappointment and failure. Take, for example, a new study that reviewed six research publications that in turn evaluated daily diets of between 800 and 1,600 calories using meal-replacement products fortified with vitamins and minerals, plus at least one meal per day. Subjects had successfully lost weight when measured at the end of 3 months, then again at 1 year. Their biomarkers for cardiovascular disease and diabetes also changed for the better. What's more, the subjects using the meal-replacement products showed significantly better weight-loss results than those not using the products yet consuming the same number of calories. Where body weight is concerned, it's not just how much you eat that matters, but what you eat, as well.

Chemical Warfare

As you realize from the preceding inflammation section, the food-cancer link isn't limited to being overweight—the intrinsic nature of foods themselves can play a role. The effect of nutritional biochemistry on genetics has been a hazy, gray area until recently, when the picture cleared somewhat through investigations at a microscopic level (although it's certainly still not black and white). Plant chemicals interact with our genes in various ways: some good, some bad. But the cutting-edge research in this area is almost uniformly fascinating.

Broccoli. All vegetables have formidable cancer-fighting properties because of their phytochemicals—just to cite one of countless examples, a recent Yale study found that people who avoid vegetables increase their risk of getting colon cancer.

But not all veggies are created equal. For example, you are less likely to get certain cancers if you work broccoli into your diet. A recent study from Mount Sinai Medical Center in New York was trying to figure out why consumption of cruciferous vegetables such as broccoli is inversely related to prostate cancer risk. They found that a chemical in the veggie, sulforaphane, inhibits the initiation of prostate cancer and the growth of tumor cells. (So if you consider that eating broccoli is a pain in the butt, just imagine the alternative.) It also appears to prevent breast cancer: When added to live human cells in a lab dish, sulforaphane activated the production of special enzymes that ward off cancer.

Researchers don't have bulletproof insight into how broccoli fights cancer, but theories have emerged that make some sense. If the body doesn't get enough of the plant chemicals that come from

FOODS THAT GIVETH, FOODS THAT TAKETH AWAY

Here's a quick list of your ultimate "Do" and "Don't" foods for longevity.

Life Extenders

- Brewer's yeast
- Fatty cold-water fish, including salmon, mackerel, and black cod
- Flaxseed
- Fruits and vegetables, especially tomato and tomato products, watermelon, onions, kale, broccoli, cabbage, cauliflower, Brussels sprouts, green beans, olives, apples, citrus, pineapple, and prunes
- Green, Oolong, and black tea
- Nuts
- Oatmeal
- Red wine and grape juice
- Soy
- Seeds
- Vegetable oils
- Water
- Whole grains
- Yogurt

Life Shorteners

- Alcoholic drinks, more than two a day
- Flame grilling (high exposure)
- High-fat foods, especially saturated fats and trans fatty acids
- High-fructose corn syrup
- High-glycemic index carbs (high intake)
- Highly processed foods, such as baked goods and snack foods
- Plastic containers in the microwave
- Red meat (high intake)

something like broccoli, certain systems might not get turned off that, left unchecked, ultimately might overproduce cellular changes that lead to cancer. Maybe the sulforaphane interacts with enzymes in such a way that eventually shuts off those genes. A recent University of Illinois study showed that lightly cooked broccoli releases two or three times the sulforaphane that raw broccoli does.

Broccoli also contains the cancer fighters indoles and isothiocyanates. Indoles work against dangerously high levels of estrogen, potentially reducing the risk of breast cancer, and isothiocyanates have been associated with prevention of stomach and lung cancers.

Broccoli alternatives. If you hate broccoli, you may want to try eating cauliflower. Or Brussels sprouts and kohlrabi. All of these have the same sulforaphane, indoles, and isothiocyanates as broccoli, and getting variety in your diet can be more helpful over the long run in fighting cancer. Alternatively, watercress and turnips are high in isothiocyanates.

Cabbage. Then there's cabbage. It also belongs to the brassica family of vegetables and also contains sulforaphane, indoles, and isothiocyanates. Although green cabbage is lower in carotenoids—you can tell by its lack of dark coloring—it's another great vegetable to include in your diet. Red cabbage gives you a boost of anthocyanins, a potent antioxidant flavonoid that is also protective against heart disease and cancer.

Now, you may think that you hate cabbage, too. But what about sauerkraut and coleslaw? It's a rare guy who doesn't like at least one of these, and both are made with cabbage. Both contain the same indoles and isothiocyanates as regular, boring cabbage. So grab a Reuben sandwich (that's corned beef, cheese, and sauerkraut for all you laymen) and fight cancer, one bite at a time.

Citrus. Citrus fruits are especially important disease protectors and have proven in studies to be useful in combating a range of cancers, specifically prostate cancer, the most common cause of cancer death among men in the United States; lung cancer; cancer of the esophagus, oral cavity, and pharynx; and stomach cancer, the most common cancer worldwide. Their high levels of vitamin C may protect cell membranes and DNA from oxidative damage that can lead to cancerous changes. Vitamin C may also stunt cancer growth by altering the chemical structure of the potentially carcinogenic compound nitrite so that it becomes something safer: nitrosamine. And the vitamin's ability to synthesize collagen may hinder tumor growth.

Citrus fruits also contain coumarin and D-limonene, phytochemicals shown in several studies to increase the activity of glutathione transferase, an enzyme critical to the body's natural detoxification process.

Alliums. Garlic, onions, shallots, leeks, and chives belong to the allium family of vegetables, which contain organosulfides known as allyl sulfides. Also responsible for making your eyes tear during peeling and preparation, allyl sulfides have been shown in the lab to inhibit tumor production. Studies of human populations have shown that people who eat a lot of garlic and onions have lower risks of cancers of the stomach, colon, and other similar cancers. Allyl sulfides are found in higher amounts in the most pungent alliums, so sweet onions like Vidalias and Walla Wallas do not contain as much. Also, heat can destroy the compounds. But because most of us can't tolerate much raw onion or garlic, a quick sauté will retain more allyl sulfides than slow cooking.

Tomatoes. Tomatoes contain the phytochemicals p-coumaric acid and chlorogenic acid. During digestion, both acids interfere with the production of nitrosamines, which have been implicated in the development of stomach cancer.

Fatty fish. Back to omega 3s. Some experts point to the Mediterranean Food Guide Pyramid, which is quite fish-heavy, as one of the best anticancer eating paradigms. They are backed by a three-decade investigation showing that men who ate fish regularly had half the risk of contracting prostate cancer than did men who didn't eat fish. This is so important that my Full-Power Meal Plan in chapter 10 suggests you eat fish at least five times a week, rather than just weekly, as the Mediterranean Food Guide recommends.

Tomato Sauce. Here's a rare instance in which taking a bite out of vegetables and fruits isn't the best way to get the nutrients that are inside them.

RATING THE FRUITS

WHILE THE RECOMMENDATION OF THE 5-A-DAY FOR BETTER HEALTH PROGRAM and the Food Guide Pyramid is to eat two to four servings of fruits each day, the recommendations don't specify which fruits to eat, other than noting the need for good sources of vitamin C and beta-carotene. Although any fruit is better than none, some fruits are even better than others. To help identify the most nutritious ones, Drs. Paul LaChance and A. Elizabeth Sloan conducted research at Rutgers University and developed a rating system for the 28 most popular fresh fruits based on the average of the percent contribution to the daily value for protein, total vitamin A, thiamine, riboflavin, niacin, folate, vitamin C, calcium, and iron.

Fruit (fresh, 100 grams)	Daily Value	Fruit (fresh, 100 grams)	Daily Value
Kiwifruit	16	Raspberries	7
Papaya	14	Honeydew	6
Cantaloupe	13	Persimmon	5
Strawberries	12	Pineapple	5
Lemon, peeled	11	Banana	4
Mango	11	Blueberries	4
Orange (Florida)	11	Grape (Empress)	4
Red currants	10	Plum	4
Mandarin orange	9	Cherry	3
Avocado	8	Nectarine	3
Tangerine, sections	8	Peach	3
Apricots	7	Watermelon	3
Grapefruit, sections	7	Apple, with peel	2
Lime, peeled	7	Pear, sliced	2

How you eat fruit matters, too. The best preparation method is none—eat fruit whole and raw. Juicing, on the other hand, preserves most of the nutrients but eliminates some of the precious fiber. With premade juices, some of the nutrients have been lost through heat processing and pasteurization. Freezing retains more nutrients than any other storage method, and frozen fruits actually have a better nutrient profile than raw fruit that's been stored for too long or improperly. Canning, drying, cooking—all of these methods rob fruits of some of their vitamin C through heating and water loss.

Because vegetables and fruits contain so much water, the lycopene inside tomatoes, watermelon, and grapefruit really isn't concentrated enough to wage war against rogue cells. Rather, the amount of lycopene tested in studies that saw decreased risk for prostate cancer came from concentrated sources: tomato products like tomato soup, tomato paste, and ketchup. Whereas guys who ate, say, pasta with marinara sauce five times a week had a significantly reduced risk of cancer, guys who ate a tomato every day didn't enjoy the same protection, although it's certainly good to eat any kind of vegetable daily.

Elevating your intake of lycopene is one great nutritional strategy for stacking the deck in your favor where prostate cancer avoidance is concerned, especially when combined with daily doses of vitamin E, selenium, and various antioxidants.

Whole-wheat bread, oatmeal, and baked beans. The fiber in these three staples is key in the battle against several cancers, including colon cancer. Because the food you eat passes through your colon, bringing the toxins and contaminants of the outside world along for the ride, colon cancer is a genuine concern for all men as they age.

The seminal research in fiber science came in the 1960s, when Drs. Walker and Burkitt went around and collected the stools of native tribesmen in Africa. (Anything in the name of science, huh?) They found a tribe in Africa where intestinal problems were virtually unheard of. Intrigued, they weighed their stool and checked it for fiber. Bingo—a theory was born about the benefits of fiber, one that has been supported consistently by 40 years of subsequent research findings.

What fiber does that's so unique and so key for disease prevention is slow the absorption of chemicals, metabolites, and other things the body is trying to get rid of. By quickening the excretion process, it leaves less opportunity for things to be reabsorbed.

Fiber is particularly effective right at the site of the action: the intestinal lining. That's why risk for cancers of the intestine, rectum, and colon are all greatly reduced with a high fiber intake.

Fiber may prevent cancer through another mechanism as well. Researchers at Harvard found that cancer cells contain high levels of a protein called interleukin-6. When they treated those cells with butyrate, produced when the body breaks down fiber, it interfered with the protein's cancer-promoting function. Whole-wheat bread, oatmeal, and baked beans are all high in butyrate.

Green tea. University of Rochester researchers recently determined that a green-tea extract can help prevent the growth of cancer cells. The people in lab coats at Medical College of Ohio found that a compound called EGCG, a potent antioxidant in green tea, may help slow or stop the progression of bladder cancer. Tea has also been shown to reduce the incidence of cancers of the prostate, breast, colon, esophagus, stomach, and pancreas.

Water. Studies in Israel, Great Britain, and the United States have observed that the more fluid that people drink, the lower their risks of bladder, prostate, kidney, testicular, pelvic, and colon cancer. In some of the studies, a decrease in cancer risk was specifically associated with water intake.

Water likely reduces the risk of the various urinary tract cancers by keeping urine more dilute. In theory, this would keep toxins less concentrated, giving them less chance to be reabsorbed into the body. A similar mechanism may be at work with water and prostate and other hormone-related cancers. A connection may exist between high concentrations of hormones and these cancers, so if you keep everything more dilute, your risk might decline.

Regardless of the mechanism, a number of studies have shown a direct correlation between the quantity of fluid consumed (measured as cups per day) and the incidence of certain cancers. Basically, the more water you drink, the better. For example, a study done at Fred Hutchinson Cancer Research Center in Seattle found that men who drank four glasses of water or more a day had a 32 percent decrease in the risk of colon cancer compared with men who drank one glass or less. Although in men this was a trend rather than statistically significant, the data in women were highly significant. Because drinking more fluid—and water in particular—is a pretty benign dietary change and has been shown to be significant in other studies, I like to err on the side of more fluids here versus the risk of getting cancer.

Cancer Causers

Let's talk ketchup. Even if it does contain prostate-protecting lycopene, it won't help if it's slathered over a mound of French fries, one of the many foods that may make you more susceptible to getting cancer. As a general rule, limit your consumption of the following foods and chemicals, which studies have shown put men at significant risk for several cancers.

Acrylamides. These are particularly worrisome, potentially cancer-causing food chemicals. They may or may not occur naturally at low levels in the food supply, but levels can become elevated, perhaps dangerously so, during food preparation. These troublemakers are most commonly produced when French fries and potato chips are fried in fat, but they may also be produced when food is being microwaved in certain containers. It probably depends on how frequently you heat food in the microwave, as well as the container in which it is being heated. If you have questions about whether a certain plastic is safe, use glass. It's safer.

Dairy. A huge asterisk accompanies this entry, as calcium is a critically important nutrient. One recent study, however, has suggested a possible link between dairy products and testicular cancer. The researchers aren't really sure what the mechanism might be. One obvious variable, whole milk versus reduced-fat and fat-free milk, didn't seem to make much of a difference. Another theory is that something in cheese is at fault, and still another possible culprit getting a lot of attention is calcium itself in amounts that might turn on a cancer gene.

The amounts of dairy in question exceed the 3 to 4 cups a day recommended in many of this book's meal plans. Those studies were looking at 1,200 to 1,500 milligrams, and sometimes as much as 2,000 milligrams of calcium daily. The research is very young, but it did receive a lot of press coverage. So if you've been wondering about how much milk you can drink and stay healthy, it looks like you'll be fine with 3 to 4 cups a day. As with so many things, moderation is the key. Remember, not only is the jury out on this one, but we're still collecting evidence.

Red meat. The most popular cuts of red meat are high in total fats (see "Meet the Beef" on the next page), saturated fats, and cholesterol. This might be at the root of some of the research that shows a link between red meat consumption and colon cancer. Although the topic is still controversial, and in some studies the association only marginal, the theory is that both the total fat and the saturated fat in high-fat meats may directly cause cancer. On the other hand, a new study from Argentina has shown that if you look specifically at what types of red meats people are eating, it is the high-fat and not the lean red meats that are causing the problem. There may be confusion in the research because prior studies have not teased out this detailed level of information from the subjects. In the end, if you eat red meat, choose lean, low-fat cuts. In addition, because you need to eat so many other great sources of protein during the week, you'll probably have the opportunity to eat red meat only a couple of times a week. When you do, you should enjoy it.

It's not just the fat content by itself that's causing the problem. It could have something to do with the way the meat is prepared, especially if it's grilled. Flamed grilling isn't something you want to do on a regular basis. Some people grill out almost every day, particularly in the summer in California, where it's as much a part of the culture as earthquakes and liposuction. When you do grill outside, be sure to use lower-fat meats. It's the high fat content of the meat that grilling can alter, sometimes into carcinogenic substances. If part of your grilled meat is charred, remove that section and throw it away, feed it to your dog . . . just don't eat it.

Farm-raised salmon. After all the praise I've heaped on eating fish, this one is bound to turn a few heads. But there's an enormous difference between wild salmon and the farm-raised variety. The

MEET THE BEEF

When it comes to keeping saturated fat and cholesterol at bay, the right amount and cuts of beef, as well as their preparation, will make a big impact. Keep serving sizes between 3 and 5 ounces. On average, a 3-ounce serving of cooked lean beef contains 8.4 grams of total fat and 3.2 grams of saturated fat. Some cuts contain even less. For a 3-ounce serving of cooked meat, start with 4 ounces of uncooked, boneless meat.

Selecting the right cut of meat is important, too. Some cuts of beef are leaner than others. The leanest cuts come from the loin and round (leg) of the animal. The skinniest six cuts of beef contain fewer than 8.6 grams of total fat, 77 milligrams of dietary cholesterol, and 180 calories for each 3-ounce cooked, trimmed serving.

Skinniest 6

Top round	Top loin	Tenderloin
Eye of round	Sirloin	Round tip

Beef is also graded according to fat marbling: prime, choice, and select. Select is the leanest grade. Purchase lean cuts closely trimmed of fat, or trim them yourself at home before you cook. Leaner beef needs to be handled and prepared properly to retain moistness and tenderness. For loin cuts, cook using a dry-heat method like broiling or grilling, and serve immediately. When broiling or grilling, remember that larger pieces of meat will maintain moistness better than smaller pieces of meat. Be careful to pay attention while preparing lean cuts to avoid overcooking or charring the meat.

For less tender cuts such as round cuts, cook using a moist-heat method, or marinate to tenderize. It's the acid (vinegar, citrus juice, or wine) that tenderizes the meat, not the oil. To reduce total fat and calories, replace oil with water without losing the tenderizing effect.

To improve the tenderness of cooked meats, carve into thin slices, on the diagonal and, when possible, across the grain.

feed used for farmed salmon is from marine animals, and a concentrated source of polychlorinated biphenyls (PCBs). When consumed by the farmed salmon, the salmon become even more concentrated sources of this cancer-causing chemical.

So what do you do? Easy. Eat wild Alaskan salmon and Pacific Ocean fish. These are naturally lower in pollutants and contaminants and still high in the beneficial omega-3 fats that they have become so well known for. If you need help discerning which is which, ask your supermarket attendant (or fishmonger) to help.

A final note: One thing that doesn't appear to cause cancer, allaying some concerns, is aspartame. After studying more than 10 years of data, Europe's Scientific Committee on Food says it was unable to find any link between the artificial sweetener and cancer or other possible side effects.

Avoiding D-Day: Diabetes

We can't stress enough the importance of managing your blood-sugar levels through proper exercise and diet. Allow yourself to get too heavy and too out of shape, and you might as well beg for diabetes.

Diabetes comes in two forms:

- **Type I diabetes.** Also called juvenile or childhood diabetes, this afflicts kids and young adults, as the name suggests. This form of diabetes is an autoimmune disease, much like rheumatoid arthritis. The immune system attacks the beta cells in the pancreas that produce insulin, and the insulin-making mechanism in the pancreas shuts down completely. As far as early malfunctions go, that's right up there with losing an engine during take-off. At one time, it was thought that this error was genetically encoded in victims' bodies, but that view has been largely discarded. The source now looks to be

---

Fruit Is Not the Enemy

If you have diabetes already, should you avoid fruit because it contains sugar? Not at all. For example, the pectin in apples controls diabetes by regulating blood sugar. In fact, the natural sugars in fruit and fruit juices raise blood-sugar levels less than many refined starchy carbohydrate foods do. Clinical studies of fructose consumption in noninsulin-dependent diabetics resulted in improved metabolic control of blood sugar, or at least no changes. The more slowly metabolized fruit sugar—combined with pectin, which slows food's digestion and absorption—makes whole fresh fruit an excellent choice for the diabetic diet.

---

viral, although the jury is still out on that, too. Regardless, it has nothing to do with lifestyle. Because of the lack of insulin, untreated Type I diabetes leads to overly high blood-sugar levels and an inability to metabolize the sugar. This creates a metabolic condition called ketosis, then ketoacidosis, which leads to coma and death when left untreated.

- **Type II diabetes.** Here's the one you need to think about. Also called adult-onset diabetes, Type II targets mostly adults whose pancreas may or may not still secrete plenty of insulin. Usually, the problem is that their body cells have become resistant to receiving insulin. Because insulin is transporting sugar to those cells, getting turned away by cells is a huge problem. Having not been deposited in cells as intended, the sugar being transported collects in the bloodstream at dangerously high levels. The risks of Type II diabetes are not the same as those of Type I. If you fail to do what it takes to bring the disease under control, your symptoms progress more slowly, but ultimately you risk blindness, impotence, limb amputation, kidney failure, and heart disease. Again, left untreated for an extensive period of time or to a point where insulin is completely unavailable or ineffective, the outcome will be the same as with Type I diabetes: ketosis, ketoacidosis, coma, and death.

In the past, doctors treated Type II diabetes by overloading the body with more insulin. It was an attempt to "ambush" cells and force at least some insulin to connect with cell receptors, which at least would lower blood-sugar levels somewhat. Today, the first line of defense against Type II diabetes is meal planning for blood-sugar control, weight loss, and exercise. If this isn't successful, doctors will usually prescribe oral medications, but changing lifestyle is the most desirable treatment option.

It appears that although some people have a genetic predisposition to Type II diabetes, they're not destined to get it—unless they get fat, don't exercise, and otherwise don't take care of themselves. Lifestyle has a lot to do with Type II diabetes, and obesity is the primary risk factor for getting it. The disease certainly will turn the tables and have a huge impact on your lifestyle if you're unfortunate enough to be diagnosed with it.

No one has really been able to finger a specific food or nutrient whose consumption, or overconsumption, becomes a fairly predictable precursor of Type II diabetes, at least not in the way that saturated fat is linked with heart disease. But the growing consumption of high-fructose corn syrup may be playing an increasingly significant role. The average kid today is no stranger to guzzling rivers of high-fructose corn syrup in sodas. Combine that with a few hours daily in front of the television and, ultimately, more kids are going to get fat. This perverse equation has had a disturbing effect: shrinking

the age differentiation between Type I and Type II diabetes. Type I diabetes still occurs predominately in young people, but adult-onset diabetes could now be called teen-onset (and in some cases child-onset). A doctor I know diagnosed a 3-year-old with Type II diabetes! Approximately 50 percent of all new cases of Type II diabetes are occurring in children, which is an appalling statistic.

It's frightening to think of the metabolic and physiological consequences for children who already have Type II diabetes. By the time these kids reach 30, they're going to have chronic lifetime diseases that we're used to seeing in the elderly—the sorts of things that happen to guys in their 70s and 80s who got Type II diabetes in their 40s.

And the cost of that kind of extended healthcare for this nation is going to be extraordinarily expensive. How will our healthcare system be able to afford an entire population of sick people?

One of the most dangerous aspects of diabetes is that it increases your risk of heart disease. In fact, your entire circulatory system is pretty much ravaged by diabetes, which takes a heavy toll on what are called microvessels, the smallest tributaries for blood extended into your hands, feet, penis, and even your eyes. Eventually, gangrene in your fingers and toes can require surgery, perhaps even amputation. In extreme cases, you can go blind as well. Impotence is also common among diabetics. Want that to happen?

To combat diabetes, you need to get moving every day, and you need to eat the right things. Commit to exercise, record it, and keep track of what you've been doing. Exercise will make your insulin-resistant cells more sensitive to insulin. Resistance training will help improve blood-sugar control and lower cholesterol levels. Everything will begin to work better, and you'll feel better, too.

Now that you're feeling better because you're moving rather than melting into your couch, you should be able to think more clearly about all the foods that your body is craving: whole fruits, vegetables, beans, whole grains, nuts, and seeds. They don't take much preparation. It's just as easy to grab a piece of fruit as it is to scarf down a doughnut. The fruit will keep you healthy, but the donut—or 6 of them—will definitely turn you in the wrong direction.

One piece of great news that we've collected in the past decade is the glycemic index of foods. It's a rating based on how quickly 100 grams of a food raises your blood-glucose levels after eating, compared with 100 grams of glucose. Glucose is at the top at 100—it is absorbed very rapidly. What difference does this make? When blood sugar is raised, it stimulates an insulin response. Insulin helps remove the sugar from your bloodstream and transport it into muscle and liver cells. Blood sugar returns to normal and stays there for several hours until it begins to drop and you eat again. This is the normal, healthy response that we want. However,

when blood-sugar levels rise rapidly over and over again, too much insulin may be secreted. This constant wash of insulin over the cells of your body causes the cells to become resistant to insulin, inhibiting the transport of glucose into the cells. Give it time, and you've got Type II diabetes.

Many things affect the glycemic index of a food. Other nutrients, like fat and protein, slow absorp-

> ### Just Say Joe (and Cinnamon) to Diabetes
>
> Anyone suffering from diabetes (or even anyone simply at risk for the disease) might want to up their intake of cinnamon-infused lattes. Studies have shown that both cinnamon and coffee have properties that help fight the causes of diabetes.

SAVING THE NUTRIENTS IN YOUR FRUIT

STORING YOUR FRUITS CORRECTLY WILL MAKE A HUGE DIFFERENCE in how long they stay fresh and how good they taste. Because fruit is generally shipped unripe during most of the year, it needs to stay out of the refrigerator until it ripens. To speed ripening, place fruit in a closed paper bag on a kitchen counter. The gases produced by the fruit promote the ripening process. Check it daily so it doesn't overripen. Then make sure to store ripe fruit, except bananas, in the refrigerator.

You can minimize the loss of nutrients from your fruit by following these very simple guidelines.

- Always purchase fresh produce.
- Store fruit in its whole form, rather than cutting it up.
- Never soak produce for extended periods of time.
- When peeling and paring, remove as little as possible.
- If you purchase precut produce, refrigerate it in airtight wrappers or containers.
- Defrost fruit in the microwave to preserve the water-soluble nutrients.
- Cook fruit in large pieces to lessen the amount of exposed surface to water.
- Cook in just enough water to prevent scorching, and put a lid on the pan.

tion. Fiber slows absorption to a remarkable extent. If absorption of carbohydrates is slower rather than faster, then glucose passes into the bloodstream in a timed-release fashion and the insulin response stays well under control. Carbohydrate metabolism remains normal and healthy.

All those whole foods that I was talking about earlier in this chapter are low to moderate on the glycemic index scale, and that's where you want to target your diet. Check out the nutrition plans for losing weight in chapter 3, especially the pre-diabetes diet. Just like exercise, losing body fat will help your cells become more sensitive to insulin. But remember, stop thinking about what you can't eat next. Instead, focus on all the foods that your body needs to eat to stay healthy. Fuel yourself so that you

LONGEVITY SUPPLEMENTS

THOUGH FOOD WILL TAKE YOU A LONG WAY, a few effective supplements can aid your battle for longevity. Take these and you may be having conversations with you great-grandchildren someday.

- ■ **Vitamin E.** This is a must-have longevity supplement. Vitamin E has been shown to help prevent heart disease and slow down Alzheimer's disease, among many other benefits, yet it's almost impossible to get enough from whole-food sources like wheat germ oil, vegetable oil, nuts, seeds, and olive oil. Dose: 400 to 800 international units (IU) daily.

- ■ **Alpha-lipoic acid.** In animal studies, supplementing with this has improved metabolic activity and lowered the degree of oxidative stress by several measures. Combined with other supplements, particularly vitamin E, it also may have applications for diabetes patients. In fact, it's often prescribed in Europe to treat nerve damage associated with diabetes. Dose: 50 to 100 milligrams daily.

- ■ **Vitamin C.** If you follow the *Power Food* diets, you'll probably get enough of this antioxidant, but given its potent anti-inflammatory effect, it doesn't hurt to be safe. Dose: 500 milligrams daily.

- ■ **Grapeseed extract.** This is another free-radical fighter that shows promise in increasing the antioxidant capacity of blood. Studies have shown that a glass or two a day of red wine reduces the risk for heart disease and possibly certain cancers, and this supplement would work through a similar mechanism. Small studies have also suggested that grapeseed extract might protect blood vessels and enhance circulation. Dose: 100 milligrams daily.

- ■ **Lutein.** This antioxidant protects against macular degeneration, the leading cause of blindness in Americans over the age of 65. Good food sources of lutein include cruciferous vegetables, green leafy vegetables, bananas, berries, grapes, black currants, Mandarin oranges, starfruit, potatoes, and yellow sweet potatoes. Lutein is included in name-brand multivitamins such as Centrum, but you'll get only 250 micrograms or less in that and similar products. One unique product, I-Caps (lutein and zeaxanthin formula), does contain 4 milligrams of lutein and a number of other important nutrients

can begin to increase the amount of exercise that you are doing. It's the most positive way to change those old, unhealthy habits into new healthy habits.

Alzheimer's Disease

Oxidative stress takes a toll on the brain as well as the body. In fact, researchers are increasingly convinced that this oxidative stress plays a primary role in the pathogenesis of Alzheimer's disease, a neurodegenerative disorder of the elderly characterized by progressive memory loss and deterioration of cognitive function.

We discussed this in chapter 2, but it also needs to be discussed in the context of food and longevity. To understand how food might be able to help pre-

---

associated with eye health. Most of the studies showing efficacy used 6 milligrams. Dose: 6 milligrams daily.

- **Green tea extract.** Catechins, the active compounds in green tea, are potent antioxidants. The studies that have been done show that green tea can slow or even stop the initiation of malignant tumors. It also seems to support immune function. Dose: 300 milligrams daily.

- **Ginkgo biloba.** This improves circulation to the brain, so it might have a role to play in delaying Alzheimer's disease, which is characterized by brain-function atrophy. Another possible application is improving problems with microcirculation (brain, extremities, sex organs), which are often caused by diabetes. Dose: For microcirculation, 120 to 160 milligrams a day. For cognitive application, 240 milligrams a day. Those amounts should be divided among 2 or 3 daily doses.

- **Saw palmetto.** This is reported to decrease the activity of 5-alpha reductase, which has been implicated in prostate enlargement (and baldness) because it stimulates the conversion of testosterone to dihydrotestosterone (DHT). Saw palmetto's DHT-blocking mechanism is similar to that of the drug finasteride. Talk to your physician before self-prescribing saw palmetto. Although rare, it can cause headaches, diarrhea, and nausea. Dose: 160 milligrams taken twice daily; 320 milligrams total.

- **EPA and DHA.** In cold-water fish, these omega-3 fatty acids are phenomenal for longevity. Extracted and put into supplement form, however, something gets lost in the translation, according to several studies that show no positive effect on cholesterol. Dose: Not recommended.

- **Lycopene.** Like EPA and DHA, this phytochemical has amazing longevity capabilities in food, but that's the best place to get it—the supplement version doesn't produce the same benefits. In a study published recently in the *Journal of the National Cancer Institute*, rats who were fed a diet of tomato powder were 26 percent less likely to die of prostate cancer than rats not given any supplements. Rats given a lycopene supplement were only slightly more likely to survive than rats given no tomato products. Dose: Not recommended.

vent this disease—or at least slow it down—you need to understand what actually causes it, at least to the extent that science has figured out that medical conundrum.

The brains of Alzheimer's patients are characterized by a generalized atrophy, as well as by nerve cells that are tangled, coated with plaque, or both tangled and coated. Their brains also contain abundant amounts of a substance called beta-amyloid. When researchers place this substance in nerve cell cultures, it unleashes free radicals that attack and kill those cells. Extrapolate from that cluster of cells in one petri dish to the billions in your brain, and you can imagine how this onslaught could become both inexorable and devastating. Given that Alzheimer's is an aging disease and free radical formation increases with age, the connection makes sense.

If you paid attention previously when we wrote about free radicals—you *did* pay attention, didn't you?—you probably would theorize that antioxidants might be able to help, because they help neutralize free radicals. Lo and behold, when researchers added vitamin E, a natural antioxidant, to that petri dish, it was beta-amyloid's turn to get terminated. It seems to work on humans, too. In a study of advanced Alzheimer's disease patients conducted by the Alzheimer's Disease Cooperative Study, subjects treated with 2,000 International Units of vitamin E (and equivalents) suffered slower functional deterioration than those who didn't receive vitamin E.

The results raise the possibility that vitamin E may slow disease progression in Alzheimer's patients. The initial physiological changes of Alzheimer's probably occur years, if not decades, before symptoms appear, at which point many of those early changes—say, in nerve deterioration—have likely become fixed and extremely difficult to treat in any significant way. If sound nutrition early on can help push back that process, the symptoms shouldn't appear as quickly.

Start Now, Live Longer

The take-home lesson from this chapter is actually very positive. Except in unusual cases, most guys can live a long, healthy life without terrible risk of disease if they just take care of themselves. As time passes, you'll age, but your body will be geared up to handle most of what life has to throw its way.

One of the keys is moderation: Don't do most things, especially bad things, to an extreme. Free radicals are bouncing around in your body 24/7, and for the most part, that's okay. It's under control. Your body is designed to handle it. The problem comes when your diet, your lifestyle, or your environment is so extreme that the internal system of checks and balances breaks down, allowing free radicals to accumulate and overrun the defense mechanisms designed to control them.

Short of that happening, there's no reason you need to contract any sort of life-threatening illness through your own doing. (Alas, there's an element of randomness in human physiology and illness pathology that can't be denied or avoided.) The body is a remarkable machine in that respect. If you just take proper care of it, you can live for a really long time. Sometimes your internal programming has mistakes or internal flaws in the form of a genetic defect, which can be hard to overcome, but even there, those coding mistakes might never get expressed if you take care of yourself. Conversely, you can have the best genetics in the world, but if you don't keep the hoses clean, so to speak, things will clog up and your risk of dying prematurely will skyrocket.

The human body comes with awe-inspiring mechanisms for self-defense, almost better than we deserve. People who have smoked for 50 years can still reduce their risk of getting lung cancer and heart disease by stopping. Better to stack the odds in your favor rather than tempting fate, though. Bob Dylan once wrote, "People don't do what they believe in/They just do what's most convenient/Then they repent." That may or may not work in the spiritual realm, but if you approach your body and your diet that way, you're really pushing your luck. Don't take the attitude that you can do whatever you want until you're 50 and then make changes; often, that's too late. In fact, you might be dead before you reach that milestone. Or your health might have been so severely compro-mised that your quality of life will decline precip-itously from 50 onward.

While you attend to your stock portfolio, your 401(k), your retirement plan, and paying for your kids' college tuition, make a small investment in yourself, too, even if it's something as simple as eating more fiber. That one simple act can help pre-vent heart disease, cancer, diabetes, obesity—virtu-ally everything we just talked about in this chapter. No matter what diet or meal plan or nutrition guru you're following, you need to eat plenty of fiber. Anyone who tells you otherwise doesn't know what he or she is talking about.

THE DIABETIC-GUY MEAL PLAN

IF YOU OR SOMEONE YOU KNOW IS DIABETIC, THIS IS THE MEAL PLAN TO CHOOSE. This diet features low-to-moderate GI carbs, without any high-fructose corn syrup. Expect to get plenty of fiber, especially the soluble stuff, and a good dose of healthy fats. We'll also stress chromium. (Remember also that exercise is imperative to help fight Type-2 diabetes.)

Daily Assumptions*†

2,500 calories
250 grams carbohydrates
188 grams protein
83 grams fat

Daily Breakdown*†

4 bread
5 fruit (2 citrus, 2 berry, 1 other)
4 milk
6 vegetable (3 carotenoid,
 2 brassica, 1 allium)
8 very lean protein
6 lean protein
1 medium-fat protein
1 bean
2 nut
2 soy
7 fat

Note: Occasionally, a fat-free product, like mustard or cooking spray, is included on the menus. These do not count toward your daily breakdown but should not be overused.

*Use every day.

† Based on a 185-pound man.

THE MENU

DAY 1

Breakfast

2 bread	1 cup Shredded Wheat
1 milk	1 cup fat-free milk
1 citrus	1/2 cup orange juice
1 berry	3/4 cup fresh blueberries
1 medium-fat protein	1 egg, scrambled in a nonstick pan
1 fat	1 1/2 tablespoons ground flaxseed
	Water
	Oil-free cooking spray (for egg)

Snack

2 soy	1 cup edamame
1 carotenoid	1 cup carrot sticks
2 fat	2 tablespoons ranch dressing (for dipping)
	Water

Lunch

1 milk	1 cup fat-free milk
2 carotenoid	Salad with 1 cup romaine lettuce, 1 cup spinach
6 very lean protein	6 ounces turkey
1 bean	1/2 cup garbanzo beans
2 fat	2 tablespoons oil and vinegar (for salad)

Pre-Workout Snack

1 other fruit	1 peach
1 milk	6 ounces sugar-free yogurt
2 nut	20 peanuts

Post-Workout

SMOOTHIE

Blend until smooth.

1 milk	1 cup fat-free milk
1 citrus	$^1/_2$ cup orange juice with calcium
1 berry	$1^1/_4$ cups frozen strawberries
2 very lean protein	14 grams whey protein powder
	1 tablespoon brewer's yeast

Dinner

2 bread	1 small ear corn on the cob
	1 small whole-wheat roll
2 brassica	1 cup grilled broccoli and cauliflower
1 allium	$^1/_2$ cup grilled onions
6 lean protein	6 ounces salmon, grilled
2 fat	8 Kalamata olives
	1 teaspoon butter

DAY 2

Breakfast

Combine yogurt, fruit, and honey. Combine muffin and egg for sandwich.

2 bread	1 whole-wheat English muffin
1 milk	1 cup fat-free, unsweetened yogurt
1 citrus	$^1/_2$ cup grapefruit juice
1 berry	$1^1/_4$ cups whole strawberries
1 medium-fat protein	1 egg, hard-cooked
1 fat	$1^1/_2$ tablespoons ground flaxseed
	Water

Snack

2 soy	2 ounces soy nuts
1 carotenoid	1 cup carrot sticks
2 fat	2 tablespoons ranch dressing
	Water

Lunch

1 milk	1 cup fat-free milk
2 carotenoid	1 cup romaine lettuce, 1 cup roasted red pepper
6 very lean protein	6 ounces skinless white-meat chicken, grilled with lime juice
2 fat	2 teaspoons olive oil (for roasted vegetables)
	2 tablespoons fat-free dressing

Pre-Workout Snack

1 other fruit	1 plum
1 milk	1/2 cup cottage cheese
2 nuts	2 tablespoons roasted sunflower seeds

Post-Workout

SMOOTHIE
Blend until smooth.

1 milk	1 cup fat-free milk
1 citrus	1/2 cup orange juice with calcium
1 berry	3/4 cup frozen blueberries
2 very lean protein	14 grams whey protein powder
	1 tablespoon brewer's yeast

Dinner

2 bread	1 cup cooked pasta
2 brassica	1 cup Brussels sprouts
1 allium	1/2 cup grilled shallots, garlic (for shrimp)
1 bean	1/2 cup kidney beans
6 lean protein	6 ounces shrimp, grilled
2 fat	2 teaspoons olive oil
	2 tablespoons fat-free dressing

DAY 3

Breakfast

2 bread	2 slices whole-wheat bread
1 milk	1/2 cup cottage cheese (on bread)
1 citrus	4 ounces freshly squeezed orange juice (with pulp)
1 berry	3/4 cup blueberries
1 medium-fat protein	1 egg, cooked sunny-side up in a nonstick pan
1 fat	1 1/2 tablespoons ground flaxseed
	Water
	Oil-free cooking spray (for egg)

Snack

2 soy	2 ounces soy nuts
1 carotenoid	1 cup sliced bell pepper
2 fat	2 tablespoons creamy peppercorn dressing
	Water

Lunch

1 milk	1 cup fat-free milk
2 carotenoid	1 cup spinach or bok choy
	1 cup yellow squash, stir-fried with garlic and fresh ginger
6 very lean protein	6 ounces skinless white-meat chicken, stir-fried
1 bean	1/2 cup black beans
2 fat	2 teaspoons oil (for stir-frying)

Pre-Workout Snack

1 other fruit	1 nectarine
1 milk	1 ounce fat-free cheddar cheese
2 nut	10 cashews

Post-Workout

SMOOTHIE

Blend until smooth.

1 milk	1 cup fat-free milk
1 citrus	1/2 cup orange juice with calcium
1 berry	1 cup frozen raspberries
2 very lean protein	14 grams whey protein powder
	1 tablespoon brewer's yeast

Dinner

2 bread	1 ounce croutons (for salad)
	1 cup chicken noodle soup
2 brassica	1 cup cauliflower and broccoli, steamed
1 allium	1/2 cup onion
6 lean protein	6 ounces swordfish, grilled with ginger and scallions
2 fat	2 teaspoons olive oil (for fish)

DAY 4

Breakfast

1 citrus	$^1/_2$ cup orange juice
1 berry	1 cup raspberries
1 milk	1 cup milk ($^1/_2$ cup for French toast)

FRENCH TOAST *(See recipe directions on page 44.)*

2 bread	2 slices whole-wheat bread
1 medium-fat protein	1 egg
1 fat	$1^1/_2$ tablespoons ground flaxseed
	Water

Snack

2 soy	50 Genisoy soy crisps
2 nuts	2 tablespoons almond butter
1 carotenoid	1 cup carrot sticks
	Water

Lunch

1 milk	1 cup fat-free milk
2 carotenoid	Salad with 1 cup lettuce, 1 cup spinach
6 very lean protein	6 ounces turkey
2 fat	2 teaspoons olive oil (for cooking)

Pre-Workout Snack

1 other fruit	1 apple
1 milk	1 fat-free latte, tall
2 nuts	40 pistachios

Post-Workout

SMOOTHIE

Blend until smooth.

1 milk	1 cup milk
1 citrus	$^1/_2$ cup orange juice with calcium
1 berry	$1^1/_4$ cups frozen strawberries
2 very lean protein	14 grams whey protein supplement
	1 tablespoon brewer's yeast

Dinner

2 bread	2 small whole-grain dinner rolls
	1 cup raw chopped tomatoes cooked with chili seasoning (for chili)
2 brassica	1 cup coleslaw
1 allium	$1/2$ cup onion, garlic for seasoning
1 bean	$1/2$ cup kidney beans (add to chili)
6 lean protein	6 ounces lean beef, minced (add to chili)
2 fat	$1/4$ avocado, diced

DAY 5

Breakfast

2 bread	1 cup quick oats (not instant)
1 milk	1 cup fat-free milk
1 citrus	$1/2$ cup orange juice
1 berry	$1^1/4$ cups strawberries
1 medium-fat protein	1 egg, hard-cooked
1 fat	$1^1/2$ tablespoons ground flaxseed
	Water

Snack

2 soy	1 cup edamame
1 carotenoid	1 cup carrot sticks
2 fat	2 tablespoons ranch dressing
	Water

Lunch

Combine ingredients.

1 milk	1 cup fat-free milk
2 carotenoid	1 cup sautéed peppers
6 very lean protein	6 ounces skinless white-meat chicken, grilled with lime juice
1 bean	$1/2$ cup fat-free refried beans
2 fat	2 teaspoons olive oil (for cooking)
	2 tablespoons salsa

Pre-Workout Snack

1 other fruit	1 pear
1 milk	1 cup fat-free milk
2 nut	1 tablespoon almond butter

Post-Workout

SMOOTHIE

Blend until smooth.

1 milk	1 cup fat-free milk
1 citrus	$^1/_2$ cup orange juice with calcium
1 berry	1 cup frozen blackberries
2 very lean protein	14 grams whey protein powder
	1 tablespoon brewer's yeast

Dinner

2 bread	1 small pita
	$^1/_2$ cup couscous
2 brassica	1 cup broccoli slaw
1 allium	Onion, shallots, garlic (add to couscous)
6 lean protein	6 ounces fresh trout (stuffed with $^1/_2$ cup couscous)
2 fat	4 tablespoons reduced-fat vinaigrette

DAY 6

Breakfast

2 bread	2 slices multigrain bread, toasted
1 milk	1 cup fat-free milk
1 citrus	$^1/_2$ cup orange juice
1 berry	1 cup raspberries
1 medium-fat protein	1 egg, hard-cooked
1 fat	$1^1/_2$ tablespoons ground flaxseed
	Water

Snack

2 soy	50 Genisoy soy crisps
2 fat	2 tablespoons peanut butter
1 carotenoid	1 cup sliced bell pepper
	Water

Lunch

1 milk	1 cup fat-free milk
2 carotenoid	$^1/_2$ cup carrots, $1^1/_2$ cups spinach
6 very lean protein	6 ounces turkey
2 fat	2 tablespoons balsamic vinaigrette (for spinach and carrots)

Pre-Workout Snack

1 other fruit	½ large banana
1 milk	1 cup fat-free cottage cheese
2 nuts	2 tablespoons roasted sunflower seeds

Post-Workout

SMOOTHIE

Blend until smooth.

1 milk	1 cup fat-free milk
1 citrus	½ cup orange juice with calcium
1 berry	1 cup frozen raspberries
2 very lean protein	14 grams whey protein powder
	1 tablespoon brewer's yeast

Dinner

2 bread	2 slices rye bread
2 brassica	1 cup coleslaw
1 allium	½ cup chopped onion (mix into tuna)
1 bean	½ cup fava beans
6 lean protein	6 ounces tuna in olive oil, drained
2 fat	2 tablespoons reduced-fat mayonnaise

DAY 7

Breakfast

2 bread	2 cups Kashi
1 milk	1 cup fat-free milk
1 citrus	½ cup grapefruit juice
1 berry	1 cup blackberries
1 medium-fat protein	1 egg, hard-cooked
1 fat	1½ tablespoons ground flaxseed
	Water

Snack

2 soy	1 cup edamame
1 carotenoid	1 cup radishes
2 fat	2 tablespoons peppercorn salad dressing
	Water

Lunch

1 milk	1 cup fat-free milk
2 carotenoid	1 cup romaine lettuce, $^1/_2$ cup carrots, $^1/_2$ cup peppers
6 very lean protein	6 ounces skinless white-meat chicken, grilled with lime juice
1 bean	$^1/_2$ cup pinto beans
2 fat	2 teaspoons oil (to cook chicken)
	2 tablespoons fat-free ranch dressing

Pre-Workout Snack

1 other fruit	17 grapes
1 milk	1 ounce fat-free cheese
2 nut	10 walnuts

Post-Workout

SMOOTHIE

Blend until smooth.

1 milk	1 cup fat-free milk
1 citrus	$^1/_2$ cup orange juice with calcium
1 berry	$^3/_4$ cup frozen blueberries
2 very lean protein	14 grams whey protein powder
	1 tablespoon brewer's yeast

Dinner

2 bread	3-inch square of corn bread
2 brassica	1 cup broccoli, steamed
1 allium	$^1/_2$ cup leeks (sautéed for salmon)
	Salad with 1 cup lettuce, $^1/_4$ cup tomato, $^1/_4$ cup cucumber
6 lean protein	6 ounces poached salmon
2 fat	1 teaspoon olive oil
	Included (in corn bread)
	2 tablespoons fat-free Caesar dressing

THE ANTI-HEART-DISEASE MEAL PLAN

IF YOU WANT TO PREVENT OR DEFEAT HEART DISEASE, a high-antioxidant diet is your priority. You'll be drinking some red wine (not to mention some tea), feasting on leafy vegetables and legumes, and upping your consumption of fiber. This diet will stress anti-inflammation while reducing your overall high-fructose corn syrup intake and upping your low-to-moderate GI carbs. Also, pay attention to how much fat you're getting— if the monounsaturated fats and omega 3s aren't on your menu, you've got a problem. That means eating fish, soy, and nuts.

THE MENU

DAY 1

Breakfast

2 bread	1 cup Shredded Wheat
1 milk	1 cup fat-free milk
1 citrus	1/2 cup orange juice
1 berry	3/4 cup fresh blueberries
1 medium-fat protein	1 egg, scrambled in a nonstick pan
2 fat	3 tablespoons ground flaxseed
	Water
	Oil-free cooking spray (for egg)

Snack

2 soy	1 cup edamame
1 carotenoid	1 cup carrot sticks
	Tea

Lunch

1 milk	1 cup fat-free milk
2 carotenoid	Salad with 1 cup romaine lettuce, 1/2 cup tomato, 1/2 cup pepper
4 very lean protein	4 ounces turkey
1 bean	1/2 cup garbanzo beans
3 fat	3 tablespoons oil and vinegar salad dressing

Pre-Workout Snack

1 other fruit	1 peach
2 nut	20 peanuts

Daily Assumptions*†

2,500 calories
313 grams carbohydrates
131 grams protein
81 grams fat

Daily Breakdown*†

5 bread
6 fruit (2 citrus, 2 berry, 2 other)
3 milk
8 teaspoons added sugar
6 vegetable (3 carotenoid, 2 brassica, 1 allium)
4 very lean protein
5 lean protein
1 medium-fat protein
8 fat
2 soy
1 bean
2 nut

Note: Occasionally, a fat-free product, like mustard or cooking spray, is included on the menus. These do not count toward your daily breakdown but should not be overused.

*Use every day.

† Based on a 185-pound man.

Post-Workout

SMOOTHIE

Blend until smooth.

1 milk	1 cup fat-free milk
1 citrus	$^1/_2$ cup orange juice with calcium
1 berry	$1^1/_4$ cups frozen strawberries
6 teaspoons added sugar	2 tablespoons honey

Dinner

3 bread	1 small ear corn on the cob
	1 whole-wheat roll
1 other fruit	1 apple
2 brassica	1 cup grilled broccoli, cauliflower
1 allium	$^1/_2$ cup grilled onions
5 lean protein	5 ounces salmon, grilled
3 fat	8 Kalamata olives
	2 teaspoons olive oil (for veggies)
2 teaspoons added sugar	2 teaspoons sugar or honey
	Tea

DAY 2

Breakfast

Combine yogurt, fruit, and flaxseed.

2 bread	1 whole-wheat English muffin
1 milk	1 cup fat-free unsweetened yogurt
1 citrus	$^1/_2$ cup grapefruit juice
1 berry	$1^1/_4$ cups fresh strawberries
1 medium-fat protein	1 egg, hard-cooked
2 fat	3 tablespoons ground flaxseed
	Water

Snack

2 nut	1 tablespoon peanut butter
1 carotenoid	1 cup carrot sticks
	Tea

Lunch

1 milk	1 cup fat-free milk
2 carotenoid	1 cup romaine lettuce, $^1/_2$ cup tomato, $^1/_2$ cup roasted red pepper
4 very lean protein	4 ounces skinless white-meat chicken, grilled with lime juice
2 fat	1 tablespoon olive oil (for roasted vegetables)
	2 tablespoons fat-free dressing

Pre-Workout Snack

| 1 other fruit | 1 plum |
| 2 soy | 2 ounces soy nuts |

Post-Workout

SMOOTHIE

Blend until smooth.

1 milk	1 cup fat-free milk
1 citrus	1/2 cup orange juice with calcium
1 berry	3/4 cup frozen blueberries
6 teaspoons added sugar	2 tablespoons honey

Dinner

3 bread	1 1/2 cups cooked pasta
1 other fruit	1 1/4 cups cubed watermelon (1 slice)
2 brassica	1 cup Brussels sprouts
1 allium	1/2 cup grilled shallots, and garlic (with shrimp over pasta)
1 bean	1/2 cup kidney beans
5 lean protein	5 ounces shrimp, grilled
3 fat	1 tablespoon oil (for shrimp)
2 teaspoons added sugar	2 teaspoons sugar or honey
	Tea
	2 tablespoons fat-free salad dressing

DAY 3

Breakfast

2 bread	2 slices whole-wheat bread
1 milk	1 cup fat-free cottage cheese (on bread)
1 citrus	4 ounces freshly squeezed orange juice (with pulp)
1 berry	3/4 cup blueberries
1 medium-fat protein	1 egg, cooked sunny-side up in a nonstick pan
2 fat	3 tablespoons ground flaxseed
	Water
	Oil-free cooking spray (for egg)

Snack

2 soy	2 ounces soy nuts
1 carotenoid	1 cup sliced bell pepper
	Tea

Lunch

1 milk	1 cup fat-free milk
2 carotenoid	1 cup spinach, bok choy
	1 cup yellow squash, stir-fried with garlic and fresh ginger
4 very lean protein	4 ounces skinless white-meat chicken, stir-fried
1 bean	$1/2$ cup black beans
3 fat	1 tablespoon oil (for stir-frying)

Pre-Workout Snack

1 other fruit	1 nectarine
2 nut	10 cashews

Post-Workout

SMOOTHIE

Blend until smooth.

1 milk	1 cup fat-free milk
1 citrus	$1/2$ cup orange juice with calcium
1 berry	1 cup frozen raspberries
6 teaspoons added sugar	2 tablespoons honey

Dinner

3 bread	4 crackers
	1 ounce croutons (for salad)
1 other fruit	1 peach
	1 cup chicken noodle soup
2 brassica	2 cups raw cauliflower, broccoli, steamed
1 allium	$1/2$ cup onion (for cauliflower and broccoli)
5 lean protein	5 ounces swordfish, grilled with ginger and scallions
3 fat	1 tablespoon oil (for fish)
2 teaspoons added sugar	2 teaspoons sugar or honey
	Tea

DAY 4

Breakfast

1 citrus	¹/₂ cup orange juice
1 berry	1 cup raspberries
1 milk	1 cup fat-free milk (¹/₂ cup for French toast)

FRENCH TOAST *(See recipe directions on page 44.)*

2 bread	2 slices whole-wheat bread
1 medium-fat protein	1 egg
2 fat	3 tablespoons ground flaxseed
	Water
	Oil-free cooking spray

Snack

2 nut	1 tablespoon almond butter
1 carotenoid	1 cup carrot sticks
	Tea

Lunch

1 milk	1 cup fat-free milk
2 carotenoid	Salad with 2 cups romaine lettuce
4 very lean protein	4 ounces turkey
3 fat	2 tablespoons low-fat dressing
	2 tablespoons sunflower seeds

Pre-Workout Snack

1 other fruit	1 apple
2 soy	1 cup edamame

Post-Workout

SMOOTHIE

Blend until smooth.

1 milk	1 cup fat-free milk
1 citrus	¹/₂ cup orange juice with calcium
1 berry	1¹/₄ cups frozen strawberries
6 teaspoons added sugar	2 tablespoons honey

Dinner

3 bread	1 hamburger bun
	1 small ear of corn
1 other fruit	1¼ cups cubed watermelon (1 slice)
2 brassica	1 cup coleslaw
1 allium	½ cup onion, garlic (for seasoning)
1 bean	½ cup baked beans
5 lean protein	5 ounces lean beef, minced (add to chili)
3 fat	⅛ avocado, diced
	1 teaspoon oil (for onion)
	Included (in coleslaw)
2 teaspoons added sugar	2 teaspoons sugar or honey
	Included (in baked beans)
	Tea

DAY 5

Breakfast

2 bread	1 cup quick oats (not instant)
1 milk	1 cup fat-free milk
1 citrus	½ cup orange juice
1 berry	1¼ cups strawberries
1 medium-fat protein	1 egg, hard-cooked
2 fat	3 tablespoons ground flaxseed
	Water

Snack

2 soy	1 cup edamame
1 carotenoid	1 cup carrot sticks
	Tea

Lunch

1 milk	1 cup fat-free milk
2 carotenoid	1 cup sautéed peppers
	2 tablespoons salsa
4 very lean protein	4 ounces skinless white-meat chicken, grilled with lime juice
1 bean	½ cup fat-free refried beans
3 fat	1 tablespoon olive oil (for cooking)

Pre-Workout Snack

1 other fruit	1 pear
2 nut	1 tablespoon almond butter

Post-Workout

SMOOTHIE

Blend until smooth.

1 milk	1 cup fat-free milk
1 citrus	$^1/_2$ cup orange juice with calcium
1 berry	1 cup frozen blackberries
6 teaspoons added sugar	2 tablespoons honey

Dinner

3 bread	1 large pita
	$^1/_2$ cup couscous
1 other fruit	1 apple
2 brassica	1 cup broccoli slaw
1 allium	$^1/_2$ cup onion, shallot, garlic (in couscous)
5 lean protein	5 ounces fresh trout (stuffed with $^1/_2$ cup couscous)
3 fat	2 tablespoons reduced-fat vinaigrette
	Included (in broccoli slaw)
	1 teaspoon oil (for onion and shallot)
2 teaspoons added sugar	2 teaspoons sugar or honey
	Tea

DAY 6

Breakfast

2 bread	2 slices multigrain bread, toasted
1 milk	1 cup fat-free milk
1 citrus	$^1/_2$ cup orange juice
1 berry	1 cup raspberries
1 medium-fat protein	1 egg, hard-cooked
2 fat	3 tablespoons ground flaxseed
	Water

Snack

2 nut	1 tablespoon peanut butter
1 carotenoid	1 cup sliced bell pepper
	Tea

Lunch

Roll vegetables and turkey in lettuce leaves.

1 milk	1 cup fat-free milk
2 carotenoid	1 cup carrot sticks
	1 cup leaf lettuce
4 very lean protein	4 ounces turkey
3 fat	¼ avocado, sliced
	2 tablespoons reduced-fat ranch dressing

Pre-Workout Snack

1 other fruit	½ large banana
2 soy	2 ounces soy nuts

Post-Workout

SMOOTHIE

Blend until smooth.

1 milk	1 cup fat-free milk
1 citrus	½ cup orange juice with calcium
1 berry	1 cup frozen raspberries
6 teaspoons added sugar	2 tablespoons honey

Dinner

3 bread	2 slices rye bread
	1 cup noodle soup
1 other fruit	1 pear
2 brassica	1 cup coleslaw
1 allium	½ cup chopped onion (mix into tuna)
1 bean	½ cup fava beans
5 lean protein	5 ounces tuna in olive oil, drained
3 fat	1 tablespoon mayonnaise (for tuna)
	Included (in coleslaw)
2 teaspoons added sugar	2 teaspoons sugar or honey
	Tea

DAY 7

Breakfast

2 bread	2 cups Kashi
1 milk	1 cup fat-free milk
1 citrus	½ cup grapefruit juice
1 berry	1 cup blackberries
1 medium-fat protein	1 egg, hard-cooked (for egg salad)
2 fat	3 tablespoons ground flaxseed
	Water

Snack

2 soy	1 cup edamame
1 carotenoid	1 cup carrots
	2 tablespoons fat-free dressing
	Tea

Lunch

1 milk	1 cup fat-free milk
2 carotenoid	Salad with 1 cup lettuce, $^1/_2$ cup tomato, $^1/_2$ cup red pepper
4 very lean protein	4 ounces skinless white-meat chicken, grilled with lime juice
1 bean	$^1/_2$ cup pinto beans
2 fat	2 tablespoons low-fat salad dressing
	2 teaspoons oil (for cooking chicken)

Pre-Workout Snack

1 other fruit	17 grapes
2 nut	10 walnuts

Post-Workout

SMOOTHIE

Blend until smooth.

1 milk	1 cup fat-free milk
1 citrus	$^1/_2$ cup orange juice with calcium
1 berry	$^3/_4$ cup frozen blueberries
6 teaspoons added sugar	2 tablespoons honey

Dinner

3 bread	$^1/_2$ cup brown rice
	3-inch square of corn bread
1 other fruit	1 cup honeydew
2 brassica	1 cup broccoli, steamed
1 allium	$^1/_2$ cup leeks and garlic
5 lean protein	5 ounces salmon, poached
3 fat	2 tablespoons low-fat Caesar dressing
	Included (in corn bread)
	1 teaspoon olive oil
2 teaspoons added sugar	2 teaspoons sugar or honey
	Tea

THE HYPERTENSIVE-GUY MEAL PLAN

THE BASIC STRUCTURE OF THIS DIET IS BUILT ON THE RESEARCH FROM THE DASH studies. Potassium, magnesium, calcium, sodium, and fiber levels meet the Dietary Approaches to Stop Hypertension guidelines. Because we still expect you to exercise, the protein levels are slightly greater than in the DASH diet. This is not a diet to lose weight on. You should have enough energy to work out, but you probably won't be building up on this diet either. If you are going to weight-train to build, rather than maintain, then increase your whole-grains and starches by 2 to 4 servings each day. That will boost your carbs and give you more energy to train harder and build muscle. The same goes for cardio work. If you're doing long-distance training, increase your carbs by the same amount to give yourself more fuel. In general, avoid alcohol and caffeine.

Daily Assumptions*†

2,500 calories
298 grams carbohydrates
174 grams protein
67 grams fat

Daily Breakdown*†

8 bread
5 fruit
4 milk
3 teaspoons added sugar
5 vegetable
8 very lean protein
5 lean protein
1 medium-fat protein
1 bean
2 nut

Note: Occasionally, a fat-free product, like mustard or cooking spray, is included on the menus. These do not count toward your daily breakdown but should not be overused.

*Use every day.

† Based on a 185-pound man.

THE DIET

DAY 1

Breakfast

2 bread	1 cup Shredded Wheat
1 milk	1 cup fat-free milk
1 fruit	3/4 cup fresh blueberries
1 medium-fat protein	1 egg, scrambled in a nonstick pan
1 very lean protein	2 egg whites, scrambled with whole egg
1 fat	1 1/2 tablespoons ground flaxseed
	Water
	Oil-free cooking spray (for eggs)

Lunch

2 bread	2 slices whole-grain bread
1 milk	1 cup fat-free milk
2 vegetable	Salad with 2 cups romaine lettuce, 1/2 cup tomato, 1/2 cup cucumber
1 fruit	1 nectarine
4 very lean protein	4 ounces turkey
1 bean	1/2 cup garbanzo beans
1 fat	1 teaspoon olive oil with added vinegar, or 1 tablespoon salad dressing

Pre-Workout Snack

1 bread	³/₄ ounce pretzels (unsalted)
1 milk	6 ounces sugar-free yogurt
2 nut	20 peanuts (unsalted)
1 vegetable	1 cup sliced vegetable sticks

Post-Workout

SMOOTHIE

Blend until smooth.

1 milk	1 cup fat-free milk
2 fruit	¹/₄ cup pineapple (frozen)
	³/₄ cup frozen strawberries
	¹/₂ cup orange juice with calcium
3 very lean protein	21 grams whey protein powder
3 teaspoons added sugar	1 tablespoon honey

Dinner

3 bread	3 ounces baked yam
	1 whole-grain dinner roll
1 fruit	1 slice watermelon
2 vegetable	1 cup broccoli and cauliflower
5 lean protein	5 ounces salmon, grilled
1 fat	8 Kalamata olives

DAY 2

Breakfast

Combine yogurt, fruit, and flaxseed. Combine muffin and egg for sandwich.

2 bread	1 whole-wheat English muffin
1 milk	1 cup fat-free, unsweetened yogurt
1 fruit	1¹/₄ cups fresh strawberries
1 medium-fat protein	1 egg, hard-cooked
1 very lean protein	2 eggs, hard-cooked (discard yolks)
1 fat	1¹/₂ tablespoons ground flaxseed
	Water

Lunch

2 bread	2 slices whole-grain bread
1 milk	1 cup fat-free milk
2 vegetable	Large salad with romaine lettuce, tomato, grilled eggplant, roasted red pepper
1 fruit	1 kiwi
4 very lean protein	4 ounces skinless white-meat chicken, grilled with lime juice
1 bean	1/2 cup kidney beans
1 fat	2 tablespoons fat-free salad dressing
	1 teaspoon olive oil (for roasted vegetables)

Pre-Workout Snack

1 bread	2 rice cakes (unsalted)
1 milk	1 cup fat-free cottage cheese
2 nut	16 almonds (unsalted)
1 vegetable	1 cup sliced bell pepper

Post-Workout

SMOOTHIE

Blend until smooth.

1 milk	1 cup fat-free milk
2 fruit	1/4 cup pineapple (frozen)
	3/4 cup frozen strawberries
	1/2 cup orange juice with calcium
3 very lean protein	21 grams whey protein powder
3 teaspoons added sugar	1 tablespoon honey

Dinner

3 bread	1 1/2 cups cooked pasta
1 fruit	1 1/4 cups strawberries
2 vegetable	1 cup ratatouille (over pasta)
	Salad with 1 cup lettuce, 1/4 cup tomato, 1/4 cup cucumber
5 lean protein	5 ounces lean ground chicken (add to ratatouille)
1 fat	2 tablespoons low-fat dressing

DAY 3

Breakfast

2 bread	2 slices whole-wheat bread
1 milk	1 cup fat-free cottage cheese (on bread; sprinkle with no-calorie sweetener and cinnamon)
1 fruit	4 ounces freshly squeezed orange juice (with pulp)
1 medium-fat protein	1 egg, cooked sunny-side up in a nonstick pan
1 very lean protein	2 egg whites, cooked with sunny-side up egg
1 fat	1 1/2 tablespoons ground flaxseed
	Water
	Oil-free cooking spray (for eggs)

Lunch

2 bread	1 cup rice
1 milk	1 cup fat-free milk
2 vegetable	2 cups Chinese vegetables, stir-fried with garlic, onion, fresh ginger
1 fruit	1/2 cup mandarin oranges
4 very lean protein	4 ounces scallops, stir-fried
1 bean	1/2 cup black beans
1 fat	1 teaspoon oil (for stir-frying)

Pre-Workout Snack

1 bread	3/4 ounce baked tortilla chips (unsalted)
1 milk	1 ounce fat-free cheddar cheese
2 nut	10 cashews (unsalted)
1 vegetable	1 cup sliced bell pepper
	1/4 cup salsa

Post-Workout

SMOOTHIE

Blend until smooth.

1 milk	1 cup fat-free milk
2 fruit	1/4 cup pineapple (frozen)
	3/4 cup frozen strawberries
	1/2 cup orange juice with calcium
3 very lean protein	21 grams whey protein powder
3 teaspoons added sugar	1 tablespoon honey

Dinner

3 bread	1 cup kidney beans (add to chili)
	2-inch square of corn bread
1 fruit	1 pear
2 vegetable	1 cup chopped cooked tomatoes with chili seasoning
	½ onion, garlic (for seasoning)
	Salad with 1 cup lettuce, ¼ cup tomato, ¼ cup cucumber
5 lean protein	2 ounces lean beef, minced (add to chili)
	1 ounce ground turkey (add to chili)
1 fat	⅛ avocado, diced

DAY 4

Breakfast

1 fruit	1 cup raspberries
1 milk	1 cup fat-free milk (½ cup for French toast)

FRENCH TOAST (*See recipe directions on page 44.*)

2 bread	2 slices whole-wheat bread
1 medium-fat protein	1 egg
1 very lean protein	2 egg whites
1 fat	1½ tablespoons ground flaxseed
	Water
	Oil-free cooking spray

Lunch

1 fruit	½ mango
1 milk	1 cup fat-free milk

FAJITAS

Combine ingredients.

2 bread	2 tortillas
2 vegetable	1 cup sautéed onions, peppers
	2 tablespoons salsa
4 very lean protein	4 ounces skinless white-meat chicken, grilled with lime juice
1 bean	½ cup fat-free refried beans
1 fat	1 teaspoon olive oil (for cooking)

Pre-Workout Snack

1 bread	$1/2$ bagel
1 milk	$1/2$ cup reduced-fat ricotta cheese
2 nut	20 pistachios (unsalted)
1 vegetable	Radishes, tomatoes, mushrooms

Post-Workout

SMOOTHIE

Blend until smooth.

1 milk	1 cup fat-free milk
2 fruit	$1/4$ cup pineapple (frozen)
	$3/4$ cup frozen strawberries
	$1/2$ cup orange juice with calcium
3 very lean protein	21 grams whey protein powder
3 teaspoons added sugar	1 tablespoon honey

Dinner

3 bread	1 ounce croutons (for salad)
	1 small multigrain roll
	1 cup chicken noodle soup
1 fruit	1 nectarine
2 vegetable	Salad with 2 cups romaine lettuce, $1/2$ cup tomato, $1/2$ cup cucumber
5 lean protein	5 ounces swordfish, grilled with ginger and scallions
1 fat	2 tablespoons fat-free salad dressing
	1 teaspoon olive oil (for fish)

DAY 5

Breakfast

2 bread	1 cup quick oats (not instant)
1 milk	1 cup fat-free milk
1 fruit	$1/2$ cup diced apples
1 medium-fat protein	1 egg, scrambled in a nonstick pan
1 very lean protein	2 egg whites, scrambled with whole egg
1 fat	$1^1/_2$ tablespoons ground flaxseed
	Water
	Oil-free cooking spray (for eggs)

Lunch

2 bread	1 cup cooked linguini
1 milk	1 cup fat-free milk
2 vegetable	Salad with 1 cup lettuce, $^1\!/_4$ cup tomato, $^1\!/_4$ cup cucumber
	$^1\!/_2$ cup marinara sauce
1 fruit	$^1\!/_2$ starfruit
4 very lean protein	4 ounces shrimp, grilled
1 bean	$^1\!/_2$ cup fava beans
1 fat	1 teaspoon olive oil (for cooking)
	Fat-free salad dressing

Pre-Workout Snack

1 bread	5 pieces melba toast
1 milk	1 cup fat-free milk
2 fat	1 tablespoon almond butter
1 vegetable	1 cup sliced carrots, celery

Post-Workout

SMOOTHIE

Blend until smooth.

1 milk	1 cup fat-free milk
2 fruit	$^1\!/_4$ cup pineapple (frozen)
	$^3\!/_4$ cup frozen strawberries
	$^1\!/_2$ cup orange juice with calcium
3 very lean protein	21 grams whey protein powder
3 teaspoons added sugar	1 tablespoon honey

Dinner

3 bread	1 large pita
	$^1\!/_2$ cup couscous
1 fruit	1 large fig
2 vegetable	Salad with 2 cups romaine lettuce, $^1\!/_2$ cup tomato, $^1\!/_2$ cup cucumber
5 lean protein	5 ounces fresh trout (stuff with fig, couscous; drizzle with mint in lime juice)
1 fat	2 tablespoons reduced-fat vinaigrette

DAY 6

Breakfast

2 bread	2 slices multigrain toast
1 medium-fat protein	1 egg, scrambled in a nonstick pan
1 very lean protein	2 egg whites, scrambled with whole egg
	Oil-free cooking spray (for eggs)

SMOOTHIE

Blend until smooth.

1 milk	1 cup fat-free milk
1 fruit	1 fresh/frozen peach
1 fat	$1^1/_2$ tablespoons ground flaxseed
	Water

Lunch

2 bread	1 whole-wheat bagel
1 milk	1 cup fat-free milk
2 vegetable	1 cup carrot sticks
	3 slices onion, tomato
1 fruit	$^1/_2$ papaya
4 very lean protein	4 ounces poached salmon
1 soy	$^1/_2$ cup edamame
1 fat	3 tablespoons reduced-fat cream cheese

Pre-Workout Snack

Wrap broccoli and cheese in tortilla, and heat.

1 bread	1 tortilla
1 milk	1 ounce fat-free shredded cheese
2 nut	20 mixed nuts (unsalted)
1 vegetable	1 cup broccoli florets

Post-Workout

SMOOTHIE

Blend until smooth.

1 milk	1 cup fat-free milk
2 fruit	$^1/_4$ cup pineapple (frozen)
	$^3/_4$ cup frozen strawberries
	$^1/_2$ cup orange juice with calcium
3 very lean protein	21 grams whey protein powder
3 teaspoons added sugar	1 tablespoon honey

Dinner

3 bread	2 slices rye bread
	½ cup macaroni salad with fat-free dressing
1 fruit	17 grapes
2 vegetable	½ cup coleslaw
	½ cup chopped vegetables (cucumbers, carrots, onions; mix into tuna)
5 lean protein	5 ounces tuna in olive oil, drained
1 fat	2 tablespoons reduced-fat mayonnaise

DAY 7

Breakfast

2 bread	2 cups Kashi
1 milk	1 cup fat-free milk
1 fruit	1 cup raspberries
1 medium-fat protein	1 egg, hard-cooked (for egg salad)
1 very lean protein	2 eggs, hard-cooked (discard yolks)
1 fat	1½ tablespoons ground flaxseed
	2 tablespoons fat-free mayonnaise (for egg salad)
	Mustard (for egg salad)
	Water

Lunch

2 bread	1 multigrain roll
1 milk	1 cup fat-free milk
2 vegetable	Sliced tomato, lettuce (for sandwich)
	½ cup radishes, celery, carrots
1 fruit	1 slice watermelon
4 very lean protein	4 ounces skinless white-meat chicken, grilled with lime juice
1 bean	½ cup pinto beans
1 fat	2 tablespoons fat-free ranch dressing (for dipping)

Pre-Workout Snack

1 bread	1 small pita
1 milk	1 ounce fat-free cheese
2 nut	10 walnuts
1 vegetable	Cucumbers, tomatoes

Post-Workout

SMOOTHIE

Blend until smooth.

1 milk	1 cup fat-free milk
2 fruit	$^1/_4$ cup pineapple (frozen)
	$^3/_4$ cup frozen strawberries
	$^1/_2$ cup orange juice with calcium
3 very lean protein	21 grams whey protein powder
3 teaspoons added sugar	1 tablespoon honey

Dinner

3 bread	1 ounce croutons
	3-inch square of corn bread
1 fruit	1 large tangerine
2 vegetable	Salad with 2 cups romaine lettuce, $^1/_2$ cup tomato, $^1/_2$ cup cucumber
5 lean protein	5 ounces poached salmon
1 fat	Included (in corn bread)
	2 tablespoons fat-free Caesar dressing

CHAPTER EIGHT

Food and Sex

FUEL YOUR PASSION (NOT TO MENTION YOUR MACHINERY) WITH INTELLIGENCE

Meet Jim. Jim is an all-around attractive guy. He's handsome. He has a good job as an account executive with a brokerage firm. He's fit, well read, and a good conversationalist. Being a guy, Jim is also a sucker for fun and good-looking women, and he has been eyeing Mary, the redhead over in marketing, for several months now. At first, he was hesitant to show his interest, so he contented himself with admiring her from afar, avoiding any moves that might cause Mary to file a restraining order. Then, one day, furtive glances exchanged across a photocopier led to flirtatious greetings as the pair passed in the hall. Next thing you know, Jim was asking for, and receiving, her cell phone number.

Now, tonight's the night. He plans to pick her up at 7:00 P.M. and then take her out to dinner at an Italian restaurant that someone-who-knows-about-such-things recommended to him. He'll then escort her to a Broadway show, and if things go well, who knows? When the final curtain falls, "playtime" may have only just begun.

As he readies himself for work, Jim wonders what he should wear, what cologne he should choose, even what he might order for dinner that night. He's thinking so far ahead, in fact, that he skips breakfast. He's nervous. Jim has had trouble relaxing in the company of young ladies in the past, especially in the bedroom, where he's had problems with maintaining erections. Please, he thinks, let tonight be different.

At 7:00, he drives to Mary's house, picks her up (she looks stunning, of course), and takes her to dinner. It's been a long day, and he feels tired and foggy-headed almost immediately when they get to the restaurant. He fights the urge to put his head down. Over light conversation, he peruses the menu and orders pork for his main entrée. "Protein makes my muscles bigger, and every woman likes muscles," he thinks. Looking over the side dishes, he orders garlic mashed potatoes. He then remembers having read something about choosing a carbohydrate source that scores low on the glycemic index, so he also orders cauliflower and Brussels sprouts. Of course, he's a little nervous, so he decides to wash everything down with a cold beer. At dessert, he orders chocolate cake and sips espresso.

After the meal, Jim still feels nervous and slightly dull-witted (as he usually does after too much caffeine and chocolate), but he tries to keep the conversation moving. They head to the theater. Throughout the play, he checks to make sure Mary is having a good time. She seems to be enjoying his company, but she winces every time he leans over to whisper something in her ear. After the play, Jim takes Mary out for a nightcap. Mary has been a bit coy during the date and he's still not convinced she likes him; he can't wait for a drink to provide a little calming buzz. Mary orders an apple martini. Determined to stay sober, Jim orders a beer, his second this evening. Things start going pretty well. Mary gets comfortable and lets on that she's been wondering for a while what it might be like to date Jim. His confidence skyrocketing (aided in part by Mary, but certainly by the beer), Jim orders another. Then another. Things begin to get a little fuzzy . . .

Suddenly, it's the next day. Jim is lying in a bed—his own bed. He's fully clothed. Mary is nowhere to be found. As he lifts himself up and assesses the damage he's done to his suit by sleeping in it, he shakes his groggy head and notices the message light blinking on his answering machine. Tentatively, he presses "Play."

"Jim, it's Mary. I hope you're doing better than you were when I put you in that cab. Listen, I appreciate what you told me last night—it's not every first date that you receive a proposal of marriage. Oh, and don't worry about throwing up on my shoes; they were an old pair. I have to admit, though, I don't see things working out for us. By the way, I promise not to repeat what you told me about your sexual dysfunction. You can trust me. Take care."

Where did Jim go wrong? Everywhere. Unfortunately, I'm not qualified to address certain problems Jim's having, but I can say this: If Jim's diet were different, at least some things would have turned out better.

For Jim or any other guy, food does more than provide a backdrop to a date. By affecting how you feel, food can have a direct impact on the way you behave and, even more important, how you perform sexually. You might be surprised to learn that the root of erectile difficulty is often plaque that has built up in arteries, inhibiting blood flow. If you've read chapter 7, you know food can fix that. And food affects your love life in more-subtle ways, too, from your breath to your smell. Because food seems to be an integral part of most dates, it gives you the opportunity to make subtle changes *as the date progresses.*

In this chapter, I'll give you the secret eating techniques that will help you have better dates, and even better sex. Along the way, we'll revisit our hapless friend Jim to see how his diet might have sabotaged his game plan.

Getting Date-Ready

Few things are as attractive as confidence, and I like to think of the following advice as your guide to gaining confidence through food. When you know you can ask a woman out without feeling too nervous, when you know you can get through a date without feeling bloated or gassy, when you know you can kiss a woman without turning her off with your breath, you'll be much more likely to date the women you want.

Food and Mood

By the time you actually go out on your date (or even better, slip between the sheets with your new girlfriend), you'd think food would be the last thing on your mind. After all, you have each other, right?

How you perform, though, has a lot to do with how you've eaten or not eaten previously. Think about Jim. He made some classic date-time blunders and ended up passing out in his clothes. Don't want to be a Jim? Follow these tips.

Breakfast and Sex

One great way to boost your sex drive and to make sure you have the energy to face a long night out is to eat breakfast that morning. Jim skipped breakfast when he should have eaten some oatmeal or Shredded Wheat along with a few eggs, cooked any way he liked. Oatmeal provides enough complex carbohydrates for you to make it through not only the workday but also the play—and beyond, if need be. Also, oats and eggs provide a nice big helping of vitamins B_6 and B_{12}, which not only keep a guy's sex drive zooming but, paradoxically, also help him stay calm in the face of stress. And in the dating game, stress can mean the difference between sealing your doom and sealing the deal.

Fortified cereals are a nice alternative if you don't have much time for breakfast, assuming they contain plenty of thiamine and riboflavin, vitamins that help you use energy efficiently. As an added bonus, these vitamins are also needed for proper functioning of the nervous system, which has obvious advantages when you and your partner get your hands all over each other. Fortified cereals are also high in niacin, a vitamin that's essential for the secretion of histamine, a chemical your body needs in order to trigger orgasms.

Caffeine

How caffeine affects dating and sex depends on your personal sensitivity to it. Jim should have remembered that it makes him nervous and skipped the chocolate cake and espresso. If you're very sensitive to caffeine or chocolate, you may get jittery, grind your teeth, and feel like you just want to hurry up and get the date over with already. If you're feeling jittery in the sack, you may not be up to performing, or you may get impatient and let yourself perform exceptionally fast. Either way, you won't please her and you may not get a second chance.

Also, caffeine is a diuretic and a cathartic (in other words, it works like a rapid-acting laxative) although usually it takes more than just a cup of coffee for that to kick in. But if you've had several cups, you could end up in the bathroom. Leave the table for the bathroom too many times during a date, and she'll wonder if you have a problem. Leave too many times while you're in bed, and she might not come back for seconds.

Alcohol

On the other hand, there is alcohol. Jim reached for a beer when he felt uncomfortable. In moderation, this may not have been such a bad idea—drink a little bit of alcohol and you decrease your inhibitions. This can improve your performance, both on the town and in the sack. But let out your inner lush and you're done—your ability to communicate will break down, and you may even black out, as Jim did.

Sexually speaking, if you are drunk, nothing is going to stand up, including your masculine machinery. Larger amounts of alcohol will definitely make you dysfunctional sexually at a given point in time. Alcohol is a toxin that impairs your ability to produce testosterone. The less T you've got, the harder it'll be to get hard. Combine that with alcohol's effect on the brain—it slows messages between your centers for arousal and your penis—and you've all but strapped on a chemical chastity belt. The lesson is, keep your drinking to a minimum on any big night.

Food and Smell

Remember how Mary reacted when Jim whispered to her during the play? She winced. No doubt it had something to do with the garlic mashed potatoes he ate at dinner. But it wasn't just his breath. Your whole body can smell from garlic, which is so strong that it actually can come out of your pores. I know a garlic lover whose ex-girlfriend hated garlic and refused to put it in his dinner when she cooked for him. He tried to get around this by sneaking a garlicky slice of pizza from time to time and masking it with some Scope. No dice: The girlfriend always smelled it on him. What he didn't learn until later was that his breath was fine, but his sweat was rife with it.

Some of the sulfur-containing vegetables have the

same effect, although with some you can cook out the sulfur, removing the offending material before it enters your body and starts stinking up the joint. Broccoli, cauliflower, and similar vegetables should all be dropped in deep water and cooked with the lid off. If you steam them, the sulfur will remain, making neither you nor the vegetables very appealing.

Food and Breath

Aside from garlic, your breath can be fouled by any number of foods. In particular, exotic curried foods, alcohol, tobacco, and onions can linger on your breath for hours.

One of the best natural antidotes to halitosis—albeit a temporary one—is the bright green herb parsley. Cooks use it to add a clean, fresh flavor to dishes, and it can do the same for your breath. If you have a sprig on the side of your plate, you might try cutting off a piece and eating it with your meal. (A word of warning, though: Get caught doing this by a woman who isn't into eating garnishes, and you might do more damage than good.) Fresh mint can also be effective in this capacity.

If your bad breath results from gum disease or tooth decay, your dentist, not your diet, needs to fix the underlying problems, although food can mask the symptoms. He or she might resort to some nutritional strategies to help, though. Any healing that needs to be done in the gums will certainly be hastened along by zinc and vitamin C. If your dentist doesn't tell you to load up on these nutrients, take it upon yourself to do so.

Another possible cause of bad breath is a food allergy, although these cases are a distinct minority among other causes. If your breath problem coincides with other allergic symptoms, have your physician explore this possibility.

Food and Flatulence

It's been said that the average person passes gas 20 times a day. While this may not be the most socially

Say "No" to Bean Problems

If beans are a problem food for you, an enzyme product called Beano might be able to help. It works just like the lactase enzymes do for people who are lactose intolerant. So what do you do if your girlfriend has invited you over for lentil stew? Take your Beano with you. It comes in liquid and tablet form, so you can either put a few droplets on your food, or take the recommended number of tablets beforehand. The product works quite well, so that should be the end of your concerns.

acceptable topic for conversation, it does reflect this reality: It's natural to have some gas. You want to control it as much as possible, obviously. If you can't, the result can be uncomfortable, unpleasant, and extremely embarrassing. If flatulence becomes frequent or painful, perhaps through bloating, you should probably look at some of the foods that are likely causing it.

Where does that gas come from, anyway? It's a by-product of your body's efforts to digest what it consumes, often from carbohydrate that enters the large intestine without having been sufficiently broken down and absorbed. If that carbohydrate reaches the bacteria in your large intestine, the bacteria digest it themselves. A by-product of their efforts is gas, including methane. Your body needs to rid itself of these by-products, and thus, you pass gas.

Heading the list of problem foods is lactose. People who lack the enzyme lactase have trouble digesting lactose (a.k.a. the sugar in milk). It hits the large intestine largely intact, and hell breaks loose in the form of flatulence. This condition is extremely common. Eventually, more than half of all people lose at least some of their ability to produce this enzyme. If you're one of them, consider using lactase-replacement enzyme products so that you can still enjoy these foods.

So-called "resistant starches"—found in cereals, breads, and crackers—are another culprit. Although these are supposed to be protective against things like colon cancer, they reach that organ without having broken down, even in those individuals with all the relevant enzymes in full functioning order.

Fiber, though good for you, can also produce gas. Insoluble fiber in particular isn't intended for digestion, so it hits the large intestine more or less intact. Fibrous foods tend to be the worst culprits: legumes, bran, dried fruits, and cruciferous vegetables— which, you'll notice, are foods that have been recommended repeatedly in *Power Food*. That's the kicker: Many of the foods that are most healthy for you produce some gas in the large intestine.

Let's look at the cauliflower and Brussels sprouts Jim ate at dinner. They're both extremely nutritious vegetables, and they're recommended throughout this book. Not here, though. Because those vegetables are loaded with fiber, they and others of their kind—beans, lentils, onions, broccoli, and cabbage—are best avoided on dates and for 24 hours before, when the last thing you want is for your gastrointestinal tract to become overactive. Better choices would have been other low-glycemic-index vegetables such as leafy greens, peas, green beans, corn, and sweet potatoes.

Through trial and error, though, you should be able to figure out how much of the gas-inducing foods you can eat at a single sitting without becoming overly gassy. The flip side is that you want to eat enough fiber so that you're not constipated.

Foods that cause people gas are highly individualized and very specific. Beans may make one guy explode and barely affect another. For some guys, it's broccoli, cauliflower, and cabbage; for others, it's onions.

Fructose, or fruit sugar, can also cause gas problems. Your body doesn't digest it as quickly as it does sucrose or glucose. In the time it takes for that fructose to be handled, bacteria go to work on it, producing carbon dioxide and sometimes methane. The result: Picture the campfire scene from *Blazing Saddles,* and you're getting warm.

AGAINST THE WIND

FOLLOW THESE TIPS TO MINIMIZE FLATULENCE.

- Cook your food well. To reduce gas caused by eating beans, soak them overnight before cooking them. Canned beans might be easier on your intestines than dried beans. Try adding Beano to your food to help digest raffinose, the sugar in beans.
- Where appropriate, puree foods before eating them.
- Cut foods into small pieces.
- Chew your food very thoroughly.
- Eat and drink slowly. Avoid gulping. Everyone swallows some air when eating, but those who swallow too much can suffer severe flatulence as a result. The mixture of that air with your gastric juices can be volatile, leading to acid reflux as well.
- Introduce high-fiber foods gradually and incrementally into your diet. But do introduce them.

In the Bedroom

The runaway success of Viagra—Pfizer sold about $1.7 billion worth of the stuff last year alone—suggests not only that a great number of men suffer from erectile dysfunction, but also that a lot of men who aren't dysfunctional, technically, are nonetheless interested in performing better in the sack. Other than eunuchs and monks, perhaps, nearly every man alive cares about potency. Valid or not, society has taught men that this is the very essence of manhood.

If you are lucky enough to get a woman into your bed, there's nothing more embarrassing than not being able to "rise" to her expectations. You already know to watch alcohol consumption. But if that's not your problem and you're contemplating the blue diamond (a.k.a. Viagra), there are a few things you should know first about food: the cheap, natural means to pumping up your shorts. Here are a few guidelines for ensuring potency, pleasure, and longevity.

Water. Any athlete needs to be adequately hydrated to have enough energy, stamina, and endurance to compete effectively. You should take the same approach to sex. Drink 9 to 11 cups of liquid daily, and be sure that 5 or 6 of those are water. Also, drink early in the day. You don't want to waste precious bedroom time excusing yourself to go to the bathroom.

Celery. Say what? Yep. The blandest of vegetables can help stir up passion between the sheets. The magic ingredients are androstenone and androstenol, which are pheromones—chemicals that naturally hook women. This all happens before they ever leave your mouth. As soon as you bite into a stalk, these molecules are released into your mouth, and then into the outside world to act on unsuspecting women through subliminal persuasion. The same molecules turn you on, too. There are other reasons to eat celery, but I particularly like this one.

Chocolate. There's something undeniably sexy about chocolate to begin with and, as it turns out, cocoa has some chemicals that might make you a better lover. The first group, methylxanthines, are stimulants that increase the sensitivity of skin. The second is a chemical called phenylethylamine, which has been dubbed the "love molecule" because it seems to be connected somehow to that state of bliss. Similar in chemical structure to amphetamine, phenylethylamine is suspected of causing the high experienced by lovers.

Vanilla. On the other hand, you could go with vanilla ice cream. It gives you a blast of libido-lifting phosphorus along with 200 milligrams of calcium. The muscles that control ejaculations need enough of the latter to fire at full force, which could conceivably intensify orgasms. As a side bonus, the people in the white lab coats have discovered that the mere scent of vanilla takes the edge off a guy, putting him in the mood for intimacy.

A final word: aphrodisiacs. Except for the foods I've listed, there isn't much to be said for so-called aphrodisiacs—foods, powders, extracts, etc., that "magically" put people in the mood for sex. Most of the historical ones have been debunked, and a good deal of the others should be. In my book (I'm a woman, remember), the best aphrodisiac is feeling good about the way you look and the way you feel. Following the diet I've designed on page 328, along with making certain lifestyle decisions like working out, is the most scientific approach to better sex.

Sex for Life

For decades, we've taken for granted that diminished sexual function comes with old age. If a guy got to 60 years and could still make the bedsprings squeak, he was fortunate; if he got to 80 and could do it, he was a mini-god. But we've had it wrong. If he watches his diet and exercise, there's little reason a guy can't celebrate his 100th birthday as nature intended: in his birthday suit, sidled up to his mate.

Review the list of conditions that have been linked to impotence, and you've got a *de facto* review of the long-term illnesses I target in *Power Foods.*

■ A 2003 study found that obese men have a higher risk for erectile dysfunction (ED). The same study found that risk factors associated with heart disease correlate with increased risk for erectile dysfunction; a follow-up review suggested that this is because hardened, clogged arteries make supplying blood to the penis more difficult.

■ Studies, including a 2000 study out of Harvard and another that year out of Belgium, link high cholesterol with an increased risk of ED. (Incidentally, this is one occasion where getting ED may be a blessing in disguise—if you get it, make sure to see a physician and get your cholesterol tested.)

■ Approximately 50 percent of men with insulin-dependent diabetes experience some degree of sexual dysfunction after the age of 55. The disease is known to cause poor circulation and peripheral neuropathy (a condition where sexual stimuli don't transmit properly to and from the brain), both of which contribute directly to erectile dysfunction.

It all comes back to foods. Eat right and your body will perform right. Abuse your body with foods and the problems start: Saturated fats build in the body, cholesterol increases, cardiovascular disease begins, and the microvessels in your penis become inhibited. Blood flow becomes a problem. Sexual function diminishes.

Of course, you can fight it. In the long term, maintaining a healthy body weight, getting regular exercise, controlling refined carbohydrates, and limiting saturated fats and cholesterol—while feasting on antioxidants, fruits, and vegetables—will help alleviate potency problems caused by blocked arteries to the penis. All the foods that help promote a healthy heart and prevent diabetes are also important for maintaining sexual function.

Beyond the suggestions I made in the last section, there are specific ways to target and improve erectile dysfunction.

Grab peaches and the blues. Peaches are chock-full of vitamin C, insufficient levels of which tend to produce lower sperm counts. And blueberries are Mother Nature's version of Viagra. They're loaded with soluble fiber, which, having been dissolved, scrubs the walls of your arteries as it travels through your bloodstream. (The other kind of fiber, which is insoluble, passes through rather than dissolving.) The phytochemicals that make blueberries blue, called anthocyanins, also help relax your blood vessels, allowing blood to flow through them more freely. Given that satisfactory erections require good circulation, you can pretty much connect the dots yourself on this one.

Liver forever. This obscure food has some sex appeal because it contains a bunch of vitamin A, which boosts fertility. In studies, guys who consumed plenty of A each day had higher sperm counts and performed better sexually than men who didn't. When you're low on A, your sperm count falls precipitously. Liver also gives you plenty of zinc, which will come in handy. Your body expels 5 milligrams of that mineral—one-third of your daily requirement—every time you ejaculate, so one banner weekend could leave you in short supply. Because liver is the toxic filter in the body of animals, I recommend eating liver from organically raised animals. And eat small portions; it is notoriously high in cholesterol.

Mind your Brazil nuts. Environmental toxins

can damage your sperm, causing mutations in the DNA inside your cells. In a nightmare scenario, this could increase your child's risk of birth defects. One way to help prevent that from happening is eating plenty of undeservedly obscure Brazil nuts. Selenium is abundant in them, and it keeps sperm cells healthy and active. When researchers in the United Kingdom had men with fertility problems increase their selenium intake, the men produced hardier, more viable sperm cells. With their high levels of vitamin E, Brazil nuts are also good at protecting sperm cells against free-radical damage.

Avoid alcohol. Alcohol also has a long-term impact on libido, beyond the short-term effects already discussed. Too much alcohol drunk over too long a time has been associated with a reduction in the long-term production of male hormones and decreased sensitivity in the male sex organs.

Zinc a lot. Zinc deficiency has been linked with lower levels of the male sex hormone testosterone, and supplementation with zinc seems to restore lost potency, not to mention fertility. Researchers think zinc boosts libido by reducing the body's production of a hormone called prolactin.

Zinc supplements are available over the counter, and it's best taken with vitamin C—and not with caffeine, which appears to affect its absorption. (If you're not deficient in zinc, however, taking more won't make a discernible difference in how you feel or perform.)

The most prominent source of zinc is red meat and the dark meat of poultry, but it's also found in grains and legumes, as well as in some fortified products, like cereals fortified with zinc. Fish and other seafood can also be a good choice; not surprisingly, the famed aphrodisiac oysters are high in zinc.

The RDA for men is 15 milligrams of zinc a day. If you don't eat red meat, take a supplement, or use any of the fortified cereals on the market, your intake could be somewhat marginal, but you still probably wouldn't be deficient, technically speaking. You certainly don't mind taking in extra—extra is okay, although there is an upper limit.

Up your folic acid. There is a positive correlation between sperm counts, semen quality, libido, and folic acid: Higher levels of folate correspond to higher sperm quality. This is important stuff. It's possible that the quality of your sperm could affect the health of your unborn children.

You get folic acid from folate. It's a water-soluble B vitamin, and it's found in dark green leafy vegetables, such as spinach and romaine lettuce, as well as broccoli, citrus fruits, beans, nuts, whole-grain breads and cereals, and products fortified with folate.

If you don't feel like you're getting enough folate from whole foods, take a supplement. Look for a good multivitamin or B-complex vitamin that has at least 400 micrograms of folic acid per serving.

Zinc and folate are best taken together for a double-whammy effect. Dutch researchers found that men with normal or below-average sperm counts who took zinc supplements *and* folic acid supplements boosted their sperm counts by 74 percent. Interestingly, the two supplements worked better together than when taken at separate times.

Be wary of soy. The link is much less clear here, but soy may also have some connection to sexual dysfunction in men. A rat-based study published in the *Journal of Urology* found that eating soy might alter male reproductive organs, triggering sexual dysfunction.

Don't get me wrong. I think guys should eat soy. It has many benefits, including the ability to protect against cardiovascular disease and prostate cancer, both of which can lead to erectile dysfunction. Just be careful not to rely too heavily on it, and you won't get the potential negative side effects. The amounts in the various menu plans in this book are healthy amounts of soy.

SEX SUPPLEMENTS (AND DRUGS)

To date, three major anti-impotence drugs have hit the market. Here's a quick rundown, along with a look at over-the-counter dietary supplements that claim to boost libido and improve sexual performance.

Viagra

What it is: A prescription drug. Technical name: sildenafil

Who makes it: Pharmaceuticals giant Pfizer

How it works: The drug manipulates enzymes in the penile tissues that help regulate blood flow. Users must take it no more than 4 hours before they have sex.

Evidence: Numerous studies have proved its efficacy and safety.

Side effects: "A lot of people get flushing," says urologist Abraham Morgental, M.D. "People [also] can get stuffy noses, sinus congestion, upset stomach, and there's the famous but uncommon [occurrence where] people see bluish-greenish tints when they look at light. But none of these things are dangerous."

Warning: "You cannot take Viagra with any form of nitrates, which are usually medically prescribed things, like nitroglycerine, that men take for heart disease," says Morgental. "Combining them can drop your blood pressure precipitously and give you a heart attack."

Where to get it: A doctor's prescription. Also widely available online.

Cialis

What it is: A prescription drug. Technical name: tadalafil

Who makes it: Pharmaceutical company Lilly Icos

How it works: Like Viagra, it stimulates blood flow to the penis, but users can take it up to 36 hours before having sex.

Evidence: Many tests and studies as required by the FDA for drug-use approval.

Side effects: Many similar to Viagra: the bluish green tint, and sometimes an erection that doesn't go away for a few hours.

Warning: Cialis, like Viagra, cannot be taken with nitrates.

Where to get it: A doctor's prescription.

Levitra

What it is. A prescription drug. Technical name: vardenafil

Who makes it: Pharmaceutical companies Bayer and GlaxoSmithKline

How it works: Like Viagra, it stimulates blood flow to the penis. Users can take it no more than 5 hours before having sex.

Evidence: Many tests and studies as required by the FDA for drug-use approval.

Side effects: Again, similar to Viagra: runny nose, tinted vision, etc.

Warning: Levitra also cannot be taken with nitrates.

Where to get it: A doctor's prescription.

Herbal potency supplements

What they are: Combinations of herbs and other substances often marketed as natural alternatives to Viagra

Who makes them: Supplement companies. Brand names include Herbal V Ultra, Horny Goat Weed, BetterMan—you get the idea.

How they work: These products usually have one main ingredient, such as horny goat weed or yohimbe, intended to improve blood flow into the penis, boost testosterone levels, or both. Usually, they also contain ingredients such as Siberian ginseng, arginine, ginkgo biloba, and saw palmetto.

Evidence: Not much that you'd want to hang your hat on, so to speak. When looking at the studies that have been published on this stuff, make sure the researchers don't have a business connection to the manufacturer, which may have commissioned the research.

Side effects: Dizziness, sleep disturbance, headaches, and heart palpitations may occur with some of these products, particularly those with yohimbe.

Warnings: Heed labels and use caution. Without referencing these products specifically, in general, avoid herbal alternatives to Viagra if you're at risk or being treated for any cardio-vascular condition, including hypertension, heart disease, and stroke; kidney or thyroid ailments; or diabetes.

Where to get them: Health-food stores, drugstores, gyms, online, etc.

THE BETTER-SEX MEAL PLAN

HERE'S THE DIET THAT'S GOING TO FIT YOUR EVERY SEXUAL NEED. Got performance anxiety? Want to do better on a date and in the sack? This diet will boost your serotonin to help you relax, while it pumps up your testosterone, helping you perform. Carbs will help with that, as well as turkey and dairy. This diet stresses low- to moderate-GI carbs like leafy greens, peas, green beans, corn, sweet potatoes, apples, pears, and grapefruit. You'll also avoid foods like beans, lentils, onions, broccoli, cabbage, cauliflower, and Brussels sprouts. (They are great low-GI choices, but they won't necessarily help when you're getting into the mood.) Of course, stay away from too much fat, alcohol, or caffeine, and make sure you drink enough water to perform at peak levels. You want plenty of endurance.

Daily Assumptions*†

2,500 calories
281 grams carbohydrates
156 grams protein
83 grams fat

Daily Breakdown*†

8 bread
4 fruit
4 milk‡
6 teaspoons added sugar
6 vegetable
6 very lean protein
6 lean protein‡
1 medium-fat protein
8 fat

Note: Occasionally, a fat-free product, like mustard or cooking spray, is included on the menus. These do not count toward your daily breakdown but should not be overused.

*Use every day.

†Based on a 185-pound man.

‡You'll notice I sometimes use cheese as a milk and sometimes as a lean protein in this diet. Because the amount of fat you get here is less important than, say, a heart-health diet, I'm comfortable sometimes using them interchangeably.

THE MENU

DAY 1

Breakfast

2 bread	1 cup Shredded Wheat
1 milk	1 cup fat-free milk
1 fruit	$^3/_4$ cup fresh blueberries
1 medium-fat protein	1 egg, scrambled in a nonstick pan
1 very lean protein	2 egg whites, scrambled with whole egg
1 fat	$1^1/_2$ tablespoons ground flaxseed
	Water
	Oil-free cooking spray (for eggs)

Snack

Stuff pita with other ingredients.

1 bread	$^1/_2$ whole-wheat pita
1 lean protein	1 ounce part-skim cheese
1 vegetable	1 cup spinach, mushrooms, other vegetables
1 fat	2 tablespoons mixed nuts

Lunch

2 bread	2 slices whole-wheat bread
2 vegetable	Salad with 2 cups romaine lettuce, $^1/_2$ cup tomato, $^1/_2$ cup cucumber
3 very lean protein	3 ounces albacore tuna in water, drained
2 fat	1 tablespoon low-fat mayonnaise (for tuna)
	1 tablespoon vinaigrette

Snack

1 milk	1 cup fat-free milk
1 fruit	1 apple
1 lean protein	1 tablespoon peanut butter
1 fat	Included (in peanut butter)

Post-Workout

SMOOTHIE
Blend until smooth.

1 milk	1 cup fat-free milk
2 fruit	1/2 cup orange juice with calcium
	1/2 cup mango
	2/3 cup strawberries
2 very lean protein	14 grams whey protein powder
3 teaspoons added sugar	1 tablespoon honey

Dinner

3 bread	Medium sweet potato, baked
	1/2 cup brown rice
1 milk	Included (in yogurt)
3 vegetable	1/2 cup steamed asparagus
	Salad with 2 cups romaine lettuce, 1/2 cup tomato, 1/2 cup cucumber
3 teaspoons added sugar	1/2 cup vanilla fat-free frozen yogurt
4 lean protein	Turkey leg (dark meat), roasted
3 fat	Vinaigrette
	1/2 cup red wine

DAY 2

Breakfast

Combine yogurt, fruit, and flaxseed.

2 bread	1 whole-wheat English muffin
1 milk	1 cup fat-free unsweetened yogurt
1 fruit	1 1/4 cups fresh strawberries
1 medium-fat protein	1 egg, hard-cooked
1 very lean protein	2 eggs, hard-cooked (discard yolks)
1 fat	1 1/2 tablespoons ground flaxseed
	Water

Snack

1 bread	$^{1}/_{2}$ bagel
1 lean protein	1 ounce low-fat cheese
1 vegetable	Sliced tomato, onion
1 fat	16 to 20 mixed nuts

Lunch

2 bread	2 slices whole-grain bread
2 vegetable	Large salad with romaine lettuce, tomato, grilled eggplant, roasted red pepper
3 very lean protein	3 ounces skinless white-meat chicken, grilled with lime juice
2 fat	2 tablespoons fat-free dressing
	2 teaspoons olive oil (for roasted vegetables)

Snack

1 milk	1 cup fat-free milk
1 fat	20 pistachios
1 fruit	$^{1}/_{2}$ mango
1 lean protein	1 ounce reduced-fat ricotta cheese

Post-Workout

SMOOTHIE

Blend until smooth.

1 milk	1 cup fat-free milk
2 fruit	$^{1}/_{2}$ cup orange juice with calcium
	$^{1}/_{2}$ cup mango
	$^{2}/_{3}$ cup strawberries
2 very lean protein	14 grams whey protein powder
3 teaspoons added sugar	1 tablespoon honey

Dinner

3 bread	$1^{1}/_{2}$ cups cooked pasta
1 milk	1 cup fat-free milk
3 vegetable	2 cups ratatouille (over pasta)
	Salad with 2 cups romaine lettuce, $^{1}/_{2}$ cup tomato, $^{1}/_{2}$ cup cucumber
3 teaspoons added sugar	7 pastel after-dinner mints
4 lean protein	4 ounces lean ground beef (add to ratatouille)
3 fat	2 tablespoons ranch dressing
	1 tablespoon sunflower seeds

DAY 3

Breakfast

2 bread	2 slices whole-wheat bread
1 milk	1 cup fat-free cottage cheese (on bread)
1 fruit	4 ounces freshly squeezed orange juice (with pulp)
1 medium-fat protein	1 egg, cooked sunny-side up in a nonstick pan
1 very lean protein	2 egg whites, cooked with sunny-side up egg
1 fat	1 1/2 tablespoons ground flaxseed
	Water
	Oil-free cooking spray (for eggs)

Snack

1 bread	4 Wheat Thins
1 lean protein	1 ounce low-fat cheese
1 vegetable	1 cup diced bell pepper
1 fat	8 cashews

Lunch

2 bread	1 cup rice
2 vegetable	1 cup Chinese vegetables, stir-fried with garlic, onion, fresh ginger
3 very lean protein	3 ounces scallops, stir-fried
2 fat	2 teaspoons oil (for stir-frying)

Snack

1 milk	1 ounce reduced-fat cheddar cheese
1 fat	Included (in cheese)
1 fruit	1 cup sliced melon
1 lean protein	1 ounce ham

Post-Workout

SMOOTHIE

Blend until smooth.

1 milk	1 cup fat-free milk
2 fruit	1/2 cup orange juice with calcium
	1/2 cup mango
	2/3 cup strawberries
2 very lean protein	14 grams whey protein powder
3 teaspoons added sugar	1 tablespoon honey

Dinner

3 bread	1 cup mashed sweet potatoes
	1 slice brown bread
1 milk	1 cup fat-free milk
3 vegetable	1 cup asparagus, steamed
	Salad with 2 cups romaine lettuce, $^1/_2$ cup tomato, $^1/_2$ cup cucumber
3 teaspoons added sugar	1 tablespoon brown sugar (in potatoes)
4 lean protein	4 ounces salmon
3 fat	1 pat butter (for bread)
	1 teaspoon olive oil (for fish)
	1 tablespoon salad dressing
	Tea

DAY 4

Breakfast

1 fruit	1 cup raspberries
1 milk	1 cup fat-free milk ($^1/_2$ cup for French toast)

FRENCH TOAST (*See recipe directions on page 44.*)

2 bread	2 slices whole-wheat bread
1 medium-fat protein	1 egg
1 very lean protein	2 egg whites
1 fat	$1^1/_2$ tablespoons ground flaxseed
	Water
	Oil-free cooking spray

Snack

1 bread	1 slice multigrain bread
1 lean protein	1 ounce low-fat Swiss cheese
1 vegetable	Sprouts, tomatoes
1 fat	8 almonds

Lunch

FAJITAS

Combine ingredients.

2 bread	2 tortillas
2 vegetable	1 cup sautéed onions, peppers
	2 tablespoons salsa
3 very lean protein	3 ounces skinless white-meat chicken, grilled with lime juice
2 fat	2 teaspoons olive oil (for cooking)

Snack

LOW-FAT SHAKE

Blend ingredients.

1 milk	1 cup fat-free milk
1 fruit	1 small banana (frozen if desired)
1 lean protein	1 tablespoon natural peanut butter
	Ice cubes
1 fat	Included (in peanut butter)

Post-Workout

SMOOTHIE

Blend until smooth.

1 milk	1 cup fat-free milk
2 fruit	$\frac{1}{2}$ cup orange juice with calcium
	$\frac{1}{2}$ cup mango
	$\frac{2}{3}$ cup strawberries
2 very lean protein	14 grams whey protein powder
3 teaspoons added sugar	1 tablespoon honey

Dinner

3 bread	1 ounce croutons (for salad)
	1 cup chicken noodle soup
1 milk	1 cup fat-free milk
3 vegetable	Salad with 2 cups romaine lettuce, $\frac{1}{2}$ cup tomato, $\frac{1}{2}$ cup cucumber
	$\frac{1}{2}$ cup broccoli
	1 cup stewed tomatoes
3 teaspoons added sugar	1 tablespoon honey (for fish)
4 lean protein	4 ounces swordfish, grilled with ginger and scallions
3 fat	2 tablespoons salad dressing
	1 teaspoon sesame oil (for fish)

DAY 5

Breakfast

2 bread	1 cup quick oats (not instant)
1 milk	1 cup fat-free milk
1 fruit	1 apple, diced
1 medium-fat protein	1 egg, scrambled in a nonstick pan
1 very lean protein	2 egg whites, scrambled with whole egg
1 fat	$1\frac{1}{2}$ tablespoons ground flaxseed
	Water
	Oil-free cooking spray (for eggs)

Snack

1 bread	$^3/_4$ ounce baked tortilla chips
1 lean protein	1 ounce shredded low-fat Mexican cheese
1 vegetable	$^1/_4$ cup salsa
	1 cup sliced bell peppers
1 fat	6 peanuts

Lunch

2 bread	1 cup cooked linguini
2 vegetable	Salad with 1 cup lettuce, $^1/_4$ cup tomato, $^1/_4$ cup cucumber
	$^1/_2$ cup marinara sauce
3 very lean protein	3 ounces shrimp, grilled
2 fat	2 teaspoons olive oil (for cooking)
	Fat-free salad dressing

Snack

1 milk	1 cup fat-free milk
1 fruit	1 medium peach
1 lean protein	$^1/_2$ cup cottage cheese
1 fat	Included (in cottage cheese)

Post-Workout

SMOOTHIE

Blend until smooth.

1 milk	1 cup fat-free milk
2 fruit	$^1/_2$ cup orange juice with calcium
	$^1/_2$ cup mango
	$^2/_3$ cup strawberries
2 very lean protein	14 grams whey protein powder
3 teaspoons added sugar	1 tablespoon honey

Dinner

3 bread	1 large whole-wheat pita
	$^1/_2$ cup rice pilaf
1 milk	1 cup fat-free milk
3 vegetable	Cucumber, tomato, sprouts
	$^1/_2$ cup broccoli
	Salad with 1 cup lettuce, $^1/_4$ cup tomato, $^1/_4$ cup cucumber
3 teaspoons added sugar	2 medium figs
4 lean protein	4 ounces lean lamb, grilled with lime juice
3 fat	2 tablespoons vinaigrette
	1 tablespoon cucumber-yogurt dressing (for lamb)

DAY 6

Breakfast

2 bread	2 slices multigrain toast
1 medium-fat protein	1 egg, scrambled in a nonstick pan
1 very lean protein	2 egg whites, scrambled with whole egg
	Oil-free cooking spray (for eggs)

SMOOTHIE

Blend until smooth.

1 milk	1 cup fat-free milk
1 fruit	$^1/_4$ cup orange juice
	$^1/_2$ fresh peach
1 fat	$1^1/_2$ tablespoons ground flaxseed
	Ice cubes
	Water

Snack

Top pita with vegetables; heat.

1 bread	1 small pita
1 lean protein	1 ounce reduced-fat mozzarella
1 vegetable	$^1/_2$ cup diced tomatoes, mushrooms
1 fat	20 pistachios

Lunch

2 bread	1 whole-wheat bagel
2 vegetable	$^1/_2$ cup carrot sticks
	Onion, tomato
3 very lean protein	3 ounces smoked salmon
2 fat	2 tablespoons cream cheese

Snack

1 milk	1 ounce fat-free cheese
1 fruit	1 small orange
1 lean protein	1 ounce turkey
1 fat	$^1/_8$ avocado

Post-Workout

SMOOTHIE

Blend until smooth.

1 milk	1 cup fat-free milk
2 fruit	1/2 cup orange juice with calcium
	1/2 cup mango
	2/3 cup strawberries
2 very lean protein	14 grams whey protein powder
3 teaspoons added sugar	1 tablespoon honey

Dinner

3 bread	2 slices rye bread
	1/2 cup macaroni salad
1 milk	1 cup fat-free milk
3 vegetable	1 cup coleslaw
	1/2 cup broccoli
	1/2 cup chopped vegetables (cucumber, carrots, onion; mix into tuna)
3 teaspoons added sugar	1/2 cup orange gelatin with mandarin oranges
4 lean protein	4 ounces tuna in olive oil, drained
3 fat	6 tablespoons reduced-fat mayonnaise (for tuna, coleslaw, macaroni salad)

DAY 7

Breakfast

2 bread	1 cup Kashi
1 milk	1 cup fat-free milk
1 fruit	1 cup raspberries
1 medium-fat protein	1 egg, hard-cooked (for egg salad)
1 very lean protein	2 eggs, hard-cooked (for egg salad; discard yolks)
1 fat	1 1/2 tablespoons ground flaxseed
	Water

Snack

1 bread	5 slices melba toast
1 lean protein	1/4 cup reduced-fat ricotta
	(Stir dry onion soup mix into ricotta to make dip.)
1 vegetable	1 cup celery sticks
1 fat	6 pecan halves

Lunch

2 bread	1 multigrain roll
2 vegetable	Sliced tomato, lettuce for sandwich
	$^1/_2$ cup radishes, celery, carrots
3 very lean protein	3 ounces skinless white-meat chicken, grilled with lime juice
2 fat	2 tablespoons ranch dressing (for dipping)

Snack

1 milk	1 ounce reduced-fat cheese
1 fruit	1 kiwi
1 lean protein	1 ounce low-fat ham
1 fat	Included (in cheese)

Post-Workout

SMOOTHIE

Blend until smooth.

1 milk	1 cup fat-free milk
2 fruit	$^1/_2$ cup orange juice with calcium
	$^1/_2$ cup mango
	$^2/_3$ cup strawberries
2 very lean protein	14 grams whey protein powder
3 teaspoons added sugar	1 tablespoon honey

Dinner

3 bread	1 ounce croutons
	3-inch square of corn bread
1 milk	1 cup fat-free milk
3 vegetable	Salad with 1 cup romaine lettuce, $^1/_2$ cup tomato, $^1/_2$ cup cucumber
	$^1/_2$ cup broccoli
3 teaspoons added sugar	$^1/_2$ fresh papaya
4 lean protein	4 ounces salmon, poached
3 fat	4 tablespoons low-fat Caesar dressing
	Included (in corn bread)

CHAPTER NINE

Food and Appearance

SAVE FACE WITH THE FOODS THAT MAKE YOU LOOK YOUR BEST

Any self-respecting guy shouldn't be caught dead doing certain things. Playing air guitar springs quickly to mind, as does participating in cardio classes led by a pony-tailed, high-stepping instructor sporting a headset mike and imploring you to "get, like, totally pumped." And doing 10 minutes of power yoga and then rolling around on rubber balls to limber up may be effective flexibility training, but . . . nah.

Here's another: No self-respecting guy should throw in the towel on his appearance. No one expects you to look like George Clooney (unless you are George Clooney), but your appearance is probably important to your employers and colleagues; it's definitely important to your partner, regardless of what he or she says; and it should be important to you. This isn't an ode to narcissism, and appearance should never be the most important thing in your life—or even among the top three. But take pride in the person you present to the outside world.

Remarkably, many men don't seem to care much about that image. Study after study has shown that, by and large, women are far more concerned with their appearance then men are with theirs. But it's a fact of life (as reliable as death and taxes) that people are going to judge you by your appearance. Americans especially can be unmercifully shallow.

Admittedly, I'm not a fan of our beauty-centric ways. Outside of keeping your weight down (which I've shown is a necessity if you want to live longer), I think people should feel comfortable with how they choose to look. But my beliefs won't keep the woman of your dreams (or your boss, relatives, etc.) from judging you by your clothes, your hair, your skin, and your smile. You have to be prepared to look your best if you want to succeed. And to look your best, you'll need to eat your best. The cosmetic improvements produced by diet are less imperative than the health changes, but they can shape a man's quality of life like few things can. Do you have acne? How you eat could be causing it. Is your hair brittle or are your teeth rotting? Maybe it's time you changed your mealtime habits. At worst, eating for appearance will keep you slim and healthy; at best, it can help change your life.

The Basics of Eating to Look Good

There are five basic principles that you need to learn if food is going to have any affect on your appearance.

1. Good hydration is a must.

We can't live without water, and neither can our social lives. If you doubt me, try going a week without bathing. Your friends at work would probably start e-mailing you instead of dropping by your office, and your dating pool would dry up like a fig. If you went a month without washing your hair? Picture a captive Saddam Hussein. Now picture his social life. Any questions?

But water works its magic beneath your skin as well. If you've read chapters 6 and 7, you've already learned some lessons about water and fiber. Together, they carry toxins out of your body. What happens when the toxins stay? In addition to bladder infections and maybe even various cancers, they can hurt how you look. Your hair, skin, and nails may get dull and dry. You may break out in acne or dermatitis. Your face may become extraordinarily puffy, especially around your eyes, which in turn may be dried out and red.

Water also fills up your cells and allows protein synthesis to occur within. These proteins are, to some extent, what compose the skin. Researchers have looked at hydration's effect on skin at the cellular level, and they've found that the more water a cell contains, the less prone it is to invasion by potentially harmful bacteria. Once their structural integrity has been breached, these "cracked" skin cells are unhealthy. In other words, don't drink water and you'll get crummy-looking skin.

The important thing to remember is that your skin is an organ, just like your heart, liver, and kidneys—only larger. All of the body's other organs suffer when you become dehydrated, and skin is no different.

2. When it comes to proteins, think zinc.

The connection between skin and the protein you consume in food can't be overstated—it has a lot to do with how you look. Skin, nails, and hair are made of protein. However, if you're eating only a small amount of protein, your body will ship the protein nutrients to essential body parts first. Your hair, skin, and nails will end up deprived of their main building block, and they'll weaken and look lousy: Your hair might start to fall out. Your nails might break more easily, while your skin gets duller, dry, flaky, sore, and irritated—even infected in areas. Even your eyes will be affected: Their mucous membranes may dry out and get distorted. With marginal protein intakes, this will probably take a number of months. With total protein deficiency, early symptoms can start in a few weeks.

Another bonus: The protein sources of lean red meats, dark meat poultry, seafood, shellfish, as well as nuts, eggs, and fermented soybean paste also have high levels of the mineral zinc, which is important for hair, skin, and nail health. This isn't a green light to eat any kind of high-fat protein source. All that saturated fat will clog up your arteries and the small blood vessels that feed your skin, nails, eyes, and hair, leading to a sorry look inside and out.

3. Get your good fats.

Fats are crucial, too. The skin's natural moisture balance depends on sufficient essential fatty acids from fish oils, nuts, seeds, olives and olive oils, lecithin (from eggs), and flaxseed. These fats help maintain the integrity of membranes that are essential for the proper functioning of cells, keeping good things in and bad things out. That's one reason your skin becomes cracked, dry, scaly, and itchy when you don't consume enough of these fats.

4. **Cover the big dangers with vegetables.**

This one should be easy to understand by now. The antioxidants in dark and brightly colored fruits and vegetables, vegetable oils high in vitamin E, green tea, soybeans high in phytochemicals, the mineral selenium—all of these are critical for helping to ward off diseases and cancers of the skin and eyes. And for any vegetarians who aren't getting enough zinc from their proteins, there's a decent amount in whole grains and some in legumes, peaches, and onions.

5. **If you're eating a lot of sugar, nothing else will matter much.**

When it comes to your appearance, the white stuff is a killer. A diet high in sugar is probably deficient in other things essential for ensuring the health of skin, hair, and nails. Unhealthy diets high in sugar and fat also increase the chances that your arteries will begin to narrow. Although it won't be your biggest concern at the time, blood won't flow easily through your clogged arteries, and the nutrients and oxygen that feed the skin and carry toxins away won't reach their target. You'll be left with lousy-looking skin, eyes, hair, and nails, not to mention a heart prone to stopping without warning.

In fact, if you want to do one thing that can make you look 10 years younger, forget facelifts—just slash your sugar consumption. The impact will be profound because sugar is responsible for nearly half of all aging that goes on inside skin cells. It wreaks its havoc by binding with collagen, the protein that constitutes 75 percent of skin.

This binding process causes a chemical reaction leading to something called *glycosylation*. Here's how it works: Unperturbed, collagen molecules slide across one another with little friction. When that's happening, skin has the softness and elasticity of a baby's bottom. Once sugar attaches to collagen molecules, however, the latter start to get stuck as they try to pass, gunking up the works. Collagen is responsible for warding off wrinkles and lines, but when sugar interferes, the result is sagging skin and wrinkles. Glycosylation can also cause age spots and discolored marks on the skin by overworking *melanocytes,* the cells that provide pigment.

A Closer Look at Your Parts

Master the five rules above, and you'll probably notice some significant changes in your appearance. But we're not done yet. If you're intent on keeping your skin clear and disease-free for life, your hair thick and healthy, and your teeth stronger than diamond chips, you'll need to focus on each part specifically. Here's a look at the places you'll see the biggest changes if you mind your meals with an eye toward your appearance.

Skin Deep

If you think about what skin does—what it combats, how it heals itself—it's arguably the most miraculous construct of the human body. It's sensitive enough to register the full range of emotions prompted by a lover's touch, yet strong enough to protect you against the searing rays of the sun. What's this strange organ that shields your insides from the outside world, while letting through those things you need for survival?

Strictly speaking, your skin is about 6 pounds of water, protein, lipids, and various minerals and chemicals. All of these hang together as a tight mesh of cells that encase your body, holding your insides in and keeping the outside out. These cells are actually a lot less stable than you may think, being born and dying with such regularity that the average human body completely "changes" its skin every 27 days.

Throughout your lifetime, your skin will face a barrage from the elements. But we're not defenseless. Science and technology have combined to give us a far better understanding into protecting our skin than we had even 15 years ago. Not surprisingly, a lot of what we've learned comes back to how we eat.

Fighting Sunlight

You may wonder what food has to do with protecting you from sunlight. Quite a bit, actually. In fact, a range of whole foods, herbs, and vitamins appears not only to protect you against cancers of the skin but also to help slow some of the physical manifestations of aging.

To understand this, you have to understand how the sun damages your skin. Think of the sun like most people think of their job. On one hand, you can't live without it; on the other, it wears you down over time, stressing your body and eventually contributing to your demise. The same sun that warms us also wages war on our skin, zapping it constantly with an invisible intruder called ultraviolet radiation (UVR). Stay out in the sun too long one day, and you'll see the superficial effects of UVR in the form of a painful burn. Compare a portion of your skin that is routinely obscured from sunlight by clothing, such as your inner thigh, with a section that receives daily exposure, like the back of your hand, and you'll have a sense of what the cumulative impact is.

Ultraviolet radiation comes in three forms. UVB rays are probably the best known; these are the rays that turn the outer layers of your skin red if you neglect your sunscreen. For long-term health, though, the bigger threat is actually posed by UVA rays. Those penetrate more deeply, damaging the fibers in

> ### *Foods That Will Make You Look Better*
>
> Eat these foods to give your looks a lift.
>
> | | |
> |---|---|
> | Dark and brightly colored fruits and vegetables | Green tea |
> | | Lean red meat |
> | Dark-meat poultry | Milk |
> | Eggs | Olive oil |
> | Fiber | Seafood (especially oysters) |
> | Fish | Soy |
> | Flaxseed | Water |

the skin called elastin. As these fibers break down, skin loses its ability to snap back after stretching, leading to wrinkles. (The third kind, UVC rays, never make it through the ozone layer.) Skin would age through time even if you spent your entire life in a dark room, but as the years pass, this process can be accelerated dramatically by UVA rays, causing your skin to loosen, sag, and wrinkle prematurely. These rays also damage the blood vessels infusing these deep skin layers, making them more susceptible to everything from minor infections and inflammation to the cell mutations that predate cancer.

The damage can be inflicted early, but it almost always gathers momentum as a guy passes through his 30s and 40s. The process is cumulative, so the damage only truly reveals itself after decades, at which point it's mostly irreversible.

Eventually, that damage can take the form of a life-threatening disease. In fact, the three most common forms of skin cancer are all caused by exposure to UV radiation. Nearly half of all Americans who make it to 65 will develop skin cancer, and just having a sunburn a few times can double or triple the risk of a melanoma. More than 750,000 new cases of skin cancer are diagnosed in the United States every year, more than any type of cancer. So the next time you receive a compliment on your killer tan, think twice about the potential long-term costs of that George Hamilton–like bronzing.

For full disclosure, I must tell you the best diet in the world isn't going to protect you if your skin routinely or even occasionally endures the damaging rays of the sun without topical protection. Some sun is good for you, and a bit of tan won't hurt. Too much sun is bad, though, and a skin tone that looks radioactive is a prescription for skin cancer down the road.

You can help protect yourself by eating right. The antioxidants you eat—and not just the ones you put on your skin topically—can help you avoid cancerous skin changes. Skin protection is just one more reason to increase your intake of antioxidant-rich foods by eating at least five servings of fresh fruits and vegetables daily. In general, eating more foods that have cancer-fighting properties—cold-water fish, beans, carrots, chard, pumpkin, cabbage, garlic, broccoli, tomatoes, oranges, apricots, and cantaloupe, for example—is a great way to keep your skin from suffering malignancies.

Some nutrients seem to prevent or combat skin cancers specifically. Lignans, which are found in cereal grains, vegetables, and flaxseed, seem to prevent the spread of malignant melanoma in animals. Polyphenols, the phytochemicals found in green tea, black tea, and grapeseed extract, also appear to reduce the formation of skin tumors. Green tea extract helps soothe skin and reduce inflammation.

Milk is another food that can help your skin, as the lactic acid it contains helps moisturize. Oat extract reduces irritation. Soybean extract functions as both an antioxidant and an anti-inflammatory.

It all boils down, again, to eating a well-rounded, healthy diet complete with cold-water fatty fish, fruits, vegetables, grains, flaxseed, beans, nuts, and seeds, supplemented with additional vitamins C and E. Pretty much all of the things that I've talked about as being good for your inside are very important for your outside as well.

Fighting acne. Few guys escape their teens without waging a losing battle against zits, and for many men, the curse can continue well into adulthood. It became fashionable in the 1960s and 1970s to blame sweets like chocolates and greasy foods for acne, but researchers have since found that the causes are more complicated than that. Diet plays a role, but it's not necessarily even the lead actor.

Where sugar is, bacteria flourish, and those bacteria can cause acne. One study looked at the pimples that afflict your average teenager—not a disease state, per se—and found that a diet high in refined carbohydrate did increase the rate at which blemishes appeared. Other research done at Colorado State University suggests that the main culprit isn't chocolate bars, cheeseburgers, and pizza, but highly refined breads and cereals. Here's the rationale: When your blood sugar rises sharply in response to these carbs, your body produces more of the hormones that clog up your pores, causing infection and inflammation. The study's author notes that in countries where diets contain little or no refined sugars, acne is virtually nonexistent.

As a general rule, the things you do to keep the rest of yourself healthy are generally good for your skin, too. That certainly applies to the perils of consuming lots of refined sugars and other refined carbohydrates. They're not good for you, and they're probably not good for your skin, either. If you have problems with acne, in addition to avoiding "bad" foods, consider staying away from foods that register high on the glycemic index. Lower-GI foods deliver sugar at a slower rate and are packed with fiber. They also tend to have antioxidants that help eliminate free radicals and reduce inflammation.

Omega-3 fatty acids are good for pretty much everything else under the sun, so it probably won't surprise you to hear that they can calm unsettled skin, too. These fats are important for maintaining the integrity of cell membranes, and if membranes are kept intact rather than compromised, the risk of an infection, and hence pimples, decreases.

Fiber can also help battle acne. It helps move things quickly through your system, and when things slow down, toxins stand a better chance of being reabsorbed from the intestines. The result of that process can definitely reach the skin's surface. If you're eating a diet high in fiber, the things your body needs to get rid of are in fact being eliminated. That's going to make you healthier overall, and your skin looking much better will merely reflect that.

Star Players in the Skin Game

So what foods are best suited to provide the sort of protection I've discussed? In addition to the general categories I just covered, the following specific foods are all good bullets to have in your holster.

Halibut. This saltwater whitefish would get high marks just for its firm texture and delicately sweet taste, but its good omega-3 content also makes it a must-eat for those concerned about their skin. Omega-3 essential fatty acids keep your skin moist and healthy looking, and halibut is about as nutrient-dense as a fish can get. In addition to the lean protein it provides, here's a laundry list of other healthy nutrients it contains: vitamins A, B$_6$, and C; calcium; fiber; folate; iron; magnesium; potassium; niacin; and thiamine.

If you can't get your hands on halibut, try salmon, trout, and sardines, all excellent options for getting a healthy dose of skin-friendly omega 3s.

Whole wheat. Whole grains, including whole-wheat breads, contain a bunch of zinc. Your body needs zinc to make collagen, the fibrous protein with which skin is formed, making it key for overall skin health, elasticity, and firmness. Working in concert with vitamin A, zinc also plays an important role in repairing burned skin.

When you go to pick out grains at the supermarket, you'll encounter a bewildering array of products under an equally bewildering array of labels. Choose one that says "whole grain" somewhere on the package. In the case of whole-wheat bread, the package should say "100 percent whole wheat" somewhere on the label. (For comparison, enriched white bread has only 36 percent of the zinc found in whole-grain bread.) And whether it's brown rice, whole rye, oats, whole wheat, or something else, check to see that the whole grain in question appears first in the list of ingredients. There are numerous grains on the market, though, so there's no need to be limited to whole-wheat bread. Barley, brown rice, buckwheat, bulgur (cracked wheat), flaxseed, millet, quinoa, and triticale will all do the trick.

Cantaloupe. Its real name, muskmelon, may sound like the title of a dirty movie, but this distinguished member of the melon family receives praise in this context because nature has jam-packed it with beta-carotene, a vitamin A precursor. Vitamin A, like zinc, plays a major role in skin growth and repair. Cantaloupes include a bunch of other healthy nutrients for good measure. None of the other melons can hold a candle to cantaloupe, either. It has at least three times more vitamin C, ten times more beta-carotene, and one-third more potassium than its counterparts. No wonder Christopher Columbus thought highly enough of this fruit to bring seeds along with him on his second voyage to the New World.

Cantaloupe is now available nearly year-round. At the supermarket or fruit stand, select one that makes you want to shoot a jump shot—the rounder, the better. The skin should be yellow-gray; ideally, the raised netting surrounding it should be thick and coarse, forming an even pattern. Avoid melons with cracks, soft spots, bruises, and other signs of wear and tear. The aroma should be mild but pleasant. If a cantaloupe has a greenish tint to it, it's still a few days away from ripeness. The cantaloupes in stores

Foods That Make You Look Worse

Avoid these foods—they won't help with your appearance.

Alcohol	High-sugar foods
High-fat foods	Salty foods

are often 2 to 4 days away from this state, and keeping it at room temperature until then will make it softer and juicer.

Once you cut it open, remove the seeds from the center and scoop out the flesh. Cover and refrigerate what you don't eat. Not only does cantaloupe dry out easily, but it also absorbs the odors of surrounding foods and emits a strong odor itself.

Spinach. This summer green didn't just make Popeye big and strong—it gave his skin that smoothness that the ladies love. Actually, we have no idea how his skin tone registered with the fairer sex, but we know this: Spinach contains healthy amounts of vitamins A, B, and C; as well as the antioxidant trifecta, which guards against sun damage, dry skin, rashes, and various skin diseases. Spinach also gives you the antioxidants lutein and quercetin, more important weapons in the war against skin and eye damage.

Raw spinach is a great constituent in salads, but cooking it actually makes the antioxidant carotenoids easier for your body to absorb. Spinach can also be sautéed, steamed, or cooked in the microwave.

Pomegranates. This low-GI fruit is a concentrated source of antioxidants like vitamin C, as well as flavonoids. Indeed, research conducted at the University of California at Davis found that the polyphenols in bottled pomegranate juice gave it two to three times the antioxidant capacity of identical amounts of red wine and green tea. Drinking the

juice or eating a pomegranate can help offset the rise in glucose that normally follows a meal high in fat and calories.

Lentils. Where skin health is concerned, these smallish disk-shaped legumes pack a wallop. First, they contain large amounts of protein and antioxidants, two things seldom found jointly in abundance. They have 15 grams of fiber per cup, most of it soluble, the kind that whisks cholesterol out of your arteries. Studies show that high-fiber diets can lower blood sugar, which might keep excess sugar from compromising the collagen in skin cells. As an added bonus, all that fiber should help fill you up. That should decrease your cravings for inflammation-causing carbohydrate sources.

Lentils are packed with other beneficial nutrients such as the B vitamin folate, iron, magnesium, and zinc. They lack cholesterol, sodium, and saturated fat. Lentils are also the richest plant source of folate.

Consider legumes a good substitute for pasta. They're also good as a side dish or as a base for salads and soups.

One final consideration where skin is concerned: It is possible that food, or supplements, can actually change the color of your skin. If you drink a whole lot of carrot juice, the beta-carotene will turn you orange, or at least more of a muted yellow-orange tint than most people would consider attractive. Starting with the soles of your feet, it spreads from there to the rest of your body. It's nothing to worry about, per se, and it isn't a sign of impending toxicity. Just realize that you're going to have the slightest of orange tints about you.

Bone Health and Posture

Nutrition affects appearance in a general, systemic way through bone health, which in turn affects posture. Walking around with stooped shoulders isn't appealing to anyone, you included. Whether they're looking at someone else or at a reflection in a mirror, most people consider bad posture to be the most telling visible calling card of a guy lacking self-esteem and self-confidence.

Bad posture can also serve as an early warning signal of a higher-than-average risk for developing osteoporosis, a bone disease characterized by decreased bone mass and structural deterioration of the tissue that forms it. As bones become increasingly fragile, you become more susceptible to fractures of the hip, spine, and wrist.

Some think bone loss is a woman's concern, not a guy's. They're wrong. Medical professionals believe that osteoporosis in men has been dangerously ignored, noting that men suffer one-third of all hip fractures. Granted, this probably isn't something you'll have to deal with until you're playing with your grandkids, especially because osteoporosis tends to set in later in men than in women. Yet your susceptibility to an osteoporosis-related fracture, for example, will reflect what you're eating now, as well as what you'll be eating in your later years. After their early 30s, men and women alike begin losing about ½ percent of their bone density annually. The body is still making bone, but it's losing more than it can replace. So just as someone facing an extended stretch of deprivation can benefit from fattening up ahead of time, maximizing the amount of bone in your body *now* may mean that later, should bone thinning occur, your bones nonetheless should still be dense enough not to fracture.

This probably won't be a news flash to even the most unenlightened guy where nutrition is concerned, but having healthy bones means taking in plenty of calcium. (Lifting weights is also important.) The National Institutes of Health recommend higher levels of calcium intake than the RDA amounts—specifically, 1,200 to 1,500 milligrams for those ages 11 to 24, and 1,000 milligrams for those ages 25 to 50.

Vitamin D plays a pivotal role in bone health, too, because the body uses it to absorb calcium. Magnesium is also involved in a number of reactions in bone formation, leading some experts to equate magnesium with calcium in importance where this is concerned.

Not just any calcium will do, though. As much of it as possible should come in a form the body can absorb efficiently. Milk, yogurt, cheese, and other dairy products are particularly good in this regard because they contain key acids that heighten calcium's absorption. That presents a potential problem for the millions of guys in the United States who are lactose intolerant, meaning they can't digest milk and other dairy without incurring a major tummyache. Fortunately, there are more ways than ever to navigate your way around that. You can take calcium in supplement form, or you can seek out nondairy sources of calcium in whole foods, including dark green leafy vegetables and breads made with calcium-fortified flour.

Other foods and nutrients that appear to help with calcium absorption are the essential fatty acids found in fish, and vegetable oils. Vitamins B_6, C, and K; folic acid; and the minerals boron and potassium also play significant roles in promoting bone health through reduced calcium loss. A more obscure, overlooked nutrient that the body uses for maintaining strong bones is silicon. We refer not to the kind in your PC or inflating Hollywood starlets' chests, but rather to a nutrient, found in oatmeal and other foods, that benefits your hair, skin, and bones. A recent report in the *American Journal of Clinical Nutrition* says that eating whole grains and drinking more beer (of all things) are good ways to corral more of this mineral. Good thing, too, because silicon consumption tends to decrease in men as they age, which could contribute to bones becoming more brittle.

Other than not taking in enough calcium to support bone development and maintenance, might your diet be undermining your bone health? Absolutely. The biggest problem for bone health is simply not taking in enough calories and nutrients. Too much phosphorus, found in soda, is another problem. It'll cause you to excrete more calcium in your urine.

Joint health is also shaped by your diet, which has implications for your appearance. You might think you look great, but if you stagger into a room like you just went three rounds with Mike Tyson, you're not going to make the best possible impression.

The key factor here is weight management. If you're overweight, reducing your weight by as little as 10 percent can help to reduce the stress on your joints. As far as specific nutrients go, the same protein that dominates your skin—collagen—underpins your joints and other connective tissues. Supplements like glucosamine can also help. It works as an anti-inflammatory and can decrease the pain in your joints. Without pain, you can continue to work out on a regular basis, helping to maintain your bone health and your body weight. As long as you still have some collagen left in your joints, glucosamine may also help rebuild some of your lost collagen. This, of course, takes months and years to occur.

Food and Your Eyes

Here's another chance for you to improve your long-term health through vanity. Stay concerned about the way your eyes look, and you'll be able to avoid conditions like macular degeneration (in its early stages, your eyes may look consistently bloodshot) and glaucoma (your eyes eventually look clouded over at the pupil) in the long run, both of which are major causes of blindness.

According to the National Eye Institute of the National Institutes of Health in Bethesda, Maryland, age-related eye diseases such as macular degeneration and cataracts may be caused by insufficient antioxidants in the diet. Specifically, if you're deficient in vitamin A, you have a greater chance of developing night blindness, and your eyes may be sensitive to flashes of light.

Beta-carotene is a precursor of vitamin A, but one of your nutrition goals should be to take in the full range of the carotenoids. There's not only beta but also alpha, gamma, and delta. You can get all of them if you eat dark green leafy vegetables and orange, red, and yellow vegetables. The recommended amount of vitamin A is 5,000 IU (international units) daily.

Along with grapes and cherries, seasonal fruits such as plums and blueberries provide the best sources of these free radical—neutralizing antioxidants that are so good for eye health.

Instead of buying expensive flavored sparkling water, try taking good old-fashioned seltzer water or just plain sparkling water and mixing it with pure grape juice, with no sugar added. Fill a glass with one part grape juice to three parts water, and it tastes really good. (A glass full of pure grape juice will be excessively sweet for some people.) If you don't drink wine, it's a great way to take in all of the antioxidants provided by red grapes.

Cranberry juice is good for you, too, and for many of the same reasons. Unlike grapes, cranberries aren't naturally sweet, so cranberry juice does contain a lot of sugar. The easiest thing for guys to do is buy the low-sugar cranberry juice. The standard ones that are bottled on the shelves by companies such as Ocean Spray are fine. (Avoid cran-apple and other hybrid juices, which dilute the cranberry in the juice.) Or you can buy a small bottle of pure cranberry extract and either cook with it, put it in tea, or sweeten it yourself.

And don't forget about lutein, found in corn (another great fiber source), spinach, and cabbage. Lutein is a primary protective component of the eye medulla, a part of the retina that's extremely sensitive to light damage. In recent studies, researchers found that lutein may help prevent both medullar degeneration and cataracts.

Aesthetic Assets

The issues just covered fall under general health issues that also affect appearance to a greater or lesser extent. Your diet also affects your body in ways that are more purely aesthetic, for lack of a better term.

Food and your smile. A fruit or vegetable a day may keep away not only the doctor but also the dentures. A recent USDA study found that men with the worst diets are also the most likely to be missing teeth after age 50. Researchers attribute the men's lack of choppers and terrible gums to their diets' lack of beta-carotene, folic acid, vitamins A and C, and fiber. Specifically, there's a pretty clear link between vitamin C and gum health. Namely, those who are deficient in the foods that contain this vitamin may be prone to bleeding gums. (Smoking, drinking alcohol, illness, or anything else that robs the body of vitamin C, creating a deficiency, can also cause the same condition.)

To make sure your smile never reminds people of a medieval torture device, you should—surprise— eat a diet high in fruits and vegetables and low in manufactured sugars and other refined foods. It's important to eat whole foods consistently, too. Your mouth, teeth, and gums need to be exercised just the like the rest of your body.

You'll also want to watch what kind of water you drink. That's right—different types of water make a big difference here. Tap water has become a health boogeyman in recent years, but people forget that fluoridating the water supply was arguably the single most successful public-health venture of the 20th century. Now, with the ascent of bottled water, people may ingest fewer contaminants than before, but they are not receiving that fluoride. Most people know that fluoride is important while your teeth are developing—it's what hardens the enamel—but adults need fluoride, too. You need to have a continuous topical exposure to fluoride throughout your lifetime in order to maintain the hardness of that enamel. It's not just a matter of gargling with tap water, either—fluoride needs to enter your body through the stomach to be completely effective. Some vitamins contain fluoride, but that's not the same as having fluoride in your water or in whatever beverage you happen to be drinking.

If you simply can't stand the taste of tap water, one option is to drink tap water through a carbon-activated filtration system. Those filter out the junk that makes tap water look and smell like a day-old science experiment, but it doesn't filter out the fluoride. Another option is purchasing bottled waters with fluoride added. Those bottles tend to be tiny, though, because they're marketed mostly to kids. Fluoridated mouthwashes and toothpastes are also options, although again, you don't swallow those.

There's actually one way in which eating the *Power Food* way can harm your smile, if you don't take precautions. We suggest that you eat five or six times a day, which means that you'll be "grazing" pretty regularly. Eating that often will overwhelm the antiquated recommendation to brush twice daily. If you don't remove food particles and bacteria, they will form layers of plaque on your teeth and gums. Once these harden into tartar, your smile will dull, and you'll basically need to get that grunge sandblasted off at the dentist. Left alone, such deposits will lead to gingivitis, which will kill your social life faster than anything we can think of.

To pacify both your friends and your mouth, I

recommend you carry a travel-size toothbrush around and brush more frequently, preferably after every meal. If you can't brush your teeth, at least floss, or just rinse with some mouthwash. Some people chew sugar-free gum that claims to help reduce cavities and other dental problems. I'm not 100 percent certain the gum is effective, but it at least encourages salivation, which keeps your mouth clean. Though that may be only an improvement, it's something.

Alcohol and appearance. Liquor can have a major negative impact on your appearance. Most of us know at least one guy or woman who is perpetually loaded and has that reddish purple cauliflower skin to show for years of double-fisting, a look that testifies to alcohol's tendency to constrict blood vessels. The liver, which normally processes toxins, doesn't function as well as it should in a guy like that; blood flow isn't what it once was. If you're not getting really good blood flow to your skin, it's going to show. It's no coincidence that people with heart disease have rotten-looking skin. We're not talking about small amounts of alcohol here—even up to two drinks a day are okay—but the kind of consumption that constitutes alcohol abuse.

Hair quality, hair loss, and nutrition. First things first: Male pattern baldness, the genetically programmed sequence of hair loss that affects tens, if not hundreds, of millions of men in the United States and around the world, is not caused by nutrition. It can't be cured by nutrition, either. (If only it were that easy.) If you're losing your hair, the greatest diet in the world isn't going to make you suddenly sprout a shiny mane; and, unless you starve yourself, a bad diet isn't going to make your hair fall out if you're not genetically programmed to lose it.

Nonetheless, your hair follicles are a barometer for your long-term nutritional intake. If your diet is deficient in minerals such as iron, magnesium, zinc, and chromium, your hair will lose its luster.

The same goes for caloric and protein deficiencies. Your hair also depends on sufficient blood flow to the scalp. A diet that's friendly to the heart and circulatory system will naturally encourage this, but a poor heart-healthy diet will hurt. The follicles from which hair grows can be compromised by poor circulation, and your hair won't receive the nutrients it needs to be full and lustrous. Again, you'll have a lot more to worry about if your arteries are clogged with plaque, and you probably should be more concerned with keeping those suckers clean. But if a great mop of hair is the motivation you need to eat heart healthy, you won't hear any complaints from me.

Allergies and Food Sensitivities

Other than the potential it has to make a guy seriously fat, food probably never exerts a greater influence on appearance than when someone has a food allergy. Jeff once sat next to a woman who was allergic to peanuts—as she unwittingly ate a candy bar containing stealth nuts. Seconds later, her ears turned fire-engine red. When someone with a real food allergy eats the offending food by mistake, the results are readily apparent.

Real food allergies produce real symptoms real fast, including those throbbing earlobes. Any food theoretically has the potential to be allergenic, but the usual suspects for such things, at least in adults, are milk, eggs, soy, wheat, peanuts, shrimp, crab, lobster, crawfish, crustaceans, tree nuts, and fish. The symptoms vary as much as the foods, but typical reactions include swelling, which can affect the eyes as part of a histamine reaction; hives; and a sort of a skin rash or eczema called atopic dermatitis. If you experience any of these symptoms and aren't sure why, you shouldn't ignore them. The second or third bout could possibly turn into something very uncomfortable, if not life-threatening. See your physician and you'll keep your body—and by extension, your appearance—in good shape.

The Gestalt: Your Total Package

It wouldn't be like me to end this chapter without making one more last-ditch plea for you to watch your weight. Unless you're a doctor working in an amnesia ward, you get only one chance to make a good first impression. That impression will depend to a great extent on what you look like. As you approach someone, before details such as your face and hair have even registered, a judgment will have been passed on the breadth of your shoulder girdle relative to the size of your waist. The tiny waist that makes your shoulders look bigger than they really are is just one of a million reasons to eat smartly, and well.

It's easy to single out individual benefits of sound nutrition on appearance (better teeth, smoother skin, fuller hair, etc.), but these are footnotes to your personal gestalt—how every aspect of your body looks better, and how the whole exceeds the sum of those parts. If you've followed at least some of the advice in the first eight chapters, you probably already know what we're talking about here. Sorry if those broader shoulders, better defined arms, and smaller waist are starting to wreak havoc with your wardrobe. For our money, that's a small price to pay for furtive glances from attractive women.

THE BETTER-APPEARANCE MEAL PLAN

WHETHER YOUR COMPLEXION IS BAD OR YOU JUST LOOK "washed out," this meal plan, combined with plenty of exercise and sufficient sleep, will have you looking better in no time. Make sure to emphasize dark green, red, orange, and yellow veggies and fruits high in carotenes, which are precursors to vitamin A.

Daily Assumptions*†

2,400 calories
273 grams carbohydates
163 grams protein
73 grams fat

Daily Breakdown*†

4 bread
6 fruit
4 milk
7 vegetable
6 very lean protein
4 lean protein
1 medium-fat protein
1 bean
6 fat
2 soy

Note: Occasionally, a fat-free product, like mustard or cooking spray, is included on the menus. These do not count toward your daily breakdown but should not be overused.

*Use every day.

† Based on a 185-pound man.

THE MENU

DAY 1

Breakfast

1 bread	¹/₂ cup Shredded Wheat
1 milk	1 cup fat-free milk
2 fruit	¹/₂ cup orange juice
	³/₄ cup fresh blueberries
1 medium-fat protein	1 egg, scrambled in a nonstick pan
1 fat	1¹/₂ tablespoons ground flaxseed
	Water
	Oil-free cooking spray (for egg)

Snack

2 fat	20 peanuts
2 vegetable	2 cups carrot sticks
	Tea

Lunch

1 bread	1 small roll
1 milk	1 latte, tall, with no-calorie sweetener
2 vegetable	Salad with 2 cups romaine lettuce, ¹/₂ cup tomato, ¹/₂ cup cucumber
4 very lean protein	4 ounces turkey
1 bean	1 cup bean soup
1 fat	1 teaspoon vinegar

Pre-Workout Snack

1 fruit	¹/₂ cup unsweetened canned pears
2 soy	2 ounces soy nuts
1 milk	1 cup fat-free plain yogurt

Post-Workout

SMOOTHIE

Blend until smooth.

1 milk	1 cup fat-free milk
2 fruit	¹/₂ cup orange juice with calcium
	1¹/₄ cups frozen strawberries
2 very lean protein	14 grams whey protein powder

Dinner

2 bread	¹/₂ baked yam
	1 slice hearty whole-grain bread
1 fruit	12 cherries
2 vegetable	¹/₂ cup steamed Brussels spouts with Asian mustard
	1 baked garlic bulb (spread on bread and fish)
4 lean protein	4 ounces grilled halibut, marinated with cider, low-sodium soy sauce, garlic, ginger, sesame oil, sesame seeds
2 fat	1¹/₂ teaspoon sesame oil
	¹/₂ teaspoon sesame seeds (for fish)
	Green tea

DAY 2

Breakfast

Combine yogurt, fruit, and flaxseed.

1 bread	¹/₂ whole-wheat English muffin
1 milk	1 cup fat-free unsweetened yogurt
2 fruit	¹/₂ cup grapefruit juice
	1¹/₄ cups fresh strawberries
1 medium-fat protein	1 egg, hard-cooked
1 fat	1¹/₂ tablespoons ground flaxseed
	Water

Snack

2 fat	1 tablespoon peanut butter
2 vegetable	1 cup celery sticks
	¹/₂ cup V8 juice
	Tea

Lunch

1 bread	1 slice whole-grain bread
1 milk	1 ounce fat-free cheese (for salad)
2 vegetable	1 cup romaine lettuce, $^1/_2$ cup tomato, $^1/_4$ cup grilled eggplant, $^1/_4$ cup roasted red pepper
4 very lean protein	4 ounces skinless white-meat chicken, grilled with lime juice
1 fat	1 teaspoon olive oil (for roasted vegetables)
	2 tablespoons fat-free salad dressing

Pre-Workout Snack

1 fruit	1 plum
2 soy	1 cup edamame
1 milk	Fat-free plain yogurt

Post-Workout

SMOOTHIE

Blend until smooth.

1 milk	1 cup fat-free milk
2 fruit	$^1/_2$ cup orange juice with calcium
	$^3/_4$ cup frozen blueberries
2 very lean protein	14 grams whey protein powder

Dinner

2 bread	1 cup cooked pasta
1 fruit	1 cup honeydew
3 vegetable	1 cup Brussels sprouts
	Grilled shallots, garlic (with shrimp)
1 bean	$^1/_2$ cup kidney beans
4 lean protein	4 ounces shrimp, grilled
2 fat	2 teaspoons olive oil
	2 tablespoons fat-free dressing

DAY 3

Breakfast

1 bread	1 slice whole-wheat bread
1 milk	1 cup fat-free cottage cheese (on bread)
2 fruit	4 ounces freshly squeezed orange juice (with pulp)
	$^3/_4$ cup blueberries
1 medium-fat protein	1 egg, cooked sunny-side up in a nonstick pan
1 fat	$1^1/_2$ tablespoons ground flaxseed
	Water
	Oil-free cooking spray (for egg)

Snack

2 fat	16 to 20 mixed nuts
2 vegetable	1 cup pepper sticks, 1 cup celery sticks
	2 tablespoons fat-free dressing
	Tea

Lunch

1 bread	1/2 cup rice
1 milk	1 cup fat-free milk
2 vegetable	1 cup spinach, bok choy
	1 cup yellow squash, stir-fried with garlic, onion, fresh ginger
4 very lean protein	4 ounces chicken, stir-fried
1 bean	1/2 cup black beans
1 fat	1 teaspoon oil (for stir-frying)

Pre-Workout Snack

1 fruit	1 nectarine
2 protein	50 Genisoy soy crisps
1 milk	1 cup fat-free plain yogurt

Post-Workout

SMOOTHIE

Blend until smooth.

1 milk	1 cup fat-free milk
2 fruit	1/2 cup orange juice with calcium
	1 cup frozen raspberries
2 very lean protein	14 grams whey protein powder

Dinner

2 bread	1 ounce croutons (for salad)
	1 cup chicken noodle soup
1 fruit	12 cherries
3 vegetable	1 cup raw cauliflower, broccoli (add to tossed salad)
	1/2 cup onion (for salad)
	Salad with 1 cup lettuce, 1/4 cup tomato, 1/4 cup cucumber
4 lean protein	4 ounces swordfish, grilled with ginger and scallions
2 fat	2 teaspoons olive oil (for fish)
	2 tablespoons fat-free dressing

DAY 4

Breakfast

2 fruit	$^1/_2$ cup orange juice
	1 cup raspberries
1 milk	1 cup fat-free milk ($^1/_2$ cup for French toast)

FRENCH TOAST *(See recipe directions on page 44.)*

1 bread	2 slices extra-thin (or 1 regular slice) whole-wheat bread
1 medium-fat protein	1 egg
1 fat	$1^1/_2$ tablespoons ground flaxseed
	Water
	Oil-free cooking spray (for egg)

Snack

2 fat	1 tablespoon almond butter
2 vegetable	2 cups celery sticks
	Tea

Lunch

1 bread	$^1/_2$ cup cooked linguini
1 milk	1 cup fat-free milk
2 vegetable	Salad with 1 cup lettuce, $^1/_4$ cup tomato, $^1/_4$ cup cucumber
	$^1/_2$ cup marinara sauce
4 very lean protein	4 ounces ground turkey (in sauce)
1 fat	1 teaspoon olive oil (for cooking)

Pre-Workout Snack

1 fruit	1 apple
2 soy	1 cup edamame
1 milk	Fat-free plain yogurt

Post-Workout

SMOOTHIE

Blend until smooth.

1 milk	1 cup fat-free milk
2 fruit	$^1/_2$ cup orange juice with calcium
	$1^1/_4$ cups frozen strawberries
2 very lean protein	14 grams whey protein powder

Dinner

2 bread	1 small roll
	$^1/_2$ cup brown rice
2 fruit	$^1/_2$ cantaloupe
3 vegetable	1 cup coleslaw
	1 cup chopped tomatoes, cooked with chili seasoning
	$^1/_2$ cup onion, garlic (for seasoning)
1 protein	$^1/_2$ cup kidney beans (add to chili)
4 lean protein	4 ounces lean beef, minced (add to chili)
2 fat	$^1/_8$ avocado, diced
	Included (in coleslaw)

DAY 5

Breakfast

1 bread	$^1/_2$ cup quick oats (not instant)
1 milk	1 cup fat-free milk
2 fruit	$^1/_2$ cup orange juice
	$1^1/_4$ cups strawberries
1 medium-fat protein	1 egg, hard-cooked
1 fat	$1^1/_2$ tablespoons ground flaxseed
	Water

Snack

2 fat	16 almonds
2 vegetable	2 cups carrot sticks
	Tea

Lunch

FAJITAS

Combine ingredients.

1 bread	1 tortilla
1 milk	1 ounce fat-free shredded cheese
2 vegetable	1 cup sautéed onions, peppers
	2 tablespoons salsa
4 very lean protein	4 ounces skinless white-meat chicken, grilled with lime juice
1 protein	$^1/_2$ cup fat-free refried beans
1 fat	1 teaspoon olive oil (for cooking)

Pre-Workout Snack

1 fruit	1 pear
2 soy	50 Genisoy soy crisps
1 milk	1 cup fat-free plain yogurt

Post-Workout

SMOOTHIE

Blend until smooth.

1 milk	1 cup fat-free milk
2 fruit	$1/2$ cup orange juice with calcium
	1 cup frozen blackberries
2 very lean protein	14 grams whey protein powder

Dinner

2 bread	1 small pita
	$1/2$ cup couscous
1 fruit	2 medium figs
3 vegetable	1 cup broccoli slaw
	$1/2$ cup onion, shallots, garlic (in couscous)
4 lean protein	4 ounces fresh trout (stuffed with $1/2$ cup couscous)
2 fat	2 tablespoons reduced-fat vinaigrette
	Included (in broccoli slaw)

DAY 6

Breakfast

1 bread	1 slice multigrain bread, toasted
2 fruit	$1/2$ cup orange juice
	1 cup raspberries
1 medium-fat protein	1 egg, hard-cooked

SMOOTHIE

Blend until smooth.

1 milk	1 cup fat-free milk
1 fat	$1^1/2$ tablespoons ground flaxseed
	Water

Snack

2 fat	1 tablespoon peanut butter
2 vegetable	1 cup celery sticks, 1 cup carrot sticks
	Tea

Lunch

1 bread	1 small whole-wheat pita
1 milk	1 ounce shredded fat-free Swiss cheese
2 vegetable	1 cup carrot sticks
	2 slices onion, 3 slices tomato, 5 spinach leaves
4 very lean protein	4 ounces turkey
1 fat	1 tablespoon reduced-fat mayonnaise

Pre-Workout Snack

1 fruit	$\frac{1}{2}$ large banana
2 soy	2 ounces soy nuts
1 milk	1 cup fat-free plain yogurt

Post-Workout

SMOOTHIE

Blend until smooth.

1 milk	1 cup fat-free milk
2 fruit	$\frac{1}{2}$ cup orange juice with calcium
	1 cup frozen raspberries
2 very lean protein	14 grams whey protein powder

Dinner

2 bread	2 slices rye bread
1 fruit	1 apple
3 vegetable	1 cup coleslaw
	$\frac{1}{2}$ cup chopped onion (mix into tuna)
1 protein	$\frac{1}{2}$ cup fava beans
4 lean protein	4 ounces tuna in olive oil, drained
1 fat	1 tablespoon reduced-fat mayonnaise
	Included (in coleslaw)

DAY 7

Breakfast

1 bread	1 cup Kashi
1 milk	1 cup fat-free milk
2 fruit	$\frac{1}{2}$ cup grapefruit juice
	1 cup blackberries
1 medium-fat protein	1 egg, hard-cooked
1 fat	$1\frac{1}{2}$ tablespoons ground flaxseed
	Water

Snack

2 fat	10 walnuts
2 vegetable	1 cup V8 juice

Lunch

1 bread	1 small multigrain roll
1 milk	1 cup fat-free milk
2 vegetable	2 slices onion, 3 slices tomato, 5 spinach leaves
4 very lean protein	4 ounces skinless white-meat chicken, grilled with balsamic vinegar
1 protein	$1/2$ cup pinto beans
1 fat	1 teaspoon oil (for cooking chicken)
	1 tablespoon fat-free ranch dressing

Pre-Workout Snack

1 fruit	17 grapes
2 soy	50 Genisoy soy crisps
1 milk	1 cup fat-free plain yogurt

Post-Workout

SMOOTHIE

Blend until smooth.

1 milk	1 cup fat-free milk
2 fruit	$1/2$ cup orange juice with calcium
	$3/4$ cup frozen blueberries
2 very lean protein	14 grams whey protein powder

Dinner

2 bread	3-inch square of corn bread
1 fruit	$1/2$ mango
4 vegetable	1 cup broccoli, steamed
	Salad with 1 cup lettuce, $1/4$ cup tomato, $1/4$ cup cucumber
4 lean protein	4 ounces salmon, poached
2 fat	1 teaspoon olive oil
	2 tablespoons fat-free Caesar dressing
	Included (in corn bread)

CHAPTER TEN

The Full-Power Meal Plan

THE ALL-IN-ONE PLAN FOR THE GUY WHO WANTS EVERYTHING

The meal plans I've prescribed in the last eight chapters are exciting to me, and I hope to you, too. I'm fascinated daily by how minor tweaks in daily eating can bring widely different results, from lifting mood, to fighting inflammation, to building muscle. But not everyone needs or wants a specialty plan like the ones I've prescribed. They may be more effective overall for achieving specific results—for instance, if diabetes runs in your family and you're mainly concerned about avoiding it, you'd be hard pressed to find a better diet than my Diabetic Guy Meal Plan—but some of you (perhaps most of you) have multiple goals in mind.

In recognition of that reality, I present the Full-Power Meal Plan. It incorporates pretty much all of the health benefits in this book and delivers a 14-day nutrition plan designed to produce major results, fast. I firmly believe that it represents the best, most comprehensive diet for the vast majority of the men reading this book. This is the blueprint you should follow after you've finished the last chapter, and after you've met your specific goals. Once you get your

six-pack abs, more energy, lower blood pressure, or whatever, follow this diet until death do you part. (The long-term health chapter may be the one exception here. If you have concerns about a certain health risk, you'll probably want to build your diet around *that* chapter for the rest of your life.)

Like the nutritional programs I design for clients in my private practice, the Full-Power Meal Plan constantly balances what's practical with what's ideal. For example, *ideally,* I'd like clients to eat fresh fish five times a week. *Practically,* a stockbroker who's a bachelor and works 70 hours a week isn't going to reach that goal week in, week out. If he eats fresh fish on, say, Monday, Wednesday, and Friday, and then has a lean cut of red meat on Tuesday and some chicken on Thursday, we're cool. It still represents progress over eating McDonald's three nights a week.

Every aspect of the Full-Power Meal Plan is based on nutrition research that has documented improvements in physical and mental performance, health, and longevity, according to specific eating strategies. It also incorporates the healthiest elements of the dietary patterns from traditional Mediterranean and Asian cultures, which I think is a great way for active men to eat. Men in both of these regions have much lower rates of certain cancers, heart disease, obesity, and other chronic, degenerative diseases than their U.S. counterparts do, and more and more research suggests that differences in diet and activity account for the largest percentage of the disparity.

The Mediterranean diet and the traditional rural Asian diet are based largely on plants. Unlike Americans, people in these regions consume meat judiciously, rather than constantly. The diets of people from the southern regions of France, Italy, Portugal, and Spain are rich in grains, vegetables, fruits, lean meat, and olive oil. They have a low intake of animal products, saturated fat, and luxury breads. On the Asian side, great emphasis is placed on rice, noodles, breads, and whole grains, all with minimal processing. Fruits, vegetables, legumes, nuts, seeds, and tea are also ubiquitous in Asian cuisine. Fish is widely consumed, and red meat is not. Asian diets are even lower in saturated fat than Mediterranean diets are.

Given that it borrows heavily from Asian and Mediterranean diets, what makes the Full-Power Meal Plan unique, you may rightly ask? Here are some significant ways in which it differs from those eating styles, giving it its unique flavor, literally and figuratively. Also included below is some good advice for boosting the benefits of the Full-Power Meal Plan.

1. To gain the greatest benefits from soy, the Full-Power Meal Plan includes two daily servings of traditional soy foods like tofu, tempeh, and edamame. When convenience takes priority, you can replace them with a 14-gram soy protein fiber supplement.

2. To get the most out of the Full-Power Meal Plan, you'll need to select from a variety of fruits every day, not just the one or two you're used to eating. Two servings of citrus fruits will give you a daily boost of vitamin C. Two servings of berries will give you a whole host of phytochemicals and antioxidants to help keep your brain and your body young. Then we'll ask you to choose two more servings of pretty much any fruit imaginable. Ideally, mix it up so that each week you're eating cherries, melon, and tropical fruits like mango, pineapple, and papaya in some measure. And don't forget the staples: apples, pears, peaches, bananas, nectarines, plums, and dried fruits like raisins and apricots.

3. You'll eat a combined three servings a day of carotene-rich vegetables such as carrots, sweet potatoes, yams, tomatoes, and tomato sauce; and dark-green leafy vegetables like romaine lettuce, kale, Swiss chard, and collard greens. Don't stop there, though: Eat two servings of vegetables from the Brassica family, which includes broccoli, cauliflower, cabbage, and Brussels sprouts. For good measure, add one serving of those wonderfully pungent vegetables from the Allium family, like onions and garlic.

4. This diet is designed for guys who work out. If you're not doing so already, start lifting weights 2 to 3 days a week, doing cardio the same number of days, and doing something like a weekend sport or a hike on off days. Keep moving.

5. The Full-Power Meal Plan demands adequate hydration. Your body must replenish the fluid it loses daily. For most men, that's 9 to 11 cups of fluid a day. Luckily, when you follow this diet, you're eating an abundance of fruits and vegetables every day, and those foods contain a lot of water. In fact, you can probably get 3 to 4 cups of fluid from fruits and veggies alone. That leaves you still needing at least 5 to 7 cups of fluids. Make no fewer than 5 of them water. The rest can be milk, maybe some orange juice, and perhaps even coffee.

If you drink caffeinated beverages, don't worry about a diuretic effect kicking in until you drink more than 3 servings a day. Once you pass that threshold, add ½ cup of a noncaffeinated fluid for every additional caffeinated beverage you drink.

Alcohol, however, is dehydrating from the first sip. For every alcoholic beverage you drink, add another ½ cup of nonalcoholic fluid to your plan.

6. The Full-Power Meal Plan includes a serving of beans every day. By adding beans to your diet on a regular basis, you consume less fat and more fiber, and you increase the complex carbohydrates, vitamins, and minerals in your diet while still taking in a wholesome amount of protein. Beans can help your health immediately, and ongoing research suggests that they may have a major impact on longevity. If there's an added benefit down the road, so much the better. You'll have gotten a head start.

7. One of the most important things you can do to ensure bone health is get plenty of calcium and vitamin D from your food. That's why the Full-Power Meal Plan prescribes four servings of dairy products every day. Dairy is invaluable for its calcium and whey protein, which promote bone and cardiovascular health, not to mention muscle growth. Calcium, vitamin D, and whey also appear to play a big role in controlling obesity. Milk in particular is high in calcium and fortified with vitamin D.

8. The Full-Power Meal Plan asks you to eat several daily servings of nuts, olives, and avocados for the benefits of their healthy oils.

9. Though seafood is eaten often in both Mediterranean and Asian cultures, you need to eat it even more often in the Full-Power Meal Plan— at least five times weekly, while still leaving room to eat a variety of other good protein sources like eggs, poultry, and lean cuts of meat. The omega-3 fatty acids found in fish and other seafood assist with brain health, mood elevation, and weight management.

10. Eating a whole egg (yolk included) every day, or at least every other day, is integral to the Full-Power Meal Plan. Yolks contain lecithin and choline, which help keep your cells healthy and operating at peak efficiency, especially your brain cells.

11. The Full-Power Meal Plan includes one 4-ounce serving of skinless poultry or other lean meat every day. A variety of foods within all the food groups will ensure the widest variety of nutrient intake to promote health and prevent disease.

12. You've read a lot about sugar and high-fructose corn syrup throughout this book. In the Full-Power Meal Plan, its presence is limited to small amounts. Cutting it out completely would be severe, if not impossible. A reasonable serving of 8 teaspoons of added sugar daily allows you extra sweets without letting you go overboard. Keep in mind that 8 teaspoons means *anywhere* where sugar is added, not just where you add it. So if you eat fruited yogurts, 1 cup has 8 teaspoons of added sugar. So do a 16-ounce sports drink . . . and two Power Bars. One packet of sugar contains 1 teaspoon of the stuff, so if you drop two packets' worth in each of 4 cups of coffee, you've just hit your limit.

13. I recommend three supplements as part of the Full-Power Meal Plan:

- 14 grams of whey protein powder.
- 1½ tablespoons of ground flaxseed. This is equivalent to one fat serving, and it's incorporated into the Full-Power Meal Plan—you don't have to modify your other fat servings to include it.
- 400 to 800 international units (IU) of vitamin E. Choose a natural one labeled d-alpha tocopherol, as opposed to laboratory synthesized dl-alpha tocopherol, which has a greatly reduced potency.

Given how I've touched on most of this stuff in previous chapters, you may be ready to jump straight to the diet. If so, wonderful. However, there are a few new headliners in this diet that you may want to know more about.

Soy for Boys

Soy is hardly a staple of the average American male's diet, but in the Full-Power Meal Plan, you eat it pretty much every day. To understand why, you need a little background.

Back in 1919, scientists were trying to quantify the quality (or lack thereof) of various proteins. By studying the amino acid needs of growing rats, they came up with the Protein Efficiency Ratio (PER). The PER ranked soy protein below animal proteins because soy provides less of one essential amino acid, methionine, than the PER standard profile. What they failed to take into account is that rats need methionine in larger amounts than humans do because it supports fur growth. (How's your fur growing? I thought so.)

In 1993, a better yardstick for evaluating protein quality was developed, based on people instead of rats. According to the Protein Digestibility-Corrected Amino Acid Score, or PDCAAS, the highest score a food protein can receive is 1.0. ("PDCAAS of Selected Food Proteins" below lists the scores of selected protein sources.) Under PDCAAS, the quality of soy protein is equal to that of casein (milk protein) and egg white, which all have perfect scores.

More recent studies have suggested that PD-CAAS, though better than PER, is still too simplistic to provide a complete look at soy's effect on human tissue. For example, it's not suggested in high amounts for guys who want to build muscle or maximize postexercise muscle recovery—when it comes to building muscle, soy just doesn't have enough amino acids to do the job whey protein does. For anyone seeking the majority of benefits that proteins can provide, however, soy is an optimal addition to your protein rotation.

For starters, soy's contributions to health promotion and disease prevention have been hailed repeatedly in studies. Perhaps because of their antioxidant capabilities, the isoflavones in soy appear to protect against cancers, specifically hormone-related cancers like colon and prostate. These same compounds, combined with soy fiber, also appear to lower bad cholesterol while raising levels of its good counterpart, making cardiovascular disease less likely to occur. This effect is more pronounced when subjects consume intact soy protein than when they take amino acid formulas patterned after soy protein, suggesting that something other than the protein appears to affect the cholesterol response to soy.

PDCAAS OF SELECTED FOOD PROTEINS

Use this table to find the Protein Digestibility-Corrected Amino Acid Score of the foods you eat. The higher the number, the more readily your body uses the complete food.

Protein Source	PDCAAS	Protein Source	PDCAAS
Soy	1.00	Rolled oats	0.57
Casein	1.00	Lentils (canned)	0.52
Egg white	1.00	Peanut meal	0.52
Beef	0.92	Whole wheat	0.40
Kidney beans (canned)	0.68	Wheat gluten	0.25

Source: *Protein Quality Evaluation*, Report of the Joint FAO/WHO Expert Consultation, FAO/WHO, 1989.

Atta Soy

Beyond its nutritional value, soybeans and soy protein show promise for weight loss, another reason they're featured in the Full-Power Meal Plan. No one is 100 percent certain what the mechanism of action is. For example, the lecithin component of soy may slow stomach emptying and suppress appetite, either of which would help guys lose weight. The phytoestrogens in soy may also help in the fat-loss effort.

I've worked with guys long enough to know some of you, or maybe most of you, are going to resist eating soy. Do yourself a favor and try it. If you can't stomach edamame, give silken tofu a try. It's super-soft, nearly odorless, and blends into a smoothie without leaving lumps. You will hardly know it's there!

If even that doesn't work, go out and buy a soy protein supplement that contains soy fiber. You may not get the full range of benefits for health and weight loss that you would from the combination of soy protein, fibers, and lecithin found in soy foods like edamame, tofu, and tempeh, but it's better than cutting the tofu out completely. When you do supplement, it's better to use products based on the whole protein rather than on specific isoflavones. Soy concentrates are at least 65 percent protein (dry weight), whereas soy protein isolates are at least 90 percent protein. The fat has been removed from soy concentrates, but they still contain carbohydrate, whereas soy isolates are pure protein.

I'd urge you to stay away from soy isoflavone pills, which we still don't fully understand and which could possibly be more harmful than helpful. Although intact soy protein reduces the risk of prostate cancer, scientists are not sure whether isoflavones in a pure supplement have the same effect.

Produce Produces

There's been some confusion lately over whether fruit is as beneficial as we've historically believed. I'd like to put that confusion to rest. Consider a British study that for 17 years tracked the lifestyles and diets of 11,000 people deemed health-conscious. Within its findings was this little morsel: Members of this group had a death rate that was one-half that of the general population. When all the study's variables were analyzed statistically, a few facts about fruit were very encouraging. Eating fresh fruit daily was highly associated with significantly fewer deaths from heart disease, cerebro-vascular disease (i.e., stroke and other diseases that may lead to stroke, like carotid stenosis and aneurysms), and for all causes of death combined.

Fewer than one-fourth of all Americans consume the five servings of fruits and vegetables recommended by the National Cancer Institute as part of its "5 a Day for Better Health" program. How unfortunate. Not only is fruit the best medicine money can buy, but it also tastes great. After all, fruit is full of sugar in the form of fructose.

Ask most guys what's good about fruits, and they'll scratch their head for a second, shuffle their feet, and then maybe mention that oranges have vitamin C. True, but that's just a starting point. In fact, we could write an entire book devoted solely to the health benefits of fruit. Instead, here's the condensed version.

The important micronutrients found abundantly in fruit include beta-carotene, folate, vitamin E, potassium, magnesium, and, yes, vitamin C. The vitamins and minerals are the stuff that makes your body *go,* basically. The biochemical reactions they're involved in number in the thousands, if not tens of thousands. Researchers have fingered all of the above as playing important roles in preventing and fighting disease, which may have a lot to do with all of the fiber and phytochemicals they contain. The latter in particular have been revealed by increasingly sophisticated studies to help reduce the risk of contracting chronic diseases such as cancer, heart disease, and diabetes. (See chapter 7 for a detailed discussion of food and disease prevention.)

All of that comes in a package extremely low in calories, as the average fruit serving contains only 60. But fruit's role in fat loss involves more than just the fact that it contains virtually no fat. In experiments where subjects consumed an identical number of calories, the ones who ate more fruit lost more weight than the subjects who ate less fruit.

This may have something to do with pectin, a class of water-soluble complex carbohydrates found in the cell walls of ripe fruits such as apples, plums, and grapefruit. Pectin isn't absorbed by the human digestive tract. The food industry uses it as a thickening agent and texturizer, as well as to replace fat and sugar in low-calorie foods. Added to diets in significant amounts, pectin moderates the natural rise in blood sugar, slows the rate at which the stomach empties food, and increases feelings of fullness—all of which can help deflate that spare tire around your waist.

In pure form, as little as 5 grams of pectin a day mixed with orange juice can complement a weight-loss program when used in conjunction with a well-planned diet and exercise regimen. Apple pomace and citrus peels are the main sources of commercially acceptable pectins, but banana, lemon pulp, passion fruit rind, tamarind, papaya, guava, and other fruits are also good sources.

Much of what's been said here about fruits applies equally to vegetables: They're loaded with antioxidants and phytochemicals, you get a huge windfall of nutrients for very few calories, and you should eat as wide a variety of them as possible.

One quick word about salads, though. They

SAVING THE NUTRIENTS IN YOUR FRUIT

STORING FRUITS CORRECTLY MAKES A BIG DIFFERENCE in how long they stay fresh and how good (or bad) they taste. Most fruit is shipped unripe throughout most of the year, and it needs to be kept out of the refrigerator until it ripens. To speed that process, place your fruit in a closed paper bag and leave it on the kitchen counter. The gases produced by the fruit and trapped in the bag will promote the ripening process. Check the fruit daily so it doesn't become overripe. Once the fruit is ripe, store it in the refrigerator. (Bananas are one exception; store them at room temperature.)

Here are some other guidelines that can help you minimize the loss of nutrients from fruit.

■ Always purchase fresh produce.

■ Store fruit whole, rather than cutting it up.

■ Never soak produce for extended periods.

■ When peeling and paring, remove as little of the actual fruit as possible.

■ If you purchase precut produce, refrigerate it in airtight wrappers or containers.

■ Defrost fruit in the microwave to reduce the loss of water-soluble nutrients.

■ Cook fruit in large pieces to lessen the amount of surface exposed to water. Use just enough water to prevent scorching, and place a lid on the pan.

should form part of any nutritious diet, but equating their consumption with successful weight loss is a common mistake. A seemingly healthy Caesar salad, for example, can leave you saddled with 50 fat grams from the cheese and Caesar dressing, which typically contains mustard, olive oil, and egg yolk, along with other fatty ingredients. What's more, you'll be starving an hour later and reach for something worse.

Think of salads as an adjunct to, rather than a substitute for, your main meal. Limit the fat they contain by going easy on the dressings and other fat-laden toppings such as grated cheese and croutons. And juice them up with lean protein sources such as salmon, chicken, and beans. Protein builds muscle, and the more of that metabolically active tissue you have, the easier it will be to lose fat.

Be Berry Careful

A few final words about fruit, and they are words of caution. First, food poisoning doesn't come from just shellfish gone bad; you can get it from any food, fruit included. In fact, well-publicized outbreaks of food poisoning have been caused by fruit juices and raspberries contaminated by bacteria. These outbreaks have stirred national debate over regulatory issues pertaining to the production of nonpasteurized juices and the irradiation of imported produce.

Second, pathogens can survive in fruit juices, and pasteurization virtually eliminates the risk of bacterial contamination. Some consumers think this process diminishes the taste of fruit juices, but surely the difference isn't worth the risk. Make sure the juices you drink have undergone this process.

HANDLE WITH CARE

THE MOST COMMON SOURCE OF FOOD POISONING is the person preparing it, usually when that person doesn't wash his or her hands. In addition to washing your hands before you prepare any kind of food—which should be a given, right?—always follow these additional food-handling and safety guidelines.

- Wash fresh produce, scrub it with a brush, and rinse it thoroughly under running water.
- Peel waxed fruit, as waxes don't wash off and can seal in pesticide residues. Peel fruits such as apples, when appropriate. (Peeling removes pesticides that remain in or on the peel, but it also removes fibers, vitamins, and minerals.) Use a knife to peel an orange or grapefruit, rather than biting into it.
- When you open a can containing fruits and vegetables and don't use the entire contents, store the remainder in a glass or plastic container, not in the can.
- Keep hot foods hot and cold foods cold. Consider 60°F to 125°F to be the danger zone for food temperature because it allows for rapid growth of bacteria and production of toxins. Don't hold foods in this range for more than 2 to 3 hours.
- Throw out foods that show any signs of mold.
- When traveling outside the United States, always peel raw fruits and vegetables. Avoid any kind of raw-vegetable salads; the water used to wash the vegetables may have been contaminated. Consuming only cooked foods is generally considered the safest practice.

As for imported produce, foreign growers around the world aren't subjected to the same regulations that apply to domestic ones. Bacterial contamination is checked for at the border, but as demonstrated by a 1996 outbreak of *cyclospora* caused by Guatemalan raspberries, the process is hardly failsafe. As it's nearly impossible to know whether the fruit you purchase was grown in the United States or abroad, make sure you follow some basic guidelines for safely handling fruits. (See "Handle with Care" on previous page.)

The second cautionary note concerns fruits and medications or drugs. Pharmacists have known about these potentially dangerous interactions for years, but most consumers remain ignorant of them. In particular, citrus juices, especially grapefruit juice, are notorious for their interactions with meds. None of the following medications should be taken with any citrus juice.

- Amlodipine
- Cortisone
- Coumadin
- Cyclosporin
- Diltiazem
- Estradiol
- Feladipine
- Midazolam
- Nifedipine
- Nitrendipine
- Nisoldipine
- Terfenadine
- Theophylline
- Triazolam
- Verapimil

Exorcise Fat Demons with Exercise

The equation is simple: Diet plus exercise equals fitness and health. A lobotomy patient could figure that one out. Remove any single variable and you're left with an incomplete formula. The *Power Food* formula is no different. I can't design a meal plan that will keep you healthy and fit if you're not going to exercise.

You don't need to train for a triathlon, but you do need to hit the gym (or the bricks, pedals, etc.) with some regularity. I'm talking real exercise here, not 10-minute dog walks. This should do the trick: 2 or 3 days with the weights, 2 or 3 days of cardio, and ac-

tive rest on your day or days off, which means biking or walking somewhere instead of driving, or participating in a sport—something like that.

Learning proper techniques can be somewhat involved, depending on the exercise in question. But don't confuse educated exercise with rocket science. Just as you can trade stocks profitably without a broker if you're willing to educate yourself, you can learn how to perform exercises correctly from any number of sources, including a book, knowledgeable training partner, reputable media source, or group seminar.

The Fluid Factor

Back to what you put into your body. I've sung the praises of water throughout *Power Food,* and with good reason. It's the most abundant compound in the human body, making up about 60 percent of an adult's body weight. It fills virtually all cells, as well as the spaces separating them. All biochemical reactions occur in water, and water helps these processes along. From energy production to joint lubrication to reproduction, every system in your body depends on water to some degree.

Unfortunately, our hardwired drive to drink isn't as compelling as the same desire to eat. The human body's thirst mechanism doesn't kick in until it's already suffering mild dehydration.

The upshot of that genetic programming is that most guys don't drink enough water. In fact, one out of every three people in the United States is walking around slightly dehydrated. As discussed in chapter 6, chronic, mild dehydration can have a measurable effect on mental and physical performance, long-term health, and even muscle growth. A water deficit of just 2 to 4 percent of your body weight can reduce the intensity of your strength-training workout by as much as 21 percent, and your aerobic power by a whopping 48 percent!

Getting to that point is easier than you might

think, too. Working out at a moderate pace in a mild climate, you're probably sweating off 2 to 4 pounds of fluid an hour. That means a 150-pounder can easily lose 2 percent of his body weight in fluid, or 3 pounds, within an hour. If the exercise is more intense or the environment is more extreme, the fluid losses will be greater.

Water affects how your muscles will grow in response to those workouts, too. In well-hydrated muscle cells, protein synthesis is stimulated and protein breakdown is lessened. Muscle-cell dehydration, on the other hand, promotes protein breakdown and inhibits protein synthesis. Cell volume has also been shown to influence genetic expression, enzyme and hormone activity, and metabolic regulation.

Water also can help you lose weight. Not only is it devoid of calories, it also takes the edge off hunger so that you eat less. If you're on a high-protein diet, you need plenty of water to detoxify ammonia, a byproduct of protein being metabolized for energy. As you mobilize your stored fatty acids for use as energy, the fat-soluble toxins that have been benignly languishing in your fat cells are released into your bloodstream, where they have the chance to do damage. The more fluid you drink, the more dilute the toxins in your bloodstream are, and the more rapidly they exit your body. Good riddance.

The health benefits of water are legion, and many of them have been discussed previously in *Power Food*. To recap, proper hydration can dramatically reduce the risk of developing kidney stones, lower the chances of getting many cancers, and prevent the heart ailment mitral valve prolapse from occurring.

Design a fluid plan with the same rigor you apply to eating. To cover your minimum intake, drink 2 cups of fluid upon waking in the morning, followed by 2 more each at midmorning, lunch, midafternoon, and dinner. Make at least 5 of them water, and make sure the rest minimize caffeine and lack alcohol, because both can promote water loss. Then add what

you need to stay well hydrated before, during, and after exercise.

Keep in mind that any number of factors could bump up your minimum fluid requirements. These include high temperatures, low humidity, high altitude, exercise, dieting, illness, and travel. (So if you're traveling to Phoenix, Arizona, by plane, while you're on a diet and sick, get drinking.) Regardless, carry water and other fluids with you as a constant reminder to drink. Freeze fluids in water bottles to keep them cold during long-distance exercise. Don't forget that fruits and vegetables are great sources of water as well.

Even if you're following some or even all of those steps, monitor your hydration status just to be certain. One of the easiest ways is to check out the color of your urine, which should be relatively odorless and no darker than straw color. Anything yellower than that means you need water pronto.

Forget *Blazing Saddles*

Except for ethnic cuisines, beans play a very minor role in the American diet. What a missed opportunity. Not only is evidence mounting in favor of the health benefits of eating beans, but their "musical" side effects can now be silenced, too. (See chapter 8.)

Dried beans, a.k.a. legumes, include beans, peas, lentils . . . you get the picture. There are actually 13,000 species of legumes, but only 20 that you'd look at and say, "Ah . . . food." Those 20 species vary widely in color, size, shape, and flavor. Soybeans, peanuts, and other legumes grown for both their protein and oil content are called oilseeds. The majority, called grain legumes, are grown primarily as protein sources. These include beans, lentils, lima beans, cowpeas, fava beans, chickpeas, and common peas.

Regardless of how you classify them, legumes are among the most nutritious vegetables known to man, and they have remarkably similar nutritional profiles. For example, a ½-cup serving of most cooked beans provides 110 to 143 calories.

Beans don't include all of the essential amino acids and, hence, aren't a complete protein, critics contend. True enough (soy excluded). Because beans are rich in most essential amino acids but slightly deficient in methionine and cysteine, you need to mix them with complementary foods to complete their array of essential amino acids. Cultures around the world figured out eons ago that the key is to consume beans with grains or flour, which is why tandems such as red beans and rice, refried beans and corn tortillas, and pasta and bean soup have become dietary staples in different parts of the world. Thus combined, beans' amino acid profiles hold their own against those of animal proteins. You don't have to combine the proteins in one sitting, either. Simply eating a variety of protein sources throughout the day will do the trick.

Beans are extremely useful for guys who work out because their carbohydrate helps spare protein from being burned as fuel. They're particularly useful in this regard for guys concerned with glycemic-index issues and insulin resistance. Beans are high-fiber, low-GI foods, so they power up your body for exercise with minimal effect on insulin.

And beans are low in fat. That's right: *low in fat*. There's a lot of confusion about this, as many people believe beans are high in fat. File that theory under Nutritional Red Herrings. Except for soybeans (19 percent) and peanuts (46 percent), the fat content of legumes ranges a low-ish 0.8 to 1.5 percent. Even with those exceptions, bear in mind that the fat in beans comes mostly from unsaturated fatty acids and that they contain no cholesterol.

What beans are high in is protein. On average, 21 to 25 percent of the calories come from protein. (Soybeans are the exception. Approximately 34 percent of their calories come from protein.) Beans are also the cheapest of protein sources.

The health benefits don't end there, either. Beans are a good source of water-soluble vitamins, especially thiamine, riboflavin, niacin, and folacin. Beans also contain healthy amounts of the minerals calcium, iron, copper, zinc, phosphorus, potassium, and magnesium, although these minerals aren't as readily bioavailable in beans as they are in animal sources.

Beans are also rich in water-soluble fiber, which lowers levels of glucose and cholesterol in the blood. They contain insoluble fiber, which aids in proper functioning of the gut, in significant amounts. Fiber not only helps with weight management, it also may lessen the risk of getting colon cancer.

As for which beans to add to your diet, we refrain from singling out two or three stars because there's no compelling reason to exclude any bean from your plate. Vegans might be the one exception here, as they will almost certainly want to consume a lot of soybeans, soy-based products, or both. As discussed earlier in this chapter, soy is the most complete plant protein available.

Dairy Contrary

Dairy has received its fair share of media bashing in recent years, but the National Dairy Council, in its counterattack, is right on: Milk does a body good. In fact, after reading this, you'll never think about cutting out dairy products again.

Unless you've been living on a desert island for the past decade, you should know that osteoporosis, a disease in which one's bones become brittle, has become widespread among the nation's elderly. But you may be under the misconception that, as a guy, you really don't have to worry about it. If so, you would be wrong, as was discussed in chapter 9. It happens to men as well, and more often than you might think.

The most important things you can do to prevent osteoporosis, in random order, are:

- Maintain a regular weight-bearing exercise program.
- Maintain a healthy body weight.
- Don't smoke.
- Include plenty of calcium and vitamin D as part of your diet.

The fourth reason explains why the Full-Power Meal Plan includes four daily servings of dairy products. Milk in particular is high in calcium and fortified with vitamin D.

Because vitamin D is limited to only a handful of foods, the human body depends on sunlight to cover the rest of its needs. In fact, that's where most of your vitamin D comes from: ultraviolet energy from the sun being absorbed by the skin. If you don't already, make it a priority to get out into the sunshine for short bursts. Exposing your hands, arms, and face to the sun (sans sunscreen) for 5 to 15 minutes a day should be enough to supply your body with enough vitamin D.

Vitamin D is a quirky nutrient, as evidenced by the fact that it's also classified as a hormone. Your bones depend on it and calcium working together, performing a delicate balancing act of biochemistry, with vitamin D helping calcium regain its balance whenever it falls short. Vitamin D acts on the kidneys and intestines to maintain adequate levels of calcium and phosphorus for bone formation, and it's integrally involved in the maintenance of calcium levels in blood.

Because vitamin D is so interdependent with calcium, it plays a crucial role in helping your muscles, heart, and nervous system function properly. Vitamin D may also influence cell growth and immune function, so it shouldn't surprise you to hear that it may decrease your risk of developing certain cancers. What's more, the recent discovery of calcium's pivotal role in controlling fat metabolism makes vitamin D central to issues concerning energy balance and weight maintenance.

This groundbreaking research, conducted by teams led by Dr. Michael Zemel at the University of Tennessee, has found that human fat cells contain a gene switched on and off by the presence or absence of calcium. When calcium levels are low, the gene turns on, causing the body to produce fat and store energy, while suppressing the system that breaks down fat and burns energy. When calcium levels are abundant, this obesity gene turns off. When this happens, the body is told to go easy on the fat production, increase fat breakdown, and crank up *thermogenesis,* the burning of calories.

The antiobesity effect of dairy appears to involve more than just calcium, though. Specifically, research subjects who get their calcium from dairy products have significantly greater weight control, less fat, and more lean body mass than subjects who get theirs predominantly from supplements. One possible contributor beyond calcium is the whey found in dairy products. This high-quality protein assists with protein metabolism and helps build muscle, but it also contains so-called ACE inhibitors, which help suppress fat formation by cells.

Another key component in dairy products is the branched-chain amino acid leucine, which is involved in protein metabolism, especially when calorie intake (especially carbohydrate) is low; activity level is high, as in exercise; or both situations come into play at once. When leucine is widely available in the body, protein synthesis gets a shot in the arm, energy metabolism revs high, and levels of blood sugar and insulin stay under control. All of the above assist with losing fat, gaining muscle, and controlling body weight.

Although milk offers some fantastic nutritional benefits, another calcium source, yogurt, does some very specific things above and beyond what milk offers. In studies, subjects who get their calcium from yogurt lose more weight and more body fat than those who get theirs from other sources. One of the magic bullets in yogurt is a group of substances called probiotics. Found in cultured dairy products that contain living bacteria, probiotics promote the growth of microorganisms. Unlike the bad bugs found in food that make you sick, these bugs are normal inhabitants of a healthy human digestive tract. Their job is to help with digestion and create an environment that discourages the growth of bad bugs.

Along with their general role in keeping the digestive system humming, probiotics confer a remarkable array of benefits on the human body. They:

- Enhance immune function
- Prevent antibiotic-induced diarrhea
- Reduce the risk of infection after some surgeries
- Protect against respiratory infections
- Combat the inflammatory skin disorder eczema
- Lower blood pressure and cholesterol
- Reduce the risk of cancer and kidney stone formation

Dairy, including yogurt, helps your mind, too. Whey protein contains tryptophan, a precursor to the brain chemical serotonin, a shortage of which has been linked to depression. Serotonin also promotes restful sleep. When your outlook is positive and you sleep well, it's much easier to stick to a healthy lifestyle that includes eating well, exercising regularly, and getting adequate rest.

In addition to consuming vitamin D in the recommended amounts from fish, milk, and fortified cereals, add a margin of safety by taking a daily multivitamin/mineral supplement containing 200 to 400 international units (IU) of vitamin D. If you spend most of your time indoors or live in a northern climate, where sun exposure may be limited, bump that range up to 400 to 800. Megadosing with vitamin D isn't recommended, as it can lead to vitamin toxicity in extreme cases.

If you're lactose intolerant, don't let that keep you from following the Full-Power Meal Plan. Many guys thus afflicted still produce enough lactase enzyme to comfortably consume 2 to 3 cups of milk, spread among three daily portions and combined with meals. Hard cheese, which contains high amounts of calcium but considerably less lactose than milk, can be used in place of a milk serving. (One ounce of hard cheese is nearly equivalent in calcium and calories to 1 cup of milk.) What's more, the use of lactose-reduced dairy products and lactase enzyme supplements can reduce the symptoms of lactose intolerance, or eliminate them altogether.

Crazy about Nuts

In recent years, nuts have gotten a bad rap. Detractors point to nuts' high fat content and their effect on the 42-inch-waistband crowd. But throw out the nuts, and you're throwing out a primary source of important nutrients such as protein, calcium, copper, iron, magnesium, fiber, folate, phytochemicals (especially from almonds, chestnuts, and pistachios), and vitamins A, C, and E.

Nuts are dense foods. An ounce contains anywhere from 165 to 200 calories, including 14 to 21 grams of fat. At first glance, that's a lot of fat, but most of it is unsaturated, the kind that provides the essential fatty acids. These are important for the body's daily health: They lower LDL (bad) cholesterol levels while maintaining high HDL (good) cholesterol levels. And like all plant foods, nuts are cholesterol-free.

Nuts are especially important when you consider vitamin E, which appears to play an important role in preventing certain kinds of cancer, heart disease, and cataract formation. The main dietary sources I used of vitamin E are nuts, nut butters, seeds, avocados, olives, and vegetable oils. Cut the nuts and you're cutting a vital dietary protector.

No Fish Tale

Protein from the sea anchors the Full-Power Meal Plan. Seldom are you encouraged to increase your fat intake, but that's exactly what we ask you to do by eating fish and seafood five times a week.

By now, you know the reasons I make the case for fish: the omega-3 fatty acids that protect against heart disease, blood clots, and strokes while boosting your brainpower, calming your nerves, and even reducing arthritic pain. An added benefit of eating fish most evenings is that it helps with weight management, apparently by enhancing the efficiency of leptin, the protein circulating throughout the body that is at least partially responsible for controlling fat stores.

For those who don't presently eat much fish, the temptation may be to take fish-oil supplements and be done with it. Not so fast. Unfortunately, not enough research justifies their use, except by patients with severely high triglycerides who haven't responded well to treatment, and by those at risk for pancreatitis, or inflammation of the pancreas. An excess of these oils can cause in-

NUTRTIONAL CONTENT OF SEAFOOD

Fish (3.5-oz. portion)	Calories	Protein (g)	Fat (g)	Saturated Fat (g)	Omega 3s (g)
SALMON					
King (Chinook)	231	25.7	13.3	3.2	1.737
Sockeye (red)	216	27.3	10.9	1.9	1.230
Coho (silver)	184	27.3	7.5	1.5	1.374
Keta (chum)	154	25.8	4.8	1.0	0.804
Pink	149	25.5	4.4	0.7	1.288
WHITEFISH					
Sablefish	250	17.2	19.6	4.0	1.787
Halibut	140	26.6	2.9	0.4	0.465
Rockfish	121	24.0	2.0	0.5	0.443
Flounder	117	24.1	1.5	0.4	0.501
Cod	105	22.9	0.8	0.1	0.276
SHELLFISH					
Dungeness crab	110	22.3	1.2	0.2	0.394
King crab	97	19.3	1.5	0.1	0.413
Snow crab	90	18.4	1.3	0.2	0.44
Oysters	90	11.1	2.2	0.5	0.71
Shrimp	99	20.9	1.0	0.3	0.315
CANNED SALMON					
Sockeye (red)	153	20.4	7.3	1.6	1.156
Pink	139	19.7	6.0	1.5	1.651

ternal or external bleeding, and though you'd be unlikely to get too many from whole foods, that possibility exists with pill forms. Also, fish-oil capsules are dietary supplements and hence unregulated by the U.S. Food and Drug Administration. Fish-oil supplements are rarely pure and often contain significant concentrations of highly toxic elements.

Speaking of toxic substances, they can be found in fish as well. Pollution in the air and soil and dumping into the oceans has led to an extremely polluted environment—and toxic levels of mercury in some fish. Fish farming practices that feed chemically contaminated fish meal to salmon have led to dangerously high levels of organochloride chemicals in farm-raised salmon. Organochlorides have been proven to be cancer-causing agents. The bottom line is this: You need to edu-

cate yourself on the safest kinds of fish, and eat them. Fish is too important to leave out of your diet; on the other hand, toxins in fish are too important to ignore.

Fishing for Options

Here are some good seafood choices that are generally low in contaminants:

Anchovies	Pollock
Crab	Sardines
Halibut	Sole
Mussels	Turbot
Oysters	Wild salmon*

*If you choose farmed salmon, ask where it was farmed; Washington State and Chile have the cleanest fish.

TUNA IS TRICKY

TUNA IS BY FAR THE MOST POPULAR FISH in the U.S. market, so it deserves special attention, especially because tuna steaks and canned albacore tuna have higher average levels of methylmercury than most other fish. Pay attention to these two factors when buying tuna.

1. How big is it?

Because fish become contaminated with mercury by eating other, smaller fish contaminated with mercury, the issue becomes one of where the fish falls on the food chain. Large fish eat more fish. The fish that they eat are more highly contaminated due to the volume of other fish that they consume, so the concentration of mercury rises with the weight of the fish. Conversely, the smaller the fish, the lower the concentration of mercury in its body.

2. Where is it from?

As you'd expect, tuna caught in cleaner waters have lower levels of mercury contamination. Many of the fishing vessels that catch tuna for the large national canners most commonly found on supermarket shelves catch fish in ocean waters with higher levels of mercury content. Canned tuna from these large tuna canneries is generally high in mercury. (On a side note, these fish also tend to be larger—most weigh 40 to 50 pounds or more. Again, these fish are more dangerous.)

Eggs

Like beans, eggs have fallen into disfavor, and unjustly so. Their protein is of the highest quality. It receives a perfect score, 1.0, for bioavailability, meaning your body gets to use pretty much all of it. Most proteins can't make that boast.

The egg yolk has been particularly scorned, but that is a particularly important source of nutrients. It contains protein and iron, but the secret treasure inside the yoke is lecithin (a.k.a. phosphatidylcholine). Lecithin helps with nerve transmissions in the brain. That conductivity has a big impact on how well your noggin recognizes and remembers things.

In fact, you'd be hard-pressed to find a better snack than hard-cooked eggs. I remember my dad telling me how he used to stash the hard-cooked eggs from breakfast in his pockets while cruising from the Mediterranean Sea to the South Pacific during World War II. That way he'd have it for a snack as the day wore on. Keep the shell on until you're ready to eat, and they can go anywhere—in your lunch bag, in your desk, or even (although I don't really recommend it) in your pocket.

Skinless Poultry and Lean Meats

Variety is one of the watchwords of the Full-Power Meal Plan, and that applies in spades to protein sources. Different meats give you not only high-quality protein but also critical nutrients such as iron, zinc, vitamins B_6 and B_{12}, and thiamine. Many other foods are bereft of those.

The fat value in poultry drops significantly when you aren't eating the fat-laden skin, so strip it from your chicken and turkey either before or

Aim for tuna caught by privately owned boutique canneries in the Pacific Northwest, which catch smaller fish one at a time by trolling, rather than in a net. The canning process used by these boutique canneries is also different and results in a far superior product both in taste and nutritional content. Here are the three canneries where I buy my canned fish. They all will ship their products. Try them, and you'll never buy commercial brands again. *Note:* The first two listed have found through laboratory testing that their fish are virtually mercury-free. East Point does not laboratory test for mercury, but it catches only 10- to 17-pound tuna. East Point also has awesome canned wild Chinook salmon and fresh or canned oysters from the famous Willapa Bay, located practically on their doorstep.

Fishing Vessel St. Jude
Seattle, Washington
Web site: www.tunatuna.com
Telephone: (425) 378-0680

Cinda's Sea Maiden Harvest
Portland, Oregon
Web site: www.seamaiden.com
Telephone: (503) 245-1596

East Point Seafood Market
South Bend, Washington
Web site: www.eastpointseafood.com
Telephone: (888) 317-8459

after you start cooking. Beef is a bit harder to de-saturate, but if you look for the leanest cuts, you're on the right track. Beef is graded according to its fat marbling (prime, choice, and select), with select being the leanest grade. Trim the remaining fat before cooking. To make sure that you're eating lean meat, choose from the six skinniest cuts of beef (see page 282).

Consumers are often told to steer clear of red meat and their saturated fatty acids and cholesterol because of the link between red meat and cancer. Although eating gobs of saturated fat is indeed terrible for you, linking red meat with cancer is simplistic at best and misguided at worst. First, eating only leaner cuts can reduce saturated fats significantly. Second, red meat is a major source of conjugated linoleic acids (CLAs). These are the only natural fatty acids said by the National Academy of Science to exhibit consistent anti-cancer properties. It appears that although fatty beef and its derivatives may increase cancer risk, leaner cuts—those containing 15 percent or less fat—may be protective against the same, which is probably attributable to CLAs.

(On a side note, one factor that you shouldn't forget is the newfound concern about bovine spongiform encephalopathy, also known as BSE or Mad Cow Disease. At least one Canadian and nearly 100 Europeans have died from a human variant of the disease—called new variant Creutzfeldt-Jakob disease—and they probably contracted it from eating infected meat products. There is probably no need for you to worry about getting the disease, as long as you follow the guidelines in "Calming Mad Cow Concerns" below.)

Pork is leaner than it used to be, particularly the leanest cuts, which come from the loin and leg areas. Lamb and veal are also lower in fat content than beef. Again, select lean cuts.

Anything but Sweet

You've probably heard people talk about "empty calories," perhaps without realizing what that means, exactly. Basically, it refers to calories that offer little or no additional nutritional value. The classic example is a can of Coke, which is basically colored sugar water.

CALMING MAD COW CONCERNS

THE LIKELIHOOD OF EATING MEAT CONTAMINATED WITH MAD COW DISEASE is very rare. However, I'd recommend you take some precautions. Here are the most important ones.

- Whenever possible, eat organic, grain-fed beef. These animals cannot be fed any animal by-products and therefore won't have Mad Cow Disease.
- Avoid high-risk cow parts—parts that are more likely to have Mad Cow—infected tissue. These include brains, beef cheeks, and neck bones.
- Avoid beef sold on the bone. Instead, choose boneless cuts of meat.
- Avoid bone marrow in general.
- If you want ground beef, have the butcher grind it fresh for you. Whenever possible, grind your own meat from a boneless cut.

As that example suggests, when it comes to empty calories, sugar takes the cake. Unfortunately, the U.S. food supply is overloaded with the stuff, adding unnecessary calories to our diets and inches to our waistlines. Sugar wreaks havoc on weight control and mood alike. As we discussed earlier, some guys might even be addicted to the stuff.

One type of sugar in particular, high-fructose corn syrup, is nearly ubiquitous in processed foods and drinks. I call it the devil's candy. (If you skipped to this chapter and haven't read about the dangers of HFCS, turn to page 92 for a primer.)

The Full-Power Meal Plan reduces consumption of foods that list high-fructose corn syrup among their first three ingredients. Note the word *reduce*—you don't need to eliminate it. The body can handle a little bit of it occasionally with no problems. Wherever possible, however, replace these engineered products with whole foods. That one simple step alone will go a long way toward improving your entire diet.

Supplemental Suggestions

Supplements can't turn a poorly designed diet into a good one. Their role should be exactly as the name suggests: augmenting an otherwise healthy diet full of all the foods necessary for optimal health and maximum performance. There are reasons to believe that such augmentation is advisable. Humans no longer live in the same environment that their ancestors did, yet they still enter the world with the same factory programming. The human body doesn't get the same amount of exercise it did when men were roaming the prairies, so it doesn't get the same quantity of food it took to keep it running at peak levels back then. The environment also hits the body with stresses, like the compromised ozone layer, that

GRILLED TO PERFECTION; GRILLED FOR PROTECTION

ADMITTEDLY, THERE ARE A LOT OF GUYS WHO WON'T BE DETERRED from throwing steaks on the barbecue, no matter how glaring the connection between grilled meat and cancer. For those guys, here are some suggestions from the American Institute of Cancer Research that can help reduce the risk.

- Choose lean cuts of meat. The fat that drips onto barbecue coals burns and creates carcinogens that float back onto your food in the grill smoke. Leaner meats cut down on the drippings.
- Trim all excess fat off the meat before you grill it.
- Use tongs or a spatula to turn the meat. Using a fork might pierce the meat and allow juices and fat to drop on the fire, causing carcinogenic flame-ups.
- Avoid or clean up pieces that are heavily charred.
- Precook meat like poultry and ribs. These can be boiled, steamed, or partially cooked in the microwave and then grilled briefly for the unique flavor and aroma.
- Marinate meats prior to grilling them. This may significantly protect them from the formation of carcinogenic substances.

would have been inconceivable even 100 years ago. Plus, we live a lot longer. These are all profound changes that haven't yet been accounted for in human DNA.

In order to take in all of the nutrients we need, we either have to eat 4,000 to 5,000 calories a day and exercise like crazy, or supplement our diets with certain specific nutrients. The following products all have an important role to play in the Full-Power Meal Plan.

Whey protein. By now, you should know that not all proteins are the same. Some digest slowly, others quickly; some are retained and used by the body in many ways, and others have only a few benefits. Things get even more confusing when you start looking into supplements, where you have to sort through terminology such as concentrates, isolates, hydrolysates, microfiltration, ion exchange, and so on. Suffice it say that whey is near the top of the charts.

Once you've decided to include a protein supplement in your diet, you will likely be using it on a regular basis, which makes ease of digestion crucial. Whey protein concentrate, for example, can contain 20 to 80 percent lactose (i.e., the sugar in milk), whereas isolates should be at least 90 percent pure. Isolate-based products generally mix up thinner—like juice rather than liquid cement—and are easier to digest.

Multivitamin/mineral supplement. You won't always know if your diet is providing you with all the vitamins and minerals you need, especially

THREE OVERVALUED (FOOD) STOCKS

IT DOESN'T TAKE A ROCKET SCIENTIST TO FIGURE OUT that belly-buster sodas, street-vendor hot dogs, and Interstate rest-area Cinnabons aren't very good for you. What's trickier is figuring out which less-obvious food choices are underrated, and which are overrated. The following three foods fall squarely in the latter camp, getting better press than their nutritional content probably warrants.

White pasta. Not only is it calorically dense, but some of white pasta's nutritional value gets lost in processing. It doesn't have much fiber in it at all. This is problematic, too, because most restaurants that serve "clean" food are going to serve a lot of pasta dishes. *Better alternative:* Whole-grain pasta.

Fruit juices. The culprit here is the large amounts of sugar they contain and the fiber that's been removed, compared with the nutrient content. Although some 100 percent fruit juice is a good choice, portion control is critical. And you'd be surprised at how many calories you're getting—along the lines of 120 for 8 fluid ounces. *Better alternative:* Whole fruit.

Iceberg lettuce. Salads offer an abundance of phytochemicals and other nutrients, but iceberg lettuce offers considerably less than darker leaves. If you're relying on salads as part of a weight-loss program, be particularly wary of relying on iceberg lettuce too heavily. *Better alternative:* Romaine lettuce and other dark leafy greens.

since the roles many of them play are subtle, albeit crucial. The B vitamins, for example, help your body absorb food properly. A daily multivitamin/mineral is the cheapest insurance policy you'll ever buy.

Vitamin E. Why single out vitamin E from the others for the supplementation? Although vitamin E is found in nuts, seeds, raw wheat germ, polyunsaturated vegetable oils, and fish liver oils, in this age of fat-reduced diets it's hard to consume the minimum amounts of vitamin E recommended in the Daily Reference Intakes (15 milligrams), let alone the much higher amounts that have been shown in studies to help stave off aging and disease progression in the brain and the body. Higher amounts of vitamin E may even help reduce the delayed-onset muscle soreness produced as a result of the oxidative damage to muscle cells after exercise.

Flaxseed. This one seemingly innocuous little seed can make up for a whole host of missing things in your diet. It's high in the omega-3 fat alpha-linolenic acid, which is heavily involved in various cell functions, especially in the brain, where it influences mood and depression. The water-soluble fibers in flax help the cholesterol in bile exit the body, reducing blood cholesterol levels. The insoluble fibers help speed bowel activity and reduce constipation. Flax is also high in an indigestible fiber component called lignan, which assists with the maintenance of healthy blood-sugar levels and helps control insulin surges.

Most guys would find whole flaxseed unpalatable, and unless you're a cow or giraffe, you don't have the teeth to chew it properly. Instead, try grinding it up first. Use a small coffee grinder that you don't use for anything else, and grind the flax daily as needed. If you don't want to hassle with machinery, purchase flaxseed meal that's been preground. Add 1 tablespoon of ground flaxseed to your morning cereal or juice, to salads or yogurt, or even to a smoothie, and

you're good to go. Another alternative is to use flaxseed oil; you'll get the healthy oils but avoid the fibers that way.

Staying on the Wagon

As you move forward with the Power-Food Meal Plan, the key will be staying the course, sticking with the program, and all of those other clichés. To do that, you're going to need to learn to avoid the foods that trigger backsliding. These are the foods you eat out of craving, rather than out of genuine hunger, and they can consistently sabotage otherwise disciplined eating habits.

Though certain foods crop up repeatedly as triggers—pizza tops the short list for most individuals—triggers can be highly individualized and even peculiar. "For one [person] it may be cheese and pizza, for another it may be red meat," writes David Heber, M.D., Ph.D., in *The Resolution Diet.* "For others it is nonfat yogurt and chocolate chip cookies. . . . These are the foods that you are eating to relieve stress or boredom." He recommends replacing cheese pizza with whole-wheat pasta and tomato sauce topped with shrimp; trying roasted garlic instead of butter; eating turkey instead of beef; and adding fresh fruit while ditching cookies and cake, among other swaps.

Despite being highly individualized, as Heber's list suggests, trigger foods are, nine times out of ten, so-called comfort foods. Put another way, trigger foods are the ones we'll go out to get in the middle of a torrential rainstorm. What makes one food a likely candidate to become a trigger and another not? Trigger foods tend to be high in sugar, fat, or both. Moreover, we usually associate them with fond memories and rewards. Again, this places the consumer of those foods in a psychological comfort zone.

The connection may also be rooted in biochemistry. Some researchers believe that answering a

Bullet Points on Trigger Foods

■ To identify your trigger foods, keep a daily journal of your food and drink consumption for two weeks. Include notes on how activities, situations, and feelings affected it. Once you identify what the triggers are, you can try to short-circuit the cues that you get.

■ If cravings lead to binge eating, where you're out of control or gaining significant weight, seek the help of a qualified health professional, such as a registered dietitian or therapist specializing in disordered eating habits. Emotional problems, such as feeling lonely or inadequate, are often the real issue, not the craving itself.

■ Fortunately, food cravings aren't dangerous in most cases. Eating small amounts of the foods you crave or versions reduced in fat or sugar on a regular basis works for most people. What you don't want to do is feel deprived, especially if you're trying to lose weight, because you'll crave that item even more.

craving for a sweet and fatty food triggers the release of endorphins—brain chemicals that produce feelings of calm and pleasure. Others turn this cause-and-effect postulate upside down, contending that the body produces chemicals that trigger the cravings. In his book, Heber puts forth an evolutionary argument, saying that our cravings for those foods are a throwback to the days of the aforementioned loincloth, when long stretches of foodlessness for hunter-gatherer types made calorie hoarding an advantageous survival strategy.

Regardless, trigger foods today have precious little to do with real hunger. Oftentimes, people are simply eating out of habit. They don't even know when they're hungry, but mental states and emotions such as anxiety or boredom will trigger eating. Then there are external impacts, such as the sight and smells of food. You walk past a bagel shop and smell the bagels, so you want a bagel. Well, if you hadn't passed the store, you wouldn't have thought twice about bagels, right?

What you have to ask yourself is, "Am I really hungry?" If the answer isn't yes, keep walking.

Situations and solutions. While a predisposition to comfort foods can usually be managed, guys succumb to temptation, more often than not, as moods shade their judgment. A mood precipitated by something like a political crisis or a terrorist attack is a special situation, but simply falling into a generalized funk can have the same effect. If you feel disconnected from people, you may need to be satisfied by other stimuli. Food provides that. Situations themselves can also be powerful food triggers. Visit your favorite restaurant or bar, or spend a Sunday watching sports, and you'll probably want the foods you associate with those events: maybe a steak or a bag of chips. The key to eating better is to anticipate these moments and take steps to protect yourself from slipping.

THE FULL-POWER MEAL PLAN

HERE IT IS: THE ALL-IN-ONE, EVERYTHING-YOU-NEED MEAL PLAN. For any guy who wants total body health, the Full-Power Meal Plan provides everything necessary.

THE MENU

DAY 1

Wake Up

Water

Breakfast

2 bread	1 cup Shredded Wheat
1 citrus	1/2 cup orange juice
1 berry	3/4 cup blueberries
1 fat	1 1/2 tablespoons ground flaxseed
1 milk	1 cup fat-free milk
1 medium fat protein	1 egg (hard-cooked)
1 added sugar	1 teaspoon brown sugar (for shredded wheat)
	Water
	Oil-free cooking spray for egg, if necessary

Snack

1 carotenoid	1/2 cup V8 juice
2 nut	20 peanuts
	Water

Lunch

2 carotenoid	Large salad with 1 cup romaine, 1/2 cup carrots, 1/2 cup tomatoes, other vegetables
1 bean	1/2 cup garbanzo beans
4 very lean protein	4 ounces shrimp
2 fat	2 tablespoons oil-and-vinegar dressing or vinaigrette
1 milk	1 nonfat latte, tall, with no-calorie sweetener

Daily Assumptions*†

2,500 calories
305 grams carbohydrates
163 grams protein
73 grams fat

Daily Breakdown*†

4 bread
6 fruit (2 citrus, 2 berry, 2 other)
4 milk
8 teaspoons added sugar
6 vegetables (3 carotenoid, 2 brassica, 1 allium)
1 bean
2 soy
4 lean protein
1 medium fat protein
6 very lean protein
6 fat
2 nut

Note: Occasionally, a fat-free product, like mustard or cooking spray, is included on the menus. These do not count toward your daily breakdown but should not be overused.

*Use every day.

† Based on a 185-pound man.

Pre-Workout Snack

1 milk	$^2/_3$ cup plain nonfat yogurt
1 other fruit	$^1/_2$ cup unsweetened canned pineapple chunks and noncaloric sweetener (add to yogurt)
2 soy	$^1/_2$ cup soy nuts
	Water

Workout

Water

Post-Workout

SMOOTHIE

Blend until smooth.

1 milk	1 cup fat-free milk
1 citrus	$^1/_2$ cup orange juice
1 berry	$1^1/_2$ cups berries
2 very lean protein	14 grams whey protein powder
6 teaspoons added sugar	2 tablespoons honey

Dinner

BROCCOLI-AND-SHRIMP STIR-FRY

2 brassica	1 cup broccoli
1 allium	$^1/_2$ onion, garlic
4 lean protein	4 ounces dark meat chicken
3 fat	1 tablespoon peanut oil
2 bread	$^2/_3$ cup brown rice
1 other fruit	$^1/_2$ mango
1 teaspoon added sugar	Tea with 1 teaspoon sugar

DAY 2

Wake Up

Water

Breakfast

2 bread	1 cup cooked oatmeal
1 citrus	1/2 cup orange juice
1 berry	1 cup raspberries
1 fat	1 1/2 tablespoons ground flaxseed
1 teaspoon added sugar	1 teaspoon brown sugar
1 milk	1 cup fat-free milk
1 medium fat protein	1 scrambled egg
	Water
	Oil-free cooking spray (for egg)

Snack

2 soy	1/2 cup soy nuts
1 carotenoid	1/2 cup tomato juice

Lunch

2 carotenoid	1 cup bibb lettuce, 1/2 cup red pepper, 1/2 cup tomatoes
4 lean protein	4 ounces dark-meat chicken
1 milk	1 ounce cheese
2 fat	2 tablespoons oil-and-vinegar dressing or vinaigrette
1 bean	1/2 cup pinto beans
	Water

Pre-Workout Snack

1 milk	2/3 cup plain nonfat yogurt with noncaloric sweetener
1 other fruit	1/2 cup unsweetened canned peaches (add to yogurt)
2 nut	12 roasted almonds
	Water

Workout

Water

Post-Workout

SMOOTHIE
Blend until smooth.

1 milk	1 cup fat-free milk
1 citrus	½ cup orange juice
1 berry	1½ cups berries
2 very lean protein	14 grams whey protein powder
6 teaspoons added sugar	2 tablespoons honey

Dinner

2 bread	1 small ear corn on the cob
	1 small whole-wheat dinner roll
2 brassica	1 cup cabbage slaw
1 allium	½ onion (for salmon)
3 fat	2 teaspoons olive oil and garlic (to marinate vegetables)
	Included (in cabbage slaw)
4 lean protein	4 ounces grilled salmon
1 other fruit	1 slice watermelon
1 teaspoon added sugar	Tea with 1 teaspoon sugar

DAY 3

Wake Up

Water

Breakfast

2 bread	2 slices whole-wheat raisin bread
1 medium fat protein	1 sunny-side up egg (cook in a nonstick pan)
	Oil-free cooking spray (for egg)

MORNING SMOOTHIE
Blend until smooth.

1 milk	1 cup fat-free milk
1 citrus	½ cup orange juice
1 berry	1 cup strawberries
1 fat	1½ tablespoons ground flaxseed (or 1 teaspoon flaxseed oil)
1 teaspoon added sugar	1 teaspoon honey
	Water

Snack

1 carotenoid	1 cup mini carrots
2 nut	1 tablespoon natural peanut butter
	Water

Lunch

1 bean	1 cup bean soup
4 very lean protein	4 ounces ground turkey burger
1 milk	1 ounce cheddar cheese
2 carotenoid	1/2 cup asparagus, steamed
	1 cup leaf lettuce
2 fat	2 tablespoons oil-and-vinegar dressing or vinaigrette

Pre-Workout Snack

1 milk	1 nonfat latte, tall
1 other fruit	4 dried apricots
2 soy	1/2 cup soy nuts
	Water

Workout

	Water

Post-Workout

SMOOTHIE

Blend until smooth.

1 milk	1 cup fat-free milk
1 citrus	1/2 cup orange juice
1 berry	1 1/2 cups berries
2 very lean protein	14 grams whey protein powder
6 teaspoons added sugar	2 tablespoons honey

Dinner

4 lean protein	4 ounces lean beef (for stir fry)
2 bread	2/3 cup rice
2 brassica	1 cup raw broccoli, 1 cup raw bok choy (for stir fry)
1 allium	1/2 cup raw onion and garlic, mixed
3 fat	1 tablespoon oil (for stir fry)
1 other fruit	1/2 cup fresh pineapple
1 teaspoon added sugar	Tea with 1 teaspoon sugar
	1 cup miso soup

DAY 4

Wake Up

Water

Breakfast

2 bread	2 cups Kashi
1 citrus	$^{1}/_{2}$ cup orange juice
1 berry	$^{3}/_{4}$ cup blueberries
1 milk	1 cup fat-free milk
1 medium fat protein	1 egg (hard-cooked or cooked in a nonstick pan)
1 fat	$1^{1}/_{2}$ tablespoons ground flaxseed
1 teaspoon added sugar	1 teaspoon sugar (for Kashi)
	Water
	Oil-free cooking spray for egg, if necessary

Snack

2 soy	$^{1}/_{2}$ cup soy nuts
1 carotenoid	$^{1}/_{2}$ cup V8 juice
	Water

Lunch

4 lean protein	4 ounces dark meat chicken
1 bean	$^{1}/_{2}$ cup three-bean salad
2 carotenoid	1 cup romaine, $^{1}/_{2}$ cup carrots, $^{1}/_{2}$ cup tomatoes
2 fat	2 tablespoons oil-and-vinegar, or vinaigrette dressing
1 milk	1 cup fat-free milk
	Water

Pre-Workout Snack

1 milk	1 nonfat latte, tall
1 other fruit	1 apple, sliced
2 nut	1 tablespoon natural peanut butter

Workout

Water

Post-Workout

SMOOTHIE

Blend until smooth.

1 milk	1 cup fat-free milk
1 citrus	¹/₂ cup orange juice
1 berry	1¹/₂ cups berries
2 very lean protein	14 grams whey protein powder
6 teaspoons added sugar	2 tablespoons honey

Dinner

2 bread	²/₃ cup cooked whole-wheat pasta
4 very lean protein	4 ounces clams in tomato-garlic and olive oil sauce
2 brassica	1 cup broccoli, steamed
1 allium	¹/₂ cup cshallots, mixed with broccoli
3 fat	included (in clam sauce)
1 other fruit	1 slice or 1¹/₂ cups cubed watermelon
1 teaspoon added sugar	Tea with 1 teaspoon sugar
	Water

DAY 5

Wake Up

Water

Breakfast

2 bread	1 cup Shredded Wheat
1 citrus	¹/₂ cup orange juice
1 berry	³/₄ cup blueberries
1 fat	1¹/₂ tablespoons ground flaxseed
1 milk	1 cup fat-free milk
1 medium fat protein	1 egg (hard-cooked)
1 teaspoon added sugar	1 teaspoon sugar (for Shredded Wheat)
	Water

Snack

2 nut	20 peanuts
1 carotenoid	1 cup mini carrots

Lunch

1 bean	1 cup minestrone soup
2 carotenoid	1 cup bibb lettuce, ¹/₂ cup tomatoes, ¹/₂ cup red peppers
4 lean protein	4 ounces dark meat turkey
2 fat	2 tablespoons oil-and-vinegar or vinaigrette dressing
1 milk	1 nonfat latte, tall, with noncaloric sweetener

Pre-Workout Snack

1 milk   ²/₃ cup plain nonfat yogurt

1 other fruit   ¹/₂ cup unsweetened canned pears with no-calorie sweetener

2 soy   ¹/₂ cup soy nuts

Water

Workout

Water

Post-Workout

SMOOTHIE

Blend until smooth.

1 milk   1 cup fat-free milk

1 citrus   ¹/₂ cup orange juice

1 berry   1¹/₂ cups berries

2 very lean protein   14 grams whey protein powder

6 teaspoons added sugar   2 tablespoons honey

Dinner

2 bread   ¹/₂ baked yam or sweet potato

1 slice hearty whole-wheat bread

2 brassica   1 cup steamed Brussels sprouts with Asian mustard

1 allium   1 roasted garlic bulb (spread on bread and fish)

4 very lean protein   4 ounces grilled or broiled halibut

3 fat   2 teaspoons sesame oil (for halibut) and 1 teaspoon sesame seeds

1 other fruit   12 cherries

1 teaspoon added sugar   Tea with 1 teaspoon sugar

DAY 6

Wake Up

Water

Breakfast

FRENCH TOAST *(See recipe directions on page 44.)*

2 bread	2 slices hearty whole-grain bread
1 medium fat protein	1 egg, scrambled
1 milk	1 cup fat-free milk
1 fat	1½ tablespoons ground flaxseed
1 teaspoon added sugar	1 teaspoon maple syrup
1 citrus	½ cup orange juice
1 berry	1 cup fresh raspberries
	Cinnamon
	Water
	Oil-free cooking spray

Snack

2 soy	1 cup edamame in the shell
1 carotenoid	½ cup V8 juice

Lunch

SALAD

4 very lean protein	4 ounces tuna in water, drained
2 carotenoid	2 large sliced tomatoes
1 milk	1 ounce mozzarella
2 fat	2 teaspoons olive oil
1 bean	½ cup fava beans
	Water

Pre-Workout Snack

1 other fruit	1 medium banana, sliced
2 nut	1 tablespoon natural peanut butter
1 milk	1 cup fat-free milk

Workout

Water

Post-Workout

SMOOTHIE

Blend until smooth.

1 milk	1 cup milk
1 citrus	$^1/_2$ cup orange juice
1 berry	$1^1/_2$ cups berries
2 very lean protein	14 grams whey protein powder
6 teaspoons added sugar	2 tablespoons honey

Dinner

2 bread	$^2/_3$ cup whole-wheat couscous
2 brassica	1 cup steamed broccoli and cauliflower
1 allium	$^1/_2$ cup onions (sautéed with steak)
1 other fruit	2 dried apricots
	1 tablespoon currants
4 lean protein	4 ounces filet mignon
3 fat	1 tablespoon olive oil (for sautéing)

DAY 7

Wake Up

Water

Breakfast

2 bread	1 cup cooked oatmeal
1 citrus	$^1/_2$ cup orange juice
1 berry	$^3/_4$ cup blueberries
1 fat	$1^1/_2$ tablespoons ground flaxseed
1 teaspoon added sugar	1 teaspoon brown sugar
1 milk	1 cup fat-free milk
1 medium fat protein	1 egg, scrambled in a nonstick pan
	Water
	Oil-free cooking spray (for egg)

Mid-Morning Snack

2 soy	$^1/_2$ cup soy nuts
1 carotenoid	$^1/_2$ cup tomato juice
	Water

Lunch

4 very lean protein	4 ounces turkey (for salad)
2 carotenoid	1 cup romaine, $1/2$ cup carrots, $1/2$ cup tomatoes
1 bean	$1/2$ cup garbanzo beans
2 fat	2 tablespoon oil-and-vinegar or vinaigrette dressing
1 milk	Nonfat latte, tall

Pre-Workout Snack

1 milk	$2/3$ cup plain nonfat yogurt
1 other fruit	$1/2$ cup unsweetened canned pineapple with no-calorie sweetener
2 nut	12 almonds
	Water

Workout

	Water

Post-Workout

SMOOTHIE

Blend until smooth.

1 milk	1 cup fat-free milk
1 citrus	$1/2$ cup orange juice
1 berry	$1^{1}/2$ cups berries
2 very lean protein	14 grams whey protein powder
6 teaspoons added sugar	2 tablespoons honey

Dinner

2 bread	1 whole-wheat pita bread
4 lean protein	4 ounces salmon steak with raspberry vinegar marinade
2 brassica	1 cup broccoli, steamed
1 allium	$1/2$ cup onions
3 fat	1 tablespoon olive oil (for marinade)
1 other fruit	17 grapes
1 teaspoon added sugar	Included (in marinade)

DAY 8

Wake Up

Water

Breakfast

2 bread	2 slices whole-wheat toast
1 medium fat protein	1 hard-cooked egg
1 milk	$^1/_2$ cup cottage cheese with pinch cinnamon
1 fat	$1^1/_2$ tablespoons ground flaxseed
1 citrus	$^1/_2$ pink grapefruit
1 berry	1 cup fresh raspberries
1 teaspoon added sugar	1 teaspoon sugar (for cottage cheese)
	Water

Snack

1 carotenoid	1 cup mini-carrots
2 nut	1 tablespoon natural almond butter
	Water

Lunch

1 bean	1 cup lentil soup
4 very lean protein	4 ounces skinless white-meat chicken, grilled or broiled with lime juice
2 carotenoid	1 cup sautéed tomatoes and yellow squash
2 fat	2 teaspoons olive oil (for sautéing)
1 milk	1 cup fat-free milk

Pre-Workout Snack

1 milk	1 nonfat latte, tall
1 other fruit	1 cup cubed cantaloupe
2 soy	1 cup edamame in the shell

Workout

Water

Post-Workout

SMOOTHIE

Blend until smooth.

1 milk	1 cup fat-free milk
1 citrus	$^1/_2$ cup orange juice
1 berry	$1^1/_2$ cups berries
2 very lean protein	14 grams whey protein powder
6 teaspoons added sugar	2 tablespoons honey

Dinner

BROCCOLI-AND-LAMB STIR-FRY

2 brassica	1 cup broccoli, steamed
1 allium	$^1/_2$ onion, garlic
4 lean protein	4 ounces lamb
3 fat	1 tablespoon peanut oil (for lamb)
2 bread	$^2/_3$ cup brown rice
1 other fruit	$^1/_2$ mango
1 teaspoon added sugar	Tea with 1 teaspoon sugar

DAY 9

Wake Up

Water

Breakfast

2 bread	1 cup Shredded Wheat
1 citrus	$^1/_2$ cup orange juice
1 berry	$^3/_4$ cup blueberries
1 fat	$1^1/_2$ tablespoons ground flaxseed
1 milk	1 cup fat-free milk
1 medium fat protein	1 egg (hard-cooked)
1 teaspoon added sugar	1 teaspoon sugar (for Shredded Wheat)
	Water

Snack

2 soy	$^1/_2$ cup soy nuts
1 carotenoid	$^1/_2$ cup tomato juice

Lunch

4 very lean protein	4 ounces tuna in water, drained
2 carotenoid	1 cup bibb lettuce, $^1/_2$ cup red peppers, $^1/_2$ cup tomatoes
2 fat	2 tablespoons reduced-fat dressing
1 bean	$^1/_2$ cup navy beans
	8 black olives
1 milk	1 nonfat latte, tall

Pre-Workout Snack

1 milk	$^2/_3$ cup plain nonfat yogurt
1 other fruit	$^1/_2$ cup unsweetened canned pineapple with no-calorie sweetener
2 nuts	12 cashews
	Water

Workout

Water

Post-Workout

SMOOTHIE

Blend until smooth.

1 milk	1 cup fat-free milk
1 citrus	$^1/_2$ cup orange juice
1 berry	$1^1/_2$ cups berries
2 very lean protein	14 grams whey protein powder
6 teaspoons added sugar	2 tablespoons honey

Dinner

2 bread	Whole-wheat bun
4 lean protein	4 ounces ground sirloin
2 brassica	1 cup coleslaw
1 allium	$^1/_2$ cup grilled onion (for sirloin)
1 other fruit	1 small banana
3 fat	2 teaspoons olive oil (for sautéing onions)
	Included (in coleslaw)
1 teaspoon added sugar	Tea with 1 teaspoon sugar

DAY 10

Wake Up

Water

Breakfast

2 bread	1 cup cooked oatmeal
1 citrus	$^1/_2$ cup orange juice
1 berry	1 cup raspberries
1 fat	$1^1/_2$ tablespoons ground flaxseed
1 teaspoon added sugar	1 teaspoon brown sugar
1 milk	1 cup fat-free milk
1 medium fat protein	1 egg, scrambled in a nonstick pan
	Water
	Oil-free cooking spray (for egg)

Snack

2 nut	20 peanuts
1 carotenoid	$\frac{1}{2}$ cup V8 juice

Lunch

1 bean	1 cup lentil soup
4 very lean protein	4 ounces halibut, grilled
2 carotenoid	1 cup romaine, $\frac{1}{2}$ cup red peppers, $\frac{1}{2}$ cup tomatoes
2 fat	2 tablespoons oil-and-vinegar dressing or vinaigrette
1 milk	1 cup fat-free milk

Pre-Workout Snack

1 milk	1 cup fat-free milk
1 other fruit	1 slice watermelon
2 soy	$\frac{1}{2}$ cup soy nuts

Workout

Water

Post-Workout

SMOOTHIE

Blend until smooth.

1 milk	1 cup fat-free milk
1 citrus	$\frac{1}{2}$ cup orange juice
1 berry	$1\frac{1}{2}$ cups berries
2 very lean protein	14 grams whey protein powder
6 teaspoons added sugar	2 tablespoons honey

Dinner

4 lean protein	4 ounces turkey sausage
2 brassica	1 cup sauerkraut
1 allium	$\frac{1}{2}$ cup chopped onion (for hash browns)
2 bread	1 large potato (for hash browns)
3 fat	1 tablespoon oil (for hash browns)
1 other fruit	12 cherries
1 teaspoon added sugar	Tea with 1 teaspoon sugar

DAY 11

Wake Up

Water

Breakfast

2 bread	2 cups Kashi
1 citrus	1/2 cup orange juice
1 berry	3/4 cup blackberries
1 fat	1 1/2 tablespoons ground flaxseed
1 milk	1 cup fat-free milk
1 medium fat protein	1 egg (hard-cooked or cooked in a nonstick pan)
1 teaspoon added sugar	1 teaspoon sugar (for Kashi)
	Water

Snack

2 soy	1 cup edamame in shell
1 carotenoid	1/2 cup V8 juice

Lunch

1 bean	1 cup black bean soup
4 very lean protein	4 ounces shrimp
2 carotenoid	2 cups romaine
2 fat	2 tablespoons Caesar dressing
1 milk	1 cup fat-free milk

Pre-Workout Snack

1 milk	2/3 cup plain nonfat yogurt
1 other fruit	1/2 cup unsweetened canned peaches with no-calorie sweetener
2 nut	12 almonds
	Water

Workout

Water

Post-Workout

SMOOTHIE

Blend until smooth.

1 milk	1 cup fat-free milk
1 citrus	1/2 cup orange juice
1 berry	1 1/2 cups berries
2 very lean protein	14 grams whey protein powder
6 teaspoons added sugar	2 tablespoons honey

Dinner

2 bread	$^2/_3$ cups cooked whole-wheat pasta
4 lean protein	4 ounces meatballs in tomato-garlic sauce and olive oil (over pasta)
2 brassica	1 cup broccoli, steamed
1 allium	$^1/_2$ onion (for sauce)
3 fat	1 tablespoon olive oil (in sauce)
1 other fruit	1 nectarine
1 teaspoon added sugar	Tea with 1 teaspoon sugar
	Water

DAY 12

Wake Up

	Water

Breakfast

2 bread	2 slices whole-wheat raisin bread
1 medium fat protein	1 sunny-side up egg, cooked in a nonstick pan
	Oil-free cooking spray (for egg)

MORNING SMOOTHIE

Blend until smooth.

1 milk	1 cup fat-free milk
1 citrus	$^1/_2$ cup orange juice
1 berry	1 cup strawberries
1 fat	$1^1/_2$ tablespoons ground flaxseed (or 1 teaspoon flaxseed oil)
1 teaspoon added sugar	1 teaspoon honey
	Water

Snack

2 nut	1 tablespoon natural almond butter
1 carotenoid	1 cup mini carrots

Lunch

4 very lean protein	4 ounces chicken fajitas (no tortillas)
2 carotenoid	1 cup cooked red and green peppers
1 bean	$^1/_2$ cup vegetarian refried beans
2 fat	2 teaspoons olive oil (for sautéing peppers)
1 milk	1 cup fat-free milk

Pre-Workout Snack

1 milk	1 nonfat latte, tall
1 other fruit	4 dried apricots
2 soy	$^1/_2$ cup soy nuts
	Water

Workout

Water

Post-Workout

SMOOTHIE

Blend until smooth.

1 milk	1 cup fat-free milk
1 citrus	$^1/_2$ cup orange juice
1 berry	1$^1/_2$ cups berries
2 very lean protein	14 grams whey protein powder
6 teaspoons added sugar	2 tablespoons honey

Dinner

4 lean protein	4 ounces dark meat chicken, marinated with apple cider, soy sauce, ginger
3 fat	2 teaspoons sesame oil (in marinade)
	Included (in coleslaw)
2 brassica	1 cup red cabbage slaw
1 allium	1 clove garlic (for chicken)
2 bread	$^1/_2$ acorn squash
	1 slice whole grain bread
1 teaspoon added sugar	1 teaspoon maple syrup (on squash)
1 other fruit	1 pear

DAY 13

Wake Up

Water

Breakfast

FRENCH TOAST (*See recipe directions on page 44.*)

2 bread	2 slices hearty whole-grain bread
1 medium fat protein	1 egg
1 milk	1 cup fat-free milk ($^1/_2$ cup for French toast)
1 fat	1$^1/_2$ tablespoons ground flaxseed, cinnamon
1 teaspoon added sugar	1 teaspoon maple syrup
1 citrus	$^1/_2$ cup orange juice
1 berry	1 cup fresh raspberries
	Water
	Oil-free cooking spray

Snack

2 soy	¹/₂ cup soy nuts
1 carotenoid	¹/₂ cup V8 juice

Lunch

1 bean	1 cup lentil soup
4 very lean protein	4 ounces ground turkey burger
1 milk	1 ounce cheddar cheese
2 carotenoid	1 cup asparagus, steamed
2 fat	1 tablespoon thousand island dressing
	1 teaspoon olive oil (for asparagus)

Pre-Workout Snack

1 milk	1 nonfat latte, tall
1 other fruit	1 apple, sliced
2 nut	1 tablespoon natural peanut butter

Workout

Water

Post-Workout

SMOOTHIE

Blend until smooth.

1 milk	1 cup fat-free milk
1 citrus	¹/₂ cup orange juice
1 berry	1¹/₂ cups berries
2 very lean protein	14 grams whey protein powder
6 teaspoons added sugar	2 tablespoons honey

Dinner

BROCCOLI-AND-SALMON STIR-FRY

2 brassica	1 cup broccoli, steamed
1 allium	¹/₂ cup onion, garlic
4 lean protein	4 ounces salmon
3 fat	1 tablespoon peanut oil
2 bread	²/₃ cup brown rice
1 other fruit	¹/₂ mango
1 teaspoon added sugar	Tea with 1 teaspoon sugar

DAY 14

Wake Up

Water

Breakfast

2 bread	1 cup cooked oatmeal
1 medium fat protein	1 egg, hard-cooked
1 citrus	$^1\!/_2$ cup orange juice
1 berry	$^3\!/_4$ cup blackberries
1 fat	$1^1\!/_2$ tablespoons ground flaxseed
1 teaspoon added sugar	1 teaspoon sugar
1 milk	1 cup fat-free milk
	Water

Snack

1 carotenoid	1 cup mini-carrots
2 nut	1 tablespoon natural almond butter
	Water

Lunch

4 very lean protein	4 ounces skinless white-meat chicken, grilled with lime juice
1 milk	1 ounce cheese
1 bean	$^1\!/_2$ cup garbanzo beans
2 fat	1 slice or 2 teaspoons crumbled bacon
2 carotenoid	2 cups romaine
	2 tablespoons fat-free Caesar dressing
	Water

Pre-Workout Snack

1 milk	1 nonfat latte, tall
1 other fruit	1 pear
2 soy	1 cup edamame in the shell

Workout

Water

Post-Workout

SMOOTHIE

Blend until smooth.

1 milk	1 cup fat-free milk
1 citrus	½ cup orange juice
1 berry	1½ cups berries
2 very lean protein	14 grams whey protein powder
6 teaspoons added sugar	2 tablespoons honey

Dinner

2 bread	1 whole-wheat pita bread, toasted

TURKEY STIR-FRY

4 lean protein	4 ounces dark meat turkey
2 brassica vegetables	1 cup broccoli, steamed
1 allium	½ cup onions, tomatoes, mushrooms
3 fat	1 tablespoon olive oil
1 other fruit	17 grapes
1 teaspoon added sugar	Tea with 1 teaspoon sugar

CHAPTER ELEVEN

Food and Your Future

SO YOU'VE COMMITTED TO A
MEAL PLAN—NOW WHAT?

More muscle, less fat. A stronger, more reliable heart. Increased energy. Improved overall health. More years to spend among the living, and a better mind and body to enjoy those years. Those sound like some pretty good reasons to eat more healthfully. And after paging through *Power Food,* you have the tools to get the job done. The question now is this: Do you know where to go from here?

Starting today, your greatest challenge will be developing and maintaining consistency. That means following a nutrition plan, like the one outlined in these pages, that you can stick with. Adherence means not carrying huge, unrealistic expectations. If you expect to prepare and eat six meals a day, every day, you'll soon realize that the simple processes of cooking and eating take up a lot of your time—time that you might not have. You'll have to make some concessions to convenience if you're going to stick with the program.

In this chapter, I'm going to review some things, throw a couple of new curves your way, and tie it all together for you. Let's start with an idea I've discussed before and hammer it home once more: A diet based primarily on whole foods such as fish, poultry, nuts, fresh fruits, and vegetables is essential for long-term health. As you'll recall, whole foods either haven't been modified from their natural state, or, if they have, the alteration has been ever so slight. In contrast, processed foods have been modified significantly. A lot happens to a potato between the time it is harvested in a field and when you reach for it in French-fried form at McDonald's. When fresh vegetables are canned, they pick up a lot of sodium. And who knows whether that cellophane-wrapped pink-frosted coconut pastry you got at 7-11 has any actual coconut inside?

Processing is designed to keep mass-produced foods looking and tasting fresh. After all, some of those Little Debbie snack pies will be sitting on the shelf for a long while before they're eaten. That durability comes at a price: The more processed a food is, the less nutritious it's likely to be, even when it has been "enriched" with nutrients.

Processed foods tend to be dense in calories and lacking in things like fiber, so the benefit of enriching them is overshadowed.

Bear in mind that dietary supplements and so-called engineered foods, like energy bars, are also processed. "Engineered" implies a little more forethought and sophistication than processed, and that's a useful distinction—a well-balanced meal-replacement shake is a lot different than a bag of Cheetos or Wonder Bread. The advantage here, and it's significant, is convenience and portability. If your flight is delayed and you can reach into your briefcase for a protein/energy bar rather than hitting a nearby Cinnabon stand, you've saved yourself from a heaping portion of saturated fats and high-glycemic index carbs and replaced it with a healthy dose of protein. Many of these engineered products are also terrific for feeding your muscles before or after your workouts, when the nourishment you need is hard to find.

Still, you shouldn't substitute supplements for whole foods. Despite all the research that goes into developing these engineered foods, they're not superior to, nor do they replace, fruits, vegetables, meat, dairy, and other whole foods. Whole foods are the holy grail of sound nutrition for a host of reasons. Here are just a few.

■ Whole foods don't contain artificial sugars, hydrogenated oils, manufactured fats, colorings, and other undesirables commonly found in processed foods—and in factories, apparently. Does it surprise you to learn that diethyl-glucol, a cheap chemical often used as a thickener and as a substitute for eggs, is a constituent part of antifreeze? Or that ethyl-acetate, found in pineapple ice cream and factory-produced candy and snacks, has been used as an industrial-strength cleaning agent for textiles?

■ Whole foods do contain whole grain complex carbohydrates, whereas their processed counterparts are loaded with simple sugars. Released slowly and steadily into the bloodstream over the course of hours, whole grain complex carbs are the best source of long-lasting energy.

■ Whole foods don't contain sodium-based preservatives. In $\frac{1}{2}$ cup of fresh green beans, you'll get only 3 milligrams of sodium. There are 400 milligrams in the same amount of green beans once they've been canned.

■ Whole foods do contain loads of vitamins, minerals, and other antioxidants needed to defend against the potentially harmful effects of the rogue molecules known as free radicals. Modern food-processing methods and an extended shelf life can strip many natural nutrients from foods.

■ Whole foods do contain water. Many guys don't get enough of that substance as it is. If you're eating more than five servings of fruits and vegetables daily, you're getting a couple of extra cups of fluid for good measure.

■ Whole foods do contain plenty of phytochemicals, which scientists are starting to realize play a profoundly important role in fighting and preventing diseases, particularly cancer. These, like vitamins and minerals, often end up on the cutting room floor when food meets processing machine. For example, anywhere from 50 to 100 percent of the healthy phytonutrients found in extra-virgin olive oil get removed in the bleaching and refining that produces refined safflower oil.

■ Whole foods do contain plenty of fiber, both soluble and insoluble. The former comes mostly from beans and oats; the latter, from fruits, vegetables, and grains. By the time produce has been peeled, cored, cut, shredded, or chopped, a lot of that fiber is gone. Similarly, when wheat is refined, the germ and hull are removed. That eliminates not only most of the fiber but also the protein, B vitamins, vitamin E, lipids, and sterols. For example, enriched wheat bread has 79 percent less fiber per serving than whole-wheat bread.

Many natural foods contain literally thousands of these healthy substances, many of which science is only now beginning to understand. When a lab creates a bar, powder, or other engineered food product that contains protein, carbohydrates, creatine, or whatever, you're missing out on all those unheralded nutrients and components. Also, because engineered foods don't contain a lot of bulk from things like fiber, they don't fill you up very fast. That's great if you're a 16-year-old defensive lineman trying to pack on size for football. Otherwise, it makes it really easy for you to overeat.

The Whole Truth

If whole foods are going to fill your new eating patterns, you need to figure out ways to fit them into your life. After all, when you're in the middle of a workday, nine times out of ten it will be easier to purchase Pop-Tarts from the office vending machine than to retrieve a piece of fresh fruit, or yogurt with granola, or edamame and green tea. That's the whole problem—unless, that is, you plan ahead. With that in mind, try these strategies for fitting whole foods into your fit lifestyle.

"Forage" as little as possible. Each month, set aside an allotment of time to buy the bulk of your food (excluding items that perish weekly or biweekly, like milk and eggs). Compile your list throughout the month, based on the food you reasonably expect to consume. When you go on this monthly shopping spree, you should have two goals: 1) to buy food in a large enough quantity that you won't need more of that food until the next month, and 2) to spend less money by buying in those larger quantities.

Here are some useful tips when shopping.

■ Find a place where you can buy quality meat inexpensively, and buy boned chicken breast, fish fillets, and lean beef in bulk. Your local supermarket may or may not be the best bet. Compare prices there with those at butcher counters and discount clubs. Have these wrapped in portions for the freezer so that you can easily pop them out of the freezer and cook just enough for a meal.

■ Buy fresh vegetables such as spinach, lettuce, carrots, cauliflower, and broccoli.

■ Buy frozen and canned vegetables as well, for those times when you run out of fresh vegetables. Frozen vegetables in particular are nearly as nutritious as their fresh counterparts; plus they will easily keep for an entire month, even considerably longer. Canned vegetables are okay but aren't nearly as healthy as fresh and frozen veggies. As I mentioned, they're also packed in salt. Read labels. Know what you're getting.

■ Buy grains and complex carbs in bulk. Make certain you're well stocked with brown rice, whole-wheat pasta, yams, winter squash, potatoes, and oatmeal. Most grains will keep well over a month without spoilage.

■ Buy fruit. Keep in mind that oranges and apples will keep longer than grapes, peaches, and bananas. Also, buy canned and frozen fruit with no sugar added to keep a month-long supply of fruit on hand while avoiding spoilage. Frozen fruits are great choices for smoothies.

As mentioned, eggs and milk won't keep an entire month. Pick those up at supermarkets, convenience stores, or mini-markets as needed.

Storage after forage. Once you've purchased your food, store it the way you'll use it. Store chicken and beef in the freezer in the quantities in which you'll cook them. Store some meat in individual servings for when you're at home and want a fresh-cooked meal, and store the rest in quantities that can be cooked assembly-line style (see opposite). Freeze servings that you don't plan to cook in the next day or two. Food that will be cooked the next day can be placed in the refrigerator to avoid freezing and thawing, without risking spoilage.

Fresh produce such as apples, bananas, onions, tomatoes, and potatoes can be kept on the counter or in a cupboard until cooked or eaten. Peaches, bananas, and avocados continue to ripen after purchase, so watch them for their point of optimal usage. Overripe bananas can be added to protein shakes.

Fresh broccoli, cabbage, carrots, and cauliflower can be refrigerated until needed. Within a week or so of your shopping trip, prepare and consume the fresh vegetables that are most likely to spoil.

Use assembly-line cooking techniques. Twice a week, set aside a few hours to do the bulk of your cooking. This will reduce overall cooking time, and you won't have to eat food that's been sitting in your refrigerator for six days, as you would if you cooked only one day a week. See "Tool Chest" below for some of the things you need to make this happen.

Break up your food preparation into three cate-gories: proteins, starchy carbs, and fibrous carbs. That way all you need to do is mix and match these three components to create awesome meals on the go.

■ **Prepare your protein.** Protein foods require the most planning. Cook all the chicken breasts, fish, and red meat that you will need for all the "quick-prep" and "on-the-go" meals you'll need until you cook again. These meats should be grilled or baked in the oven. For example: Use any Pyrex cooking dish with a cover. Preheat the oven to 350°F. Season four or five breasts in the pan, cover, and cook for 45 minutes to an hour. Check each breast to make sure it's completely cooked. Make sure to cover and refrigerate any food you don't plan on eating immediately.

Eggs can be hard-cooked and then refrigerated, making them an excellent on-the-go whole-food protein source.

TOOL CHEST

WHAT FOLLOWS ARE A FEW BASIC TOOLS YOU'LL NEED to help you eat the *Power Food* way.

■ A large, reliable refrigerator/freezer. Brand-new quality refrigerators and freezers are surprisingly inexpensive—you can get a good one for under $500. If you're currently using an unreliable, older model, the new one may be more energy efficient, saving you money on your electric bill. A new fridge may also keep you from losing a few hundred dollars' worth of food by avoiding the death of your old model. Separate compartments for fruit and vegetables can provide different temperatures throughout to preserve different types of food for as long as possible.

■ A microwave oven. Nothing can speed the preparation of good nutritious meals more than a microwave oven.

■ A fridge at work. If your workplace doesn't have a refrigerator, get yourself a small portable cooler and some frozen cold packs to keep food and drinks fresh and cold during the day.

■ An abundant supply of durable plastic containers. They'll come in handy for holding individual servings or meals.

■ Pyrex pans. They're the best utensil for baking your delicious, healthy meals.

■ **Prepare your complex carbs.** Prepare a large quantity of rice, baked potatoes, and sweet potatoes. Starchy carbs like winter squash and potatoes are good sources of complex carbohydrates, as are yams, brown rice, and oatmeal. They provide slow-burning energy so that fewer calories will take you farther during the day. Refrigerate your leftovers.

■ **Cook a variety of vegetables.** Vegetables such as spinach, cauliflower, and broccoli can be pre-cooked, too. Steaming is one of the most healthful ways of cooking, but boil sulfur-containing cruciferous veggies like cauliflower and broccoli with the lid off. Boiling costs you a few more nutrients, but it will make the sulfur-containing vegetables taste much better. Cook vegetables individually, or mix them together, depending on your preference. Refrigerate your leftovers.

If you can't cook, now is as good a time as any time to start learning. You don't have to be Wolfgang Puck to cook good food, and the benefits to learning go beyond all the money you'll save eating out less. In a study done at Tufts University, subjects who dined out were significantly fatter than those who cooked and ate at home. Restaurants are much less concerned about your health than you are; hence the insanely large portions in restaurants, the use of fattening sauces, and so on.

Don't be intimidated by the kitchen. If you start slowly and master a few quick and healthy dishes, you'll be amazed at how quickly you'll progress from there. For starters, try this: Slice up chicken breasts or defrost some uncooked shrimp; dice onions, peppers, mushrooms, and zucchini; chop some garlic. Sauté the garlic in olive oil until lightly browned in a frying pan or wok and throw everything else in with teriyaki sauce; throw it over some Uncle Ben's minute brown rice.

Congrats. You just cooked your first *Power Food* dish.

This Is Your Lifestyle

Success is more than just procuring, preparing, and storing food in an efficient manner, although that will help you succeed. As you take the lessons learned in *Power Food* out into the real world, you need to make other aspects of your life mesh with your diet:

Reduce your stress. As advice goes, "Reduce your stress" sounds pretty useless. Who doesn't want anxiety excised from their life? No one I know. You must realize that, if you're stressed, taking the time to eat right may be a lot harder. First of all, you won't be thinking about your diet when you're worried about work, your relationship, or anything else. And second, stress naturally leads us to those "comfort" foods.

Luckily, if you start eating right, food itself can help that stress disappear, making it easier to eat better, and so on.

You'll be keeping your brain cells well nourished; promoting the secretion of serotonin, the neurotransmitter responsible for maintaining an elevated mood state; and decreasing your chances of suffering from depression. Healthy fats from fish, flaxseed, olives and olive oil, avocados, nuts, and mixtures of carbohydrate and protein-containing meals all work together to help you cope with stress.

Focus on rest and recovery. Rest and recovery are vastly underappreciated and a crucial part of a healthy lifestyle. Again, when you're rested and feeling good, you'll be more likely to stick with your health plan. Sleep at least 8 hours a night.

Get regular dental checkups, and see your physician when you are ill. No matter what your food goal, this is a good idea. If you're young and healthy, you may not see a doctor or dentist regularly. If you don't and you're within shouting distance of 30—on either side—it's time to start. Even though the historical recommendation to have annual physical exams is still commonly a popular notion, the American College of Physicians, the American Medical Association, the U.S. Preventive Services Task Force (USPSTF), and the U.S. Public Health Service have all agreed that routine annual checkups for healthy adults should be abandoned in favor of a more selective approach to preventing and detecting health problems.

In other words, just showing up at the doctor's office with no specific goal in mind is not very effective health care. On the other hand, making sure that you get to the doctor when you don't feel up to snuff may make a huge difference in your health; scheduling screenings for cholesterol, colon, and prostate cancer may save your life. These interventions can help your physician identify unknown conditions before they become serious.

If you are overhauling your diet, it is also a great time to measure your blood pressure, resting heart rate, and other bodily indicators. Track these numbers over time, just as you might track how much you weigh or can bench. Compare the results from one checkup to the next. Take note of large shifts between checkups. Look for trends, like a number moving in one direction for three consecutive tests or more. This is one of the best preventative health measures a guy can undertake.

An initial blood workup is particularly good for tracking cholesterol, which I've discussed in several chapters. Your doctor should test you for what's called a lipid profile, which measures LDL ("bad") cholesterol, HDL ("good") cholesterol, and triglycerides, the fats circulating in your blood. You want HDL to be high, and your LDL, total cholesterol, and triglycerides to be low.

According to the Academy of General Dentistry, regardless of your age, you should see your dentist twice a year at 6-month intervals. Dental health is important for body health. A chronic low-grade infection like gum disease can have a shockingly big impact on the rest of your body, as discussed in chapter 6. Bacteria can enter the bloodstream through microscopic lacerations and promote blood clots. Cavities, abscesses, and other dental infections can also increase the risk of suffering a cardiovascular-related death. Mouth tissues may also reflect symptoms of other problems. Many diseases can be diagnosed in their early stages through an oral examination.

Don't Go to Extremes or Expect Immediate Results

Whatever your goal, adjust your calorie consumption gradually and moderately. Depending on your goal, you shouldn't be increasing or decreasing your calorie consumption by more than 20 percent at a time.

Another thing: No one expects you to eat every single item in every single meal plan in this book in the exact order and amounts. For some of you, that's a recipe for failure. As long as you're working out and eating better, you'll meet your goals eventually. The closer you follow the meal plans, the more progress you'll make. But if you eat only half of the things you're supposed to eat, you haven't failed. On the contrary—you'll be much better off than when you started. Will you progress as fast as the guy who follows the program lock, stock, and barrel? Of course not. But you'll be headed in the right direction.

In the same way, your diet won't transform you completely overnight (although you'll be surprised by how rapidly good stuff starts happening). You're not going to be a grouch on Tuesday and then have a disposition like Mr. Rogers on Wednesday, all because of what you ate the night before. Nor would you want to. As your blood sugar becomes less volatile, though, you'll be much less likely to fly off the handle in response to the stresses of everyday life.

The same thing goes with the aesthetics of your body. That spare tire around your waist won't become a washboard overnight. It's an imperfect process. After, say, 6 weeks of trying to put on size, take a gut check, literally. Most calories you add in search of size are absorbed as fuel for workouts and muscle growth. If your build is slight, if you have a slower-than-normal metabolism, or if you've been slacking off a bit in the gym, you may be witnessing gains where you don't want them: around the waist, where men are genetically predisposed to store fat. It's not a big deal; your body has entered an anabolic (growth) phase, and you're almost guaranteed to gain a bit of fat along with that new muscle. If you're uncomfortable with your belt-tightening, however, try pulling back the reins on your eating a bit. For whatever reason, maybe you're one of those guys who need to add only 250 or 300 calories a day to gain size, rather than 500.

THE LAST WORD ON ALCOHOL

WE DON'T WANT TO LET YOU GO BEFORE ONE LAST CALL where alcohol is concerned. If you don't drink, skip this. If you drink even occasionally, though, the more you know about alcohol and its effects on the body, the better off you'll be. It's no coincidence that ethanol, the intoxicating agent in booze, is also used in rocket fuel. Alcohol can blow up your waistline and your life if you don't respect its potency.

Low doses of alcohol give you a buzz that has earned a drink like beer the nickname "liquid courage." Tension dissipates, inhibitions drop, and your motor reflexes begin to slow as well. The first time you get down from your bar stool to use the men's room, you may feel a bit uncoordinated. Drink a few more, and your speech will slur, you may become drowsy, and your personality may change palpably. Keep right on drinking, and you eventually may find yourself vomiting en route to losing consciousness.

The rate at which these things happen is highly individual and circumstance-specific, depending on how big you are, how fast you drink, whether you're mixing drinks, how much food is in your stomach, and a whole host of other factors. In the end, what it boils down to is the concentration of alcohol in your blood.

When consumed in small amounts daily, alcohol seems to have some beneficial health effects on some people. For example, alcohol seems to protect against heart disease, probably by raising HDL ("good") cholesterol. Wine appears to offer a double whammy because the grapes from which it is made contain powerful antioxidants like resveratrol, which also lowers levels of LDL ("bad") cholesterol. It also contains saponins, plant compounds that attach themselves to cholesterol molecules, preventing their absorption. Red wines in particular contain these phytonutrients in large quantities. (Much of the research has studied wine, but scientists are starting to compile similar results for beer and distilled spirits.)

Although alcohol's effect on the heart grabs most of the headlines, a recent study that spanned 10 years found that moderate drinking (one drink per day in this case) may substantially reduce the risk of getting diabetes. The same researchers found that heavy drinking has the opposite effect, increasing susceptibility to diabetes.

The benefits of moderate drinking apply more to middle-aged men than to the fake-ID crowd, if only because cardiovascular health becomes more of an issue as you age. Con-

Learn How to Cheat Healthfully

Not being a perfectionist means cheating once in a while, too. Physically and psychologically, you need an occasional day to rest from the rigors of dieting. Loosening the reins on a strict diet now and then can actually help you stay on track in the long run.

Then there are the holidays, which for many guys amounts to a month-and-a-half-long cheating session. It's easy to do what's convenient and then repent with resolution come New Year's Day. Part of what turns Thanksgiving and Christmas into a

versely, the risk of alcohol contributing to an accident-related injury, which is the greatest risk to drinkers under the age of 30, decreases over time.

As of yet, though, the evidence isn't compelling or uniform enough to recommend that you include alcohol in your diet expressly for health reasons. What it does mean is that if you enjoy a glass or two of wine with dinner, or unwind with an occasional beer after work, you're probably enjoying a nice little health windfall as well.

One reason that praise for alcohol is always somewhat equivocal is that negative effects can arise even from moderate alcohol consumption. For starters, alcohol contains 7 calories per gram. A 5-ounce glass of wine gives you around 100 calories, and "dessert" wines pack about 220 because of their higher sugar and alcohol content. A 12-ounce bottle of beer is good for 150 to 200 calories, and even "light" and low-carb alternatives contain 100 or so. Distilled spirits vary by alcohol content and run from 64 (80 proof) to 82 calories (100 proof) *per ounce*. Add mixers, and the calories rise. Two piña coladas are good for 1,052 calories. Ouch.

And then there's the pesky issue of alcohol abuse. Long-term heavy drinking can lead to a litany of health problems, including addiction; brain damage, including shrinkage; neurological damage; blood-clotting abnormalities; cirrhosis and liver failure; vitamin deficiencies, particularly of vitamin B_1 (thiamine); heightened cancer risk; and every malady associated with obesity, as drinking rivers of alcohol will likely make you really fat. (Unless all you do is drink, rather than eat: That's the classic gaunt, malnourished look of an alcoholic.)

For men, moderate drinking means two alcoholic beverages or fewer per day. (A drink equals 5 ounces of wine, a 12-ounce beer, or 1.5 ounces of distilled spirits, such as gin, rum, or vodka.) That doesn't mean that you can do without it all week, throw back eight beers on Sunday, and average it all out. In fact, an Australian study found that drinking more than nine drinks just one day a week doubled the risk of heart attacks in men. And the symptoms of a hangover—headache, nausea, diarrhea, fatigue, dehydration, and body aches—should suggest to you that binge drinking isn't having a friendly impact on your insides.

Look for some guidance from Uncle Sam on alcohol in January 2005. That's when the new U.S. Dietary Guidelines will be finalized after a thorough review of the scientific findings on alcohol.

waistline wipeout is the tendency to replace the good stuff you normally eat and drink with less healthy alternatives. One day you're reaching for a V8 to wash down celery sticks covered with all-natural peanut butter, and the next moment your hand is diving furtively into a canister of caramel popcorn in the office kitchen.

Part of avoiding those pitfalls, or getting back on track once they've occurred, is reversing the bad substitutions. Try some or all of these more healthful choices.

- Drop the doughnuts and eat a whole-wheat English muffin smeared with peanut butter and jelly.
- Walk past the holiday cookies and grab a handful of peanuts.
- Say no to the mixed drinks and have fruit juice or a diet cola.
- Replace French fries with baked sweet-potato fries.
- Have oranges instead of candy.

If you know you're going to eat too much over the holidays, another option is to use that time to gain muscle. Let's face it: For many guys, good intentions notwithstanding, there's little chance of you reining in your hunger during that time. Come Christmas, you may fit better in a Santa Claus suit than you do in your work suits. Because you're going to eat like a horse over the holidays anyway, consider exploiting it. Prodigious eating can be more than a road to ruin; it can also be a way to gain size if you're so lacking. Just make sure that along with the extra food, you get in a few extra workout sessions.

Speaking of roads to ruin, travel is another sinkhole that can swallow even the most carefully planned diets. Hitting the road—or, especially, going airborne—can seriously hinder your progress. No longer should your diet be at the mercy of the travel industry. Taking snacks along is a great starting

place. Airline security can be strict, but most airports still allow packaged food through customs. So consider packing protein bars, granola, or even bags of nuts and dried fruit for emergency snacking.

In the air, you might want something a little healthier than the mystery food they're serving for lunch. Carriers that do serve meals will have special food for vegans and passengers with high cholesterol or other dietary needs. Most people are aware of this service, yet fewer than 2 percent of airline meals are special-ordered. Airlines typically require only 24 hours advance notice for this service. Make a special-meal request when you book your flight. You can also take lunch into your own hands and pick up a turkey sandwich on whole wheat to take on board. (This is especially smart when you're flying a cheapie airline that doesn't serve meals. You'll be the envy of your seatmates.)

At your destination, hit a market and stock your hotel fridge. When abroad, be forewarned: The quality of the food and water isn't always up to par with the United States. Canned foods and bottled water are usually your safest bets. Avoid uncooked food, such as raw fruits and vegetables, and instead stick to cooked veggies and meats. Always ask for things well done and served either very hot or very cold.

Remember, too, that drinking plenty of water is one of the best ways to keep your body from losing its way on a trip. Airplane air is as dry as a desert, so drink even more water than you normally would. Unless you positively need a stiff Jack-and-Coke to endure flying, avoid the ultra-dehydrating in-flight alcohol consumption.

The Checkout Checklist

Before I let you go, let's run through a final checklist, shall we? No matter what else you implement from what you read in *Power Food,* the following eight steps will allow you to build muscle, gain energy, and lose fat. These are all keepers.

1. **Eat enough calories.** The total number of calories you eat, as opposed to the type of calories you eat, is by far the most important consideration in weight management and general health. The composition of your diet matters, too, but eating fewer calories than you expend during the day is the absolute key to losing fat weight. For that reason, the most effective weight-loss programs combine a moderate reduction in calories with regular physical activity. In a nutshell, the key to fat loss is moving a whole lot more and eating a little bit less.

   If you've ever eaten a *whole* lot less—say, fewer than 1,200 calories a day—you probably remember feeling lousy. That kind of dieting slows down your metabolism—something you want to avoid at all costs. As you should know by now, your body can still function on relatively few calories, but you won't perform at peak levels. To stay healthy, your body requires a minimum of 1,500 to 1,600 calories a day. If you try to exercise on fewer than that, you won't be able to work out at a high enough intensity for long enough to gain the weight-control or muscle-building benefits of exercise. Over time, your body will trade muscle for fat. As a result, your metabolic rate will slow even more, and no matter how much you diet, you won't lose fat.

   Remember, it takes muscle to burn fat. You need to eat enough calories to fuel your strength and cardio workouts, as well as the process of muscle maintenance, repair, and growth. When you don't, your body recruits protein as an energy fuel, preventing it from doing its primary job.

2. **Eat enough protein.** Not only is protein required for the maintenance, replacement, and growth of your body's tissues, it's also used to make the hormones that regulate your metabolism, maintain water balance, protect against disease, transport nutrients in and out of cells, carry oxygen, and regulate blood clotting. There's no getting around it: If you don't eat enough protein, you simply won't achieve your goals (unless your goals are to become fat and weak).

   Your protein consumption should be roughly 0.8 gram per pound of body weight per day. If you don't eat animal-based foods (i.e., if you're a vegan), add 10 percent to this amount, since plant-based proteins tend to lack the full array of amino acids.

3. **Eat enough carbohydrates.** Don't be misled by the fad diets that are all the rage now. Carbohydrate is the energy that fuels strength training, and if you want to train hard and long, you're going to need plenty of that fuel. Don't get so focused on carbs that you shortchange protein and healthy fats, but make sure to eat the recommended amounts. When you combine intense cardio work with a good strength-training program, your body needs 2.0 to 2.3 grams of carbohydrate per pound of body weight per day.

4. **Don't have a fat phobia.** One of the points I've drilled home is that the so-called essential fats—linoleic and linolenic acid—aren't made by the body in sufficient amounts. You must acquire them from food. Essential fats are required for the maintenance of cell membranes, healthy arteries, and nerves; the lubrication and protection of joints; healthy skin; the absorption of fat-soluble nutrients; and the breakdown and metabolism of cholesterol.

   The fat in your body not only protects your organs but also provides exercise fuel. In fact, it's your body's preferred fuel during aerobic exercise lasting longer than 20 minutes. During strength training, however, your body prefers to burn carbohydrate for energy, since that process doesn't require oxygen. When you're lifting a weight for a set, oxygen isn't available to the muscle rapidly enough to use fat as a fuel source.

That's not to say that resistance training won't help you burn fat. On the contrary: One of the advantages of combining strength training and aerobic exercise is that the better trained you become, the more efficient your body becomes at burning fat as fuel. And the more fat you can break down and burn, the more defined you'll look.

You now know that the type of fat in your diet influences both your blood cholesterol levels and your risk of developing heart disease and cancer, so choose the heart-healthy monounsaturated fats and omega-3 fats such as high-fat fish and shellfish; olive, peanut, and canola oils; avocados; nuts; and seeds as your main sources. Next in importance come polyunsaturated fats from all other vegetable sources. Finally, permit very limited amounts of saturated and hydrogenated (trans) fats, whether from animal sources (meats, butter, and milk) or plant-based sources (baked goods, crackers, chips, and other "convenience" foods).

Saturated and trans fats should be avoided for the most part, regardless of your body weight. Even if you're skinny and just happen to be interested in your health, it's not reasonable to eat large amounts of saturated fat. From a weight-loss perspective, it doesn't make any difference whether it's olive oil or animal lard—it still contains 9 calories per gram, and a fat is a fat is a fat where calories are concerned. From a health perspective, though, it makes a huge difference. There's no reason to single out saturated fat for attack if you're interested exclusively in losing weight, but if you're interested in losing weight and doing it in a healthy way, you certainly want to limit saturated fat.

Once you've taken in all the protein and carbohydrates you need, the remainder of your calories should come from fat. You haven't heard us talk much about percentages for these macronutrients, and with good reason. They're way overrated. Your percentages can look wonderful on paper, but if you're not eating enough calories, you're not giving your body what it needs. What's important is getting enough protein to build muscle and enough carbohydrate to fuel your workouts, as well as enough fat to provide your essential fatty acids and absorb your fat-soluble vitamins.

5. **Drink plenty of fluids.** You encountered water as a theme in every chapter of *Power Food*. That's because water does so many good things for your body. It flushes out toxins, reduces the risk of kidney stones, allows your brain to think clearly, helps keep heart attacks and strokes away, helps build muscle, and even assists with fat loss—fluids help you feel full, allowing to control your appetite better.

If those benefits aren't sexy enough for you, consider that water also helps you get better erections by increasing blood flow everywhere, including your penis.

As I've discussed, if the human body were a consumer product, its natural thirst mechanism would have prompted a factory recall long ago. By the time your body tells your brain to tell you to drink, it's already parched. That's why you need to drink *before* you become thirsty. Even mild dehydration will limit your mental and physical performance. If it becomes chronic, dehydration can have health consequences ranging from troublesome to dire.

Drink 1 quart (4 cups) of fluid for every 1,000 calories of food you eat, and a minimum of 9 cups of water daily. That doesn't include the extra fluid you need for exercise. Being well hydrated keeps your body's circulatory system functioning properly, transporting oxygen- and nutrient-rich blood to the working muscles while at the same time helping remove lactic acid accumulation more efficiently, which means faster recovery and better growth. So 2 hours before you exercise, drink at least 2 cups of water or sports drink, and then drink 4 to 8 ounces of cool liquid every 15 to 20 minutes during the session. Afterward, drink at least 2 to 3 cups of fluid for every pound of body weight you just lost.

Because alcoholic beverages can have a dehydrating effect, don't count these as part of your day's drinking. In fact, occasionally replace that glass of wine with a cup of water instead. If you drink more than three caffeinated beverages daily, follow the same guidelines. Otherwise, feel free to count your cup of java toward your total fluid intake. You also need more fluid when it's hot, when humidity is unusually high or low, and when you're at high altitudes, including air travel.

6. **Get your timing right.** Nutritionists have known for some time now that eating small meals frequently promotes fat burning, whereas infrequent feeding frenzies favor fat storage. The same strategy also helps you build and preserve muscle, since your body spends more of its day in an anabolic state. That may explain the results of a study of boxers performed at Nagoya University in Japan. When following a low-calorie diet, the boxers sacrificed less muscle when their meals were spread among six meals rather than two.

Ideally, you should eat five or six times a day—more if your daily caloric needs exceed 3,000. Also, gradually taper the size of your meals during the day so that the smaller ones come later.

Research has increasingly shown us the importance of timing not only your meals but also your nutrients. Even something as seemingly innocuous as the protein you consume before bed can be tweaked to increase protein synthesis and muscle building. Casein, found abundantly in cottage cheese and yogurt, is a "slow-release" protein, making it great for distribution over the course of what amounts to an 8-hour fast. Most of the aminos in whey are discharged quickly, which makes them less effective overnight, but great immediately after lifting weights, when your body can make good use a sudden influx.

The "windows" before and after you exercise are particularly critical. Roughly 2 hours before working out, eat a small meal containing both carbohydrates and protein, along with a bit of fat. This combination will help reduce the damage hard exercise does to your muscle tissue. Some well-trained strength athletes also have 100 to 200 milligrams of caffeine (equal to 1 cup of coffee or two cans of soda) before exercise to help promote fat burning and decrease their perception of exercise intensity. Whether you want to go there is up to you.

To promote muscle building and glycogen replenishment, consume at least 10 grams of carbohydrate and 20 grams of protein immediately after exercising. Wait too long and you significantly reduce your body's ability to store glycogen.

After that initial post-workout feeding, eat again within 2 hours. If it's impractical to eat a meal the moment you finish that last rep, consider using supplements such as a combined carb-protein drink and sports bars (sports bars are my last resort). Don't forget the water.

7. **Supplement when necessary.** In addition to filling the void immediately after training, supplements can support health and performance more generally. No one size fits all when it comes to taking supplements—it depends on what your goals are, among other things. See individual chapters for recommendations, and refer to "Supplement Dollars and Sense" on page 412 for

(continued on page 415)

SUPPLEMENT DOLLARS AND SENSE

THE SUPPLEMENT INDUSTRY'S RESEARCH AND DEVELOPMENT LABS have developed some useful products in recent years, but as the pace of new-product introductions has accelerated, the amount of money you can spend on supplements has increased, too. In fact, heading off to your local health food store and buying a representative sample of what you see advertised in fitness magazines could quickly make your monthly supplement investment resemble a car payment.

Unless you just won the lottery, this no doubt presents a dilemma. However, by doing your homework and applying some common sense and logic to your supplement strategy, you can almost always either save money or get more bang from the same buck.

Prioritize

Once you've established a realistic monthly budget for supplements, the first step is to sort through the myriad products available to identify those best suited to meet your needs. If your goal is to add some muscle to your frame gradually, A-list supplements should be creatine, glutamine, protein powder, or branched-chain amino acids; a sports drink for during your workout; and an exercise recovery drink for after your workout.

If your goal is to eat more frequently and conveniently, consider adding a daily high-calorie meal-replacement shake or two to the mix. As their name suggests, meal replacements are designed to provide a nutritionally complete substitute for meals, so if you use them for that purpose—rather than as a source of extra calories and protein for weight gain—you're spending less than you would otherwise on food. Don't regularly replace more than one meal each day with these products. You'll be missing out on too many important nutrients.

For those whose primary interest is losing weight, store shelves spill over with so-called magic pills, most of which are marketed as some variation of the catch-all phrase "fat burner." Rather than going for a quick fix, however, give priority to supplements that support the changes in body composition (i.e., more muscle, less fat) that you're trying to achieve with your diet and workouts. A good place to start is with branched-chain amino acids, which not only have beneficial effects on muscle building and preservation but also appear to optimize fat loss under calorie-restricted conditions.

Regardless of your goal, give priority to supplements that would be difficult to reproduce from natural sources. For example, a banana gives you 33 grams of carbohydrate, but you'd have to ingest 2.2 pounds of red meat to get the 5 grams of creatine found in 1 tablespoon of a typical powder. If you can't afford supplements, you certainly can't afford to buy steak every night, and that amount of red meat would give you unhealthy doses of saturated fat and cholesterol as well.

The one supplement that everyone should take is a good multivitamin/mineral that includes the recommended daily allowance (RDA) of chromium. In contrast to supplements that try to "blitz" your body into a growth state, a multivitamin/mineral amounts to a preventive defense, ensuring that any deficiencies resulting from your diet or training are covered.

Compare Prices and Avoid Overlap

Armed with a budget and your supplement wish list, you can start doing the legwork. Take the time to compare prices and learn how to read labels, so you know what you're comparing. One benefit of understanding labels is the ability to identify redundancies—not only identical ingredients, but similar ones. If you're already using a protein powder, for example, you can probably do without one of their constituent parts, branched-chain amino acids.

Also, educate yourself about the amounts of supplements that your body can actually use. An average-size guy doesn't have much use for more than 50 grams of protein at a time, so it doesn't make sense to pay extra for powders supplying more than that in a single serving. That tendency to load supplements with megadoses of nutrients also means that if your build is smaller than average or if you simply need to stretch your supplement dollar during a given month, you can usually reduce the recommended dose as necessary.

Another way to save money is by purchasing products that manage to kill two or more birds with one stone. Be wary of products that take a "kitchen sink" approach to supplementation, focusing instead on those that combine elements more selectively.

Retail vs. Mail Order

The ability to browse through a store and compare labels is one of the advantages of shopping for supplements at retail outlets, which range from national chains to independently owned and operated stores. Shopping retail also allows you to enlist the help of a salesperson, although the knowledge of such individuals can range from extensive to nonexistent. (Salespeople can also have an inherent bias, often toward the house brand.) Convenience is another advantage of retail: If you run out of a particular supplement, you can replace it almost immediately.

Conventional wisdom holds that shopping retail is more expensive than mail order, but don't assume that to be the case. Instead, arrive at your own conclusions by comparing a series of retail prices for one item with mail-order prices for the same product. If you prefer buying retail, you can save money there as well through special offers such as the GNC Gold Card.

(continued)

SUPPLEMENT DOLLARS AND SENSE (CONT.)

In contrast to retailers, distributors and wholesalers typically fulfill orders through the mail rather than over a store counter. These organizations offer products from numerous manufacturers through a variety a channels, including catalogs, magazine ads, and, increasingly, the Internet. Because mail-order firms typically have lower overhead costs than retail establishments, in theory they can accept lower profit margins on sales. More often than not, this translates into lower prices for consumers.

Of course, mail-order firms can also charge an identical or even higher price than a retailer for a given product and simply enjoy a higher margin. Either way, it pays to compare prices. When weighing the pros and cons of mail order, also factor additional costs such as shipping and handling into your overall price. Some distributors offer free delivery via Federal Express.

Regardless of where you buy your supplements, another great way to save money is to hook up with some like-minded friends and buy your supplements as a group. Not only can you then purchase the largest sizes available, which usually offer the best value, but you can also divide the contents among group members if necessary. Some manufacturers even offer group discounts.

Last, be careful with Internet and mail-order purchases. Check quality control on the products. Don't buy something that comes in from outside the United States. Inquire about good manufacturing processes and possibilities of contamination.

Supplement Strategies

- Set a realistic monthly budget.
- Determine the goals you have for your body's health and aesthetics, and identify those supplements that can best help you achieve them.
- Learn to read labels so you know what you're buying and can avoid redundancies.
- Go to www.consumerlab.com to see what they say about the quality of the various brands and the reliability of the product claims.
- Assuming you need them, give priority to supplements like creatine that would be difficult to reproduce from natural food sources.
- Plan your purchases in advance.
- Seek the best deal on the supplements you want. Compare retail prices with mail order.
- Purchase in bulk amounts whenever possible, hooking up with friends to buy as a group if necessary.
- Use the most efficient serving size. If you're smaller than average, for example, you can probably save money by reducing your serving size accordingly.
- Use what you buy. If you don't like the way something tastes, mix it with different fruits or juices until you come up with a combination that you find palatable.

(continued from page 411)

advice on cost-effective ways to acquire what you need.

8. **Practice patience.** Good things come to those who wait. Although you'll feel better and see at least some visible changes quickly, big changes come every 6 to 12 weeks, depending on what your diet was like to begin with. (As I've said before, keep a log along the way. The best way to change old habits into new ones is to write things down.) Patience should come from the knowledge that this is the last major diet change you'll ever make. You'll be eating right for the rest of your healthy and fit life.

Go Forth and Conquer

As you prepare to move forward, I recommend two additional strategies for getting yourself on the right track. First, make sure you've read all (or at least most) of *Power Food*. The subjects covered have been as complex at times as they are far-reaching, and you'll get the most out of it if you've read it all. That way, you'll see the big picture instead of just a few snapshots. Of course, you'll need to revisit the book periodically. It contains a lot of information, and getting the most out of it will require repeat visits.

Second, now that you've absorbed all this information, think even harder than you did initially about what you *really* want to get out of it. No

doubt, one or more of the chapter-heading benefits grabbed your attention initially, but whether you want to get bigger or smaller, healthier or more energetic, you're setting a unique course for individual change and improvement. In doing so, you'll be developing the personal mindset that you can control your own destiny.

What can sound nutrition give you in addition to everything I've talked about thus far in *Power Food*? Only you can know that for sure, but I can give you some ideas. For some guys, the discipline it brings to one part of life spills over into all other aspects. For many, healthy eating creates or enhances self-esteem. Others use it as a form of therapy to turn their lives around after major trauma or setback, whether personal or professional.

Once those changes have taken hold, you won't think in terms of diets anymore. You'll think, "I've made these changes to the way I eat, and these are sustainable changes." In the end, that's what it's all about. The guy who's lost 1,000 pounds over 10 years—losing, gaining, losing, gaining, losing—isn't the winner here. It's the guy who loses 20 or 30 once, for good.

We hope this has provided some insight into what you can expect from nutrition and *Power Food*. Whatever brought you to this book, I can assure you that nutrition can be a force for positive change in your own life.

So put it down and get started!

Appendix

SERVING SIZES

Food Groups	Description	Serving Size
BEANS, LEGUMES		
	Aduki, black, garbanzo, navy, pinto, white, etc., cooked	$^1/_2$ cup
BREADS, CEREALS, STARCH VEGETABLES		
	Cereals, cooked	$^1/_2$ cup
	Corn bread	$1^1/_2$-inch square
	Corn, cooked	$^1/_2$ cup
	Corn on the cob, large	$^1/_2$ cob
	Kashi cereal	1 cup
	Matzoh	$^3/_4$ oz
	Pasta, couscous, cooked	$^1/_3$ cup
	Peas, green	$^1/_2$ cup
	Plantain	$^1/_2$ cup
	Popcorn, popped	3 cups
	Potato , baked with skin	1 small

Food Groups	Description	Serving Size
	Potato, medium, boiled or mashed	$\frac{1}{2}$ or $\frac{1}{2}$ cup
	Pretzels	$\frac{3}{4}$ oz
	Rice, brown (preferable) or white, cooked	$\frac{1}{3}$ cup
	Rice cakes (4" diameter)	2
	Shredded Wheat	$\frac{1}{2}$ cup
	Squash, winter (acorn, butternut, pumpkin)	1 cup
	Tortilla chips, baked	15–20
	Tortilla, corn or flour (6" diameter)	1
	Whole-grain bread	1 slice or 1 oz
	Whole-grain bun, bagel, English muffin or pita	$\frac{1}{2}$
	Whole-grain pancake or waffle (4" diameter)	1
	Whole-wheat crackers	2–5
	Yam, sweet potato, plain	$\frac{1}{2}$ cup
EGGS		
	Whole	1 large
FAT-FREE AND LOWFAT DAIRY (0–1% FAT)		
	Buttermilk	8 oz (1 cup)
	Cheese	1 oz
	Cottage cheese	$\frac{1}{2}$ cup
	Milk (counts toward total fluid intake)	8 oz (1 cup)
	Yogurt, plain or with no-calorie sweetener	$\frac{2}{3}$ cup
FISH AND SEAFOOD		
	Anchovy, black cod, clams, cod, crab, flounder, halibut, herring, lobster, mackerel, oysters, rockfish, sablefish, salmon, sardines, scallops, shrimp, trout, tuna	1 oz.
FLUIDS		
Wine	Red wine may have some health benefits over white wine	4 oz.
Other	Water, non-caloric beverages	8 oz. (1 cup)
FRUITS		
Berries	Blackberries, blueberries	$\frac{3}{4}$ cup
	Raspberries	1 cup
	Strawberries	$1\frac{1}{4}$ cup whole berries

Food Groups	Description	Serving Size
Citrus	Grapefruit	$1/2$ large or $3/4$ cup sections
	Orange, lemon, lime	1 small
Juice	Apple juice/cider	$1/2$ cup
	Apricot nectar	$1/2$ cup
	Cranberry juice cocktail, reduced-calorie	1 cup
	Fruit juice blends, 100% juice	$1/3$ cup
	Grape	$1/3$ cup
	Grapefruit, orange, pineapple	$1/2$ cup
	Prune	$1/3$ cup
	Tomato	$1/2$ cup
	V8	$1/2$ cup
Others	Apple	1 small
	Applesauce	$1/2$ cup
	Apples, dried	4 rings
	Apricots, canned	$1/2$ cup
	Apricots, dried	8 halves
	Apricots, fresh	4 whole
	Bananas	1 small
	Cantaloupe	$1/3$ small melon or 1 cup cubes
	Cherries, sweet, fresh	12
	Dates	3
	Figs, dried	$1 1/2$
	Figs, fresh	2 medium
	Grapes	17 small
	Honeydew melon	1 slice or 1 cup cubes
	Kiwis	1
	Mangos	$1/2$ small or $1/2$ cup
	Nectarines	1 small
	Oranges	1 small
	Papayas	$1/2$ or 1 cup cubes
	Peaches	1 medium
	Peaches, canned	$1/2$ cup
	Pears	1 medium

Food Groups	Description	Serving Size
	Pears, canned	$\frac{1}{2}$ cup
	Pineapple, canned	$\frac{1}{2}$ cup
	Pineapple, fresh	$\frac{3}{4}$ cup
	Plums	2 small
	Plums, dried (prunes)	3
	Raisins	2 Tbsp
	Tangerines	2 small
	Watermelon	1 slice or $1\frac{1}{4}$ cups cubed

OILS AND FATS

Food Groups	Description	Serving Size
Oils	Olive, sesame, canola, peanut, corn, safflower, soybean	1 tsp
Fats	Almonds, cashews	6 nuts
	Avocado, medium	2 Tbsp ($\frac{1}{8}$ cup)
	Black olives	8 large
	Cream cheese, reduced-fat	$1\frac{1}{2}$ Tbsp
	Cream cheese, regular	1 Tbsp
	Cream, half-and-half	2 Tbsp
	Green stuffed olives	10 large
	Kalamata olives	4
	Mayonnaise, soy-based, reduced-fat	1 Tbsp
	Mayonnaise, soy-based, regular	1 tsp
	Mixed nuts (50% peanuts)	6 nuts
	Peanut, almond, cashew butter	$\frac{1}{2}$ Tbsp
	Peanuts	10 nuts
	Pecans	4 halves
	Pumpkin, sesame, or sunflower seeds	1 Tbsp
	Salad dressing, reduced-fat	2 Tbsp
	Salad dressing, regular	1 Tbsp
	Sour cream, reduced-fat	3 Tbsp
	Sour cream, regular	2 Tbsp
	Tahini or sesame paste	2 tsp
	Walnuts	4 halves

Food Groups	Description	Serving Size
POULTRY AND LEAN MEATS		
	Beef: USDA Select or Choice grades trimmed of fat, including: round, sirloin, flank steak, tenderloin, roast (rib, chuck, rump), steak (T-bone, porterhouse, cubed), ground round	1 oz.
	Game: pheasant, venison, buffalo, ostrich, rabbit	1 oz.
	Lamb: roast, chop, or leg	1 oz.
	Pork: Canadian bacon; canned, cured, or boiled ham; center loin chop; fresh ham; tenderloin	1 oz.
	Skinless, chicken, turkey, duck, goose (well-drained of fat)	1 oz.
	Veal: lean chop, roast	1 oz.
SOY		
	Beans, cooked	$^1/_2$ cup
	Edamame, cooked in shell	$^1/_2$ cup
	Soy milk	1 cup
	Soy nuts	1 oz or $^1/_4$ cup
	Tempeh	$^1/_4$ cup
	Tofu	4 oz or $^1/_2$ cup
SUPPLEMENTS		
	Ground flaxseed	$1^1/_2$ Tbsp
	Vitamin E, natural d-alpha tocopherol	400–800 IU
	Whey, isolated protein	7 grams
VEGETABLES (NON-STARCHY)		
Allium family	Onions, garlic, shallots, chives	1 cup raw or $^1/_2$ cup cooked
Brassica family	Broccoli, cauliflower, cabbage, Chinese cabbage, Brussels sprouts	1 cup raw or $^1/_2$ cup cooked
Carotenoid	Carrots, dark green leafy, tomatoes, yellow squash, peppers	1 cup raw or $^1/_2$ cup cooked

Selected Bibliography

Chapter 2

Benkelfat, C., M. A. Ellenbogen, P. Dean, R. M. Palmour, and S. Young. "Mood-lowering Effect of Tryptophan Depletion." *Archives of General Psychiatry* 51 (1994):687–97.

Blumenthal, et al. (eds.) Herbal Medicine. Expanded Commission E Monographs, American Botanical Council, 2000.

Bucci, L. "Selected herbals and human exercise performance." *American Journal of Clinical Nutrition* 72(2suppl) (2000): 624S–36S.

Christensen, L., K. Krietsch, B. White, and B. Stagner. "Impact of a Dietary Change on Emotional Distress." *Journal of Abnormal Psychology* 94, no.4 (1985):565–79.

Colantuoni, C., et al. "Evidence that intermittent, excessive sugar intake causes endogenous opioid dependence," *Obesity Research* 10 no. 6 (2002): 478–88.

Colantuoni, C., et al. "Excessive sugar intake alters binding to dopamine and mu-opioid receptors in the brain," *Neuroreport* 2001 12, no. 16:3549–52.

Curzon, G. "Effects of Food Intake on Brain Transmitter Amine Precursors and Amine Synthesis." In *Psychopharmacology and Food*, edited by M. Sandler and T. Silverstone, 59–70.Oxford: Oxford University Press, 1985.

Delgado, P. L., L. H. Price, H. L. Miller, R. M. Salomon, G. K. Aghajanian, G. R. Heninger, and D. S. Charney. "Serotonin and the Neurobiology of Depression: Effect of Tryptophan Depletion in Drug-free Depressed Patients." *Archives of General Psychiatry* 51 (1994):865–74.

Drevon, C. A. "Marine Oils and Their Effects." *Nutrition Reviews* 50, no. 4 (1992):38–45.

Fernstrom, J. D., and R. J. Wurtman. "Brain Serotonin Content: Increase following Ingestion of Carbohydrate Diet." *Science* (1971):1023–25.

Fulder, S. "Ginseng: useless root or subtle medicine?" *New Scientist*, 1977;73:138–39.

Grandjean, A. C., et al. "The effect of caffeinated, non-caffeinated, caloric and non-caloric beverages on hydration." *Journal of the American College of Nutrition* 19 (2000): 591–600.

Grundman, M. "Vitamin E and Alzheimer disease: the basis for additional clinical trials." *American Journal of Clinical Nutrition* 71, no. 2 (Feb 2000): 630S–36S.

Hibbeln, J. R. "Fish Consumption and Major Depression (letter)." *Lancet* 351, no. 9110 (1998):1213.

Li, TSC. "The range of medicinal plants influencing mental and physical performance," In Watson, D. H. (ed.) *Performance Functional Foods*. Woodhead Publishing Ltd., Cambridge, England, 2003.

Linde, K., et al. "St John's wort for depression—an overview and meta-analysis of randomised clinical trials." *British Medical Journal* 313 (Aug 3 1996):253–58.

Maes, M., and H. Meltzer. "The Serotonin Hypothesis of Major Depression." In *Psychopharmacology: The Fourth Generation of Progress*, edited by F. E. Bloom and D. J. Kupfer. New York: Raven Press, 1995.

Markus, C. R., B. Olivier, G. Panhuysen, J. Van De Gugten, M. Alles, H. Westenberg, D. Fekkes, H. Koppeschaar, E. H. F. De Haan. "The Bovine Protein Alpha-Lactalbumin Increases the Plasma Trp/LNAA, and in Vulnerable Subjects It Raises Brain Serotonin Activity, Reduces Cortisol and Improves Mood under Stress." *American Journal of Clinical Nutrition* 71 (2000):1536–44.

Markus, C. R., B. Olivier, and E. H. F. de Haan. "Whey Protein Rich in Alpha-lactalbumin Increases the Plasma Trp/LNAA Ration, and Improves Cognitive Performance in Stress-vulnerable Subjects." *American Journal of Clinical Nutrition* 75 (2002):1051–56.

Markus, C. R., G. Panhuysen, L. I. Jonkman, and M. Bachman. "Carbohydrate Intake Improves Cognitive Performance of Stress-prone Individuals under Controllable Laboratory Stress." *British Journal of Nutrition* 82 (1999):457–67.

Markus, C., et al. "Does carbohydrate-rich, protein-poor food prevent a deterioration of mood and cognitive performance of stress-prone subjects when subjected to a stressful task?" *Appetite*, 1998;31(1): 49–65.

NeuhäuserBerthold, M., et al. "Coffee consumption and total body water homeostasis as measured by fluid balance and bioelectrical impedance analysis." *Annals of Nutrition and Metabolism* 41 (1997): 29–36.

Olivier, G., J. Wardle, and L. Gibson. "Stress and Food Choice: A Laboratory Study." *Psychosomatic Medicine* 62 (2000):853–65.

Oomah, B. D. "Ginkgo biloba and Alzheimer's disease," In Watson, D. H. (ed.) *Performance Functional Foods*. Woodhead Publishing Ltd., Cambridge, England, 2003.

Perkins, et al. "Association of antioxidants with memory in a multiethnic elderly sample using the Third National Health and Nutrition Examination Survey." *American Journal of Epidemiology* 150, no. 1 (Jul 1 1999): 37–44.

Rosenthal, N. E., M. J. Genhart, B. Caballero, F. M. Jacobsen, R. G. Skwerer, R. D. Coursey, S. Rogers, and B. Spring. "Psychobiological Effects of Carbohydrate- and Protein-rich Meals in Patients with Seasonal Affective Disorder and Normal Controls." *Biological Psychiatry* 25 (1989):1029–40.

Sahelian, R. *Mind Boosters: A Guide to Natural Supplements That Enhance the Mind, Memory and Mood.* New York: St. Martin's Press, 2000.

Stoll, A. L., G. S. Sachs, B. M. Cohen, B. Lafer, J. D. Christensen, and P. F. Renshaw. "Choline in the Treatment of Rapid-cycling Bipolar Disorder: Clinical and Neurochemical Findings in Lithium-treated Patients." *Biological Psychiatry* 40, no. 5 (1996):382–88.

Wells, A., N. W. Read, and I. A. Macdonald. "Effects of Carbohydrate and Lipid on Resting Energy Expenditure, Heart Rate, Sleepiness and Mood." *Physiology & Behavior* 63, no. 4 (1998):621–28.

Wurtman, R. J. "Nutrients Affecting Brain Composition and Behavior." *Integrative Psychiatry* 5 (1987):226–57.

Young, S. N., S. E. Smith, R. O. Pihl, F. R. Ervin. "Tryptophan Depletion Causes a Rapid Lowering of Mood in Normal Males." *Psychopharmacology* 87 (1985):173–77.

Chapter 3

Deutz, R. C., D. Benardot, D. E. Martin, and M. M. Cody. "Relationship between Energy Deficits and Body Composition in Elite Female Gymnasts and Runners." *Medicine and Science in Sports and Exercise* 32, no. 3 (March 2000):659–68.

Foster, G. D., H. R. Wyatt, J. O. Hill, B. G. McGuckin, C. Brill, B. S. Mohammed, P. O. Szapary, D. J. Rader, J. S. Edman, and S. Klein. "A Randomized Trial of a Low-Carbohydrate Diet for Obesity." *New England Journal of Medicine* 348, no. 21 (2003):2082–90.

Elliott, S. S., N. L. Keim, J. S. Stern, K. Teff, and P. J. Havel. "Fructose, Weight Gain, and the Insulin Resistance Syndrome." *American Journal of Clinical Nutrition* 76 (2002):911–22.

Minehira, K., V. Bettschart, H. Vidal, N. Vega, V. Di Vetta, V. Rey, P. Schneiter, and L. Tappy. "Effect of Carbohydrate Overfeeding on Whole Body and Adipose Tissue Metabolism in Humans." *Obesity Research* 11 (2003):1096–103.

Raben, A., T. H. Vasilaras, A. C. Moller, A. Astrup. "Sucrose Compared with Artificial Sweeteners: Different Effects on Ad Libitum Food Intake and Body Weight after 10 Weeks of Supplementation in Overweight Subjects." *American Journal of Clinical Nutrition* 76 (2002):721–29.

St. Jeor, S. T., B. V. Howard, T. E. Prewitt, V. Bovee, T. Bazzarre, R. H. Eckel. "Dietary Protein and Weight Reduction: A Statement for Healthcare Professionals from the Nutrition Committee of the Council on Nutrition, Physical Activity, and Metabolism of the American Heart Association." *Circulation* 104, no. 15 (October 9, 2001):1869–74.

Teegarden, D. "Calcium Intake and Reduction in Weight or Fat Mass." *Journal of Nutrition* 133 (2003):249S–251S.

Yunsheng, M., E. R. Bertone, E. J. Stanek III, G. W. Reed, J. R. Hebert, N. L. Cohen, P. A. Merriam, and I. S. Ockene. "Association between Eating Patterns and Obesity in a Free-living US Adult Population." *American Journal of Epidemiology* 158 (2003):85–92.

Zemel, M. B. "Mechanisms of Dairy Modulation of Adiposity." *Journal of Nutrition* 133 (2003):252S–256S.

Chapter 4

Anonymous. "Physiological and Health Effects of Oral Creatine Supplementation." *Medicine and Science in Sports and Exercise* 32 (2000):706–17.

Arciero, P. J., N. S. Hannibal, B. C. Nindl, C. L. Gentile, J. Hamed, M. D. Vukovich. "Comparison of Creatine Ingestion and Resistance Training on Energy Expenditure and Limb Blood Flow." *Metabolism* 50, no. 12 (2001):1429–34.

Bemben, M. G, D. A. Bemben, D. D. Loftiss, and A. W. Knehans. "Creatine Supplementation during Resistance Training in College Football Athletes. *Medicine and Science in Sports and Exercise* 33, no. 10 (2001):1667–73.

Børsheim, E., K. D. Tipton, S. E. Wolf, and R. R. Wolfe. "Essential Amino Acids and Muscle Protein Recovery from Resistance Exercise." *American Journal of Physiology – Endocrinology & Metabolism* 283, no. 4 (October 2002):E648–E657.

Bouche, C., Rizkalla, S. W., Luo, J., Vidal, H., Veronese, A., Pacher, N., Fouquet, C., Lang, V., Slama, G. "Five-week, low-glycemic index diet decreases total fat mass and improves plasma lipid profile in moderately overweight nondiabetic men." *Diabetes Care* 2002, no. 25:822–28.

Brilla, L. R., and V. Conte. "Effects of a Novel Zinc-Magnesium Formulation on Hormones and Strength." *Journal of Exercise Physiology Online* 3, no. 4 (1999):26–36.

Butterfield, G. E. "Whole-body protein utilization in humans. *Medical Science Sports Exercise* 19, no. 5 Suppl (1987): S157–65.

Casey, A., and P. L. Greenhaff. "Does Dietary Creatine Supplementation Play a Role in Skeletal Muscle Metabolism and Performance?" *American Journal of Clinical Nutrition* 72 (2000):S607–S617.

Jacobs, P. L., E. T. Mahoney, K. A. Cohn, L. F. Sheradsky, and B. A. Green. "Oral Creatine Supplementation Enhances Upper Body Extremity Work Capacity in Persons with Cervical-level Spinal Cord Injury." *Archives of Physical Medicine and Rehabilitation* 83, no. 1 (2002):19–23.

Jowko, E., P. Ostaszewski, M. Jank, J. Sacharuk, A. Zieniewicz, J. Wilczak, and S. Nissen. "Creatine and Beta-hydroxy-beta-methylbutyrate (HMB) Additively Increase Lean Body Mass and Muscle Strength during a Weight-training Program." *Nutrition* 17, nos. 7–8 (200 ?):558–66.

Kreider, R.B., R. Klesges, K. Harmon, P. Grindstaff, L. Ramsey, D. Bullen, L. Wood, Y. Yi, and A. Almada. "Effects of Ingesting Supplements Designed to Promote Lean Tissue Accretion on Body Composition during Resistance Training." *International Journal of Sports Nutrition* 6, no. 3 (1996):234–46.

Kreider, R. B., R. C. Klesges, D. Lotz, M. Davis, E. Cantler, K. Harmon-Clayton, R. Dudley, P. Grindstaff, L. Ramsey, D. Bullen, L. Wood, and A. Almada. "Effects of Nutritional Supplementation during Off-season College Football Training on Body Composition and Strength." *Journal of Exercise Physiology Online* 2, no. 2 (1999):24–39.

Lemon, P. W. "Do Athletes Need More Dietary Protein and Amino Acids?" *International Journal of Sports Nutrition* 5 (1995):S39–S61.

Lemon, P. W. "Is Increased Dietary Protein Necessary or Beneficial for Individuals with a Physically Active Lifestyle?" *Nutrition Review* 54 (1996):S169–S175.

Lemon, P. W. "Protein Requirements of Strength Athletes." In *Sports Supplements*, edited by J. Antonio and J. R. Stout, 301–15. Philadelphia: Lippincott Williams and Wilkens, 2001.

Manore, M. M. "Effect of Physical Activity on Thiamine, Riboflavin, and Vitamin B-6 Requirements." *American Journal of Clinical Nutrition* 72 (2000):S598–S606.

Okuda, T., Koishi, H., Koh, H., Waki, M., Kurata, M., Nambu, S. "Relationship between protein intake and nitrogen balance in obese patients on low energy diet." *Journal of Nutritional Science and Vitaminology* 33 no. 3 (1987): 219–26.

Rodriguez, V. M., Portillo, M. P., Pico, C., Macarulla, M. T., Palou, A. "Olive oil feeding up-regulates uncoupling protein genes in rat brown adipose tissue and skeletal muscle." *American Journal of Clinical Nutrition* 75 (2002): 213–20.

Schroder, H., E. Navarro, J. Mora, D. Galiano, and A. Tramullas. "Effects of Alpha-tocopherol, Beta-carotene and Ascorbic Acid on Oxidative, Hormonal and Enzymatic Exercise Stress Markers in Habitual Training Activity of Professional Basketball Players." *European Journal of Nutrition* 40, no. 4 (2001):178–84.

Sen, C. K. "Antioxidants in Exercise Nutrition." *Sports Medicine* 31, no. 13 (2001):891–908.

Skov, A. R., Toubro, S., Bulow, J., Krabbe, K., Parving, H. H., Astrup, A. "Changes in renal function during weight loss induced by high vs. low-protein low-fat diets in overweight subjects." *International Journal of Obesity* 23, no. 1:1170–77.

Slater, G., D. Jenkins, P. Logan, H. Lee, M. Vukovich, J. A. Rathmacher, and A. G. Hahn. "Beta-hydroxy-beta-methylbutyrate (HMB) Supplementation Does Not Affect Changes in Strength or Body Composition during Resistance Training in Trained Men. *International Journal of Sports Nutrition Exercise Metabolism* 11, no. 3 (2001):384–96.

Todd, K. S., Butterfield, G. E., Calloway, D. H. "Nitrogen balance in men with adequate and deficient energy intake at three levels of work. *Journal of Nutrition* 114, no. 11 (1984): 2107–18.

Van Dale, D., J. Schrijver, and W. H. Saris. "Changes in Vitamin Status in Plasma during Dieting and Exercise." *International Journal for Vitamin and Nutrition Research* 60, no. 1 (1990):67–74.

Volek, J. S., N. D. Duncan, S. A. Mazzetti, R. S. Staron, M. Putukian, A. L. Gomez, D. R. Pearson, W. J. Fink, and W. J. Kraemer. "Performance and Muscle Fiber Adaptations to Creatine Supplementation and Heavy Resistance Training." *Medicine and Science in Sports and Exercise* 31, no. 8 (1999):1147–56.

Vukovich, M.D., G. Slater, M. B. Macchi, M. J. Turner, K. Fallon, T. Boston, and J. Rathmacher. "Beta-hydroxy-beta-methylbutyrate (HMB) Kinetics and the Influence of Glucose Ingestion in Humans." *Journal of Nutritional Biochemistry* 12, no. 11 (2001):631–39.

Willoughby, D.S., and J. Rosene. "Effects of Oral Creatine and Resistance Training on Myosin Heavy Chain Expression." *Medicine and Science in Sports and Exercise* 33, no. 10 (2001):1674–81.

Ziegenfuss, T.N., L. M. Lowery, and P. W. Lemon. "Acute Fluid Volume Changes in Men during Three Days of Creatine Supplementation." *Journal of Exercise Physiology Online* 1, no. 3 (1998).

Chapter 5

Boirie, Y., et al. "Slow and fast dietary proteins differently modulate postprandial protein accretion." *Proceedings of the National Academy of Sciences* 94 (1997): 14930–35.

Bujko, J., Schreurs, V. V., Koopmanschap, P. E., Furstenberg, E., Keller, J. S. "Benefit of more but smaller meals at a fixed daily protein intake." *Z Ernahrungswiss* 36, no. 4 (1997): 347–49.

Charlier, C., Desaive, C., Plomteux, G. "Human exposure to endocrine disrupters: consequences of gastroplasty on plasma concentration of toxic pollutants." *International Journal of Obesity* 26, no. 11 (Nov 2002): 1465–68.

Doherty, M. "The effects of caffeine on the maximal accumulated oxygen deficit and short-term running performance." *International Journal of Sport Nutrition* 8 (1998): 95–104.

Graham, T. E., et al. "Caffeine vs. coffee: coffee isn't an effective ergogenic aid." *Medicine and Science in Sports and Exercise* 27 (1995): S224.

Graham, T. E, et al. "Caffeine and exercise: metabolism and perfor-mance." *Canadian Journal of Applied Physiology* 19 (1994): 111–38.

Graham, T. E., Spriet, L. L. "Caffeine and exercise performance." *Sports Science Exchange* 9 (1996): 1–6.

Jackman, M., et al. "Metabolic catecholamine and endurance re-sponses to caffeine during intense exercise." *Journal of Ap-plied Physiology* 81 (1996): 1658–63.

Koopman, R., D. L. Pannemans, A. E. Jeukendrup, A. P. Gijsen, J. M. Senden, D. Halliday, W. H. Saris, L. J. Van Loon, and A. J. Wagenmakers. "The Combined Ingestion of Protein and Car-bohydrate Improves Protein Balance During Ultra Endurance Exercise." *American Journal of Physiology Endocrinology Me-tabolism* (May 27, 2004).

Lemon, Peter W.R. "Beyond the Zone: Protein Needs of Active In-dividuals." *Journal of the American College of Nutrition* 19, no. 90005 (2000):S513–S521.

Lemon, P., Tarnopolsky, M., MacDougall, J., Atkinson, S. "Protein requirements and muscle mass/strength changes during in-tensive training in novice bodybuilders." *Journal of Applied Physiology* 73, no. 2 (1992): 767–75.

Lindinger, M. I., et al. "Caffeine attenuates the exercise-induced increase in plasma [K+] in humans." *Journal of Applied Phys-iology* 74 (1993): 1149–55.

Lukaski, H. C. "Vitamin and Mineral Status: Effects on Physical Performance." *Nutrition* 20, nos. 7–8 (July/August 2004):632–44.

Pelletier, C., Doucet, E., Imbeault, P., Tremblay, A. "Associations between weight loss-induced changes in plasma organochlo-rine concentrations, serum T(3) concentration, and resting metabolic rate." *Toxicological Sciences* 2002 67, no. 1:46–51.

Saunders, M. J, Kane, M. D., Todd, M. K. Effects of a carbohy-drate-protein beverage on cycling endurance and muscle damage. Med Sci Sports Exerc 2004; 36(7): 1233–1238.

Spriet, L. L. "Caffeine and performance." *International Journal of Sport Nutrition* 5 (1995): S84–S99.

Tarnopolsky, M. "Protein Requirements for Endurance Athletes." *Nutrition* 20, nos. 7–8 (July/August 2004):662–68.

Tarnopolsky, M., et al. "Evaluation of protein requirements for trained strength athletes." *Journal of Applied Physiology* 73, no. 5 1992): 1986–95.

Vandenberghe, K., et al. "Caffeine counteracts the ergogenic ac-tion of muscle creatine loading." *Journal of Applied Physiology* 80, no. 2 (1996): 452–57.

Von Duvillard, S. P., W. A. Braun, M. Markofski, R. Beneke, and R. Leithauser. "Fluids and Hydration in Prolonged Endurance Performance." *Nutrition* 20, nos. 7–8 (July/August 2004):651–56.

Weir, J., et al. "A high carbohydrate diet negates the metabolic ef-fect of caffeine during exercise." *Medicine and Science in Sports and Exercise* 19 (1987): 100–105.

Chapter 6

Blair, S. N. "Revisiting fitness and fatness as predictors of mortality." *Clinical Journal of Sport Medicine* 13, no. 5 (Sep 2003): 319–20.

Bodkin, N. L., Alexander, T. M., Ortmeyer, H. K., Johnson, E., Hansen, B. C. "Mortality and morbidity in laboratory-main-tained Rhesus monkeys and effects of long-term dietary re-striction." *Journals of Gerontology Series A: Biological Sciences and Medical Sciences* 58 (2003): 212–19.

Calle, E. E., Rodriguez, C., Walker-Thurmond, K., Thun, M. J. "Overweight, obesity, and mortality from cancer in a prospec-tively studied cohort of U.S. adults." *New England Journal of Medicine* 348 (2003): 1625–38.

Chi, Y. S., Lim, H., Park, H., Kim, H. P. "Effects of wogonin, a plant flavone from Scutellaria radix, on skin inflammation: in vivo regulation of inflammation-associated gene expression." *Bio-chemical Pharmacology* 66, no. 7 (Oct 12003): 1271–78.

Heymsfield, S. B., van Mierlo, C.A.J., van der Knaap, H.C.M., Heo, M., Frier, H. I. "Weight management using a meal replace-ment strategy: meta and pooling analysis from six studies." *International Journal of Obesity* 27 (2003): 537–49.

MacKay, D., Miller, A. L. "Nutritional support for wound healing." *Alternative Medicine Review* 8, no. 4 (Nov 2003): 359–77.

Marles, R. J., Kaminski, J., Arnason, J. T., Pazos-Sanou, L., Hep-tinstall, S., Fischer, N. H., Crompton, C. W., Kindack, D. G., Awang, D. V. "A bioassay for inhibition of serotonin release from bovine platelets." *Journal of Natural Products* 55, no. 8 (Aug 1992): 1044–56.

Micke, P., Beehm K. M., Schlaak, J. F., Buhl, R. "Oral supplemen-tation with whey proteins increases plasma glutathione levels of HIV-infected patients." *European Journal of Clinical Inves-tigation* 31, no. 2 (Feb 2001): 171–78.

Murdoch, S. "Managing the Inflammatory Response through Nu-tritional Supplements." *Athletic Therapy Today* 5 (2001).

Sano, M., Ernesto, C., Thomas, R. G., et al. "A controlled trial of selegiline, alpha-tocopherol, or both as treatment for Alzheimer's disease. The Alzheimer's Disease Cooperative Study." *New England Journal of Medicine* 336 (1997): 1216–22.

Stevens, J., Cai, J., Evenson, K. R., Thomas, R. "Fitness and fatness as predictors of mortality from all causes and from cardiovas-cular disease in men and women in the lipid research clinics study." *American Journal of Epidemiology* 156, no. 9 (Nov 1, 2002): 832–41.

Wang, F., Van Den Eeden, S. K., Ackerson, L. M., Salk, S. E., Reince, R. H., Elin, R. J. "Oral magnesium oxide prophylaxis of frequent migrainous headache in children: a randomized, double-blind, placebo-controlled trial." *Headache* 43, no. 6 (Jun 2003): 601–10.

Chapter 7

Block, G., B. Patterson, and A. Subar. "Fruit, Vegetables, and Cancer Prevention: A Review of the Epidemiological Evi-dence." *Nutrition and Cancer* 18, no. 1 (1992):1–29.

Craig, W. J. "Phytochemicals: Guardians of our health." *Journal of the American Dietetic Association* 1997; (suppl 2): S199–S204.

"Diabetes Rates Rise Six Percent in One Year," by Donald R. Hall, DrPh, Monday, December 15, 2003, ©2003, Wellsource, Inc.

Easton, M. D., Luszniak, D., Von der, G. E. "Preliminary examination of contaminant loadings in farmed salmon, wild salmon and commercial salmon feed." *Chemosphere* 46, no. 7 (Feb 2002): 1053–74.

Eynard, A. R., Lopez, C. B. "Conjugated linoleic acid (CLA) versus saturated fats/cholesterol: their proportion in fatty and lean meats may affect the risk of developing colon cancer." *Lipids in Health and Disease* 2, no. 1 (2003): 6.

Harding, A. H., L. A. Sargeant, K. T. Khaw, A. Welch, S. Oakes, R. N. Luben, S. Bingham, N. E. Day, and N. J. Wareham. "Cross-sectional Association between Total Level and Type of Alcohol Consumption and Glycosylated Haemoglobin Level: The EPIC-Norfolk Study." *European Journal of Clinical Nutrition* 56, no. 9 (September 2002):882–90.

Howard, A.A., J. H. Arnsten, and M. N. Gourevitch. "Effect of Alcohol Consumption on Diabetes Mellitus: A Systematic Review." *Annual of Internal Medicine* 140, no. 3 (February 3, 2004): 211–19.

Kaitosaari, T., Ronnemaa, T., Raitakari, O., Talvia, S., Kallio, K., Volanen, I., Leino, A., Jokinen, E., Valimaki, I., Viikari, J., Simell, O. "Effect of 7-year infancy-onset dietary intervention on serum lipoproteins and lipoprotein subclasses in healthy children in the prospective, randomized Special Turku Coronary Risk Factor Intervention Project for Children (STRIP) study." Circulation 108, no. 6 (Aug 12, 2003): 672–77, Epub 2003 Jul.

Meyer, K. A., K. M. Conigrave, N. F. Chu, N. Rifai, D. Spiegelman, M. J. Stampfer, and E. B. Rimm. "Alcohol Consumption Patterns and HbA1c, C-peptide and Insulin Concentrations in Men." *Journal of American College of Nutrition* 22, no. 3 (June 2003):185–94.

Mozaffarian, D., R. N. Lemaitre, L. H. Kuller, G. L. Burke, R. P. Tracy, D. S. Siscovick. "Cardiac Benefits of Fish Consumption May Depend on the Type of Fish Meal Consumed. The Cardiovascular Health Study." *Circulation* 107 (2003):1372.

Riboli, E., and T. Norat. "Epidemiologic Evidence of the Protective Effect of Fruit and Vegetables on Cancer Risk." *American Journal of Clinical Nutrition* 78 (September 2003):S559–S569.

Robaczyk, M. G. "Evaluation of leptin levels in plasma and their reliance on other hormonal factors affecting tissue fat levels in people with various levels of endogenous cotisol." *Annales Academiae Medicae Stetinensis* 48 (2002): 283–300.

Steinmetz, K. A., Potter, J. D. "Vegetables, fruit, and cancer prevention: a review." *Journal of the American Dietetic Association* 96 (1996): 1027–39.

Stender, S., Dyerberg, J. "Influence of Trans Fatty Acids on Health." *Annals of Nutrition and Metabolism* 48, no. 2 (2004): 61–66. Epub 2003 Dec.

Van Lieshout, E. M., Bedaf, M. M., Pieter, M., Ekkel, C., Nijhoff, W. A., Peters, W. H. "Effects of dietary anticarcinogens on rat gastrointestinal glutathione S-transferase theta 1-1 levels." *Carcinogenesis* 19, no. 11 (Nov 1998): 2055–57.

Vogt, T. M., L. J. Appel, E. Obarzanek, T. J. Moore, W. M. Vollmer, L. P.Svetkey, F. M. Sacks, G. A. Bray, J. A. Cutler, M. M. Windhauser, P. H. Lin, and N. M. Karanja. "Dietary Approaches to Stop Hypertension: Rationale, Design, and Methods." *Journal of American Dietetic Association* 99 (1999):S12–S18.

Wang, L., Liu, D., Ahmed, T., Chung, F. L., Conaway, C., Chiao, J. W. "Targeting cell cycle machinery as a molecular mechanism of sulforaphane in prostate cancer prevention." *International Journal of Oncology* 24, no. 1 (Jan 2004): 187–92.

Yeum, K. J., Aldini, G., Chung, H. Y., Krinsky, N. I., Russell, R. M. "The activities of antioxidant nutrients in human plasma depend on the localization of attacking radical species." *Journal of Nutrition* 133, no. 8 (Aug 2003): 2688–91.

Chapter 8

Constance G. Bacon, Sc.D.; Murray A. Mittleman, M.D., Sc.D.; Ichiro Kawachi, M.D., Ph.D.; Edward Giovannucci, M.D., Sc.D.; Dale B. Glasser, Ph.D.; and Eric B. Rimm, Sc.D. "Sexual Function in Men Older Than 50 Years of Age: Results from the Health Professionals Follow-up Study." *Annals of Internal Medicine* 139, no. 3 (Aug 2003): 161–68.

Henkel, R., J. Bittner, R. Weber, F. Huther, and W. Miska. "Relevance of Zinc in Human Sperm Flagella and Its Relation to Motility." *Fertility and Sterility* 71, no. 6 (June 1999):1138–43.

Markus, C., et al. "Does carbohydrate-rich, protein-poor food prevent a deterioration of mood and cognitive performance of stress-prone subjects when subjected to a stressful task?" *Appetite* 1998;31(1): 49–65.

Mohan, H., J. Verma, I. Singh, P. Mohan, S. Marwah, and P. Singh. "Inter-relationship of Zinc Levels in Serum and Semen in Oligospermic Infertile Patients and Fertile Males." *Indian Journal of Pathology and Microbiology* 40, no. 4 (October 1997):451–55.

Saso, L. "Effects of drug abuse on sexual response," [Article in Italian] Dipartimento di Farmacologia delle Sostanze Naturali e Fisiologia Generale, Universita degli Studi La Sapienza, P.le Aldo Moro 5, 00185 Roma. luciano.saso@uniroma1.it.

Roumeguere, T., Wespes, E. Carpentier, Y., Hoffmann, P., Schulman, C. C. "Erectile dysfunction is associated with a high prevalence of hyperlipidemia and coronary heart disease risk." *European Urology* 44, no. 3 (Sep 2003): 355–59.

Chapter 9

American Academy of Orthopedic Surgeons, "Falls and Hip Fractures," http://orthoinfo.aaos.org/fact/thr_report.cfm?Thread_ID=77&topcategory=Hip.

American Osteopathic College of Dermatology, "Acne," *Dermatologic Disease Database*, http://www.aocd.org/skin/dermatologic_diseases/acne.html.

Cordain, L., S. Lindeberg, M. Hurtado, K. Hill, S. Boyd Eaton, and J. Brand-Miller. "Acne Vulgaris: A Disease of Western Civilization." *Archives of Dermatology* 138 (2002): 1584–90.

Hammond, B. R. Jr., E. J. Johnson, R. M. Russell, N. I. Krinsky, K. J. Yeum, R. B. Edwards, and D. M. Snodderly. "Dietary Modification of Human Macular Pigment Density." *Investigative Ophthalmology & Visual Science* 38 (year?): 1795–1801.

Jugdaohsingh, R., S. H. C. Anderson, K. L. Tucker, H. Elliott, D. P. Kiel, R. P.H. Thompson, and J. J. Powell. "Dietary Silicon Intake and Absorption." *American Journal of Clinical Nutrition* 75, no. 5 (May 2002): 887–93.

Landrum, J. T., R. A. Bone, H. Joa, M. D. Kilburn, L. L. Moore, and K. E. Sprague. "A One Year Study of the Macular Pigment: The Effect of 140 Days of a Lutein Supplement." *Experimental Eye Research* 65 (July 1997): 57–62.

Marse-Perlman, Julie A., Fisher, Alicia I., Klein, Ronald, Palta, Mari, Block, Gladys, Millen, Amy E., Wright, Jacqueline D. "Lutein and Zeaxanthin in the Diet and Serum and Their Relation to Age-related Maculopathy in the Third National Health and Nutrition Examination Survey." *American Journal of Epidemiology* Vol. 153, No. 5: 424–432 (2001) The Johns Hopkins University School of Hygiene and Public Health.

Olmedilla, B., F. Granado, I. Blanco, and M. Vaquero. "Lutein, but not Alpha-tocopherol, Supplementation Improves Visual Function in Patients with Age-related Cataracts: A 2-y Double-blind, Placebo-controlled Pilot Study." *Nutrition* 19 (January 2003): 21–24.

Chapter 10

David Heber, M.D., Ph.D., *The Resolution Diet,* Avery Publishing Group, 1999.

Doreen Virtue, Ph.D., *Constant Craving,* Hay House, 1995.

Ming, M. C., Jones, J. H. "Dietary fat type and energy restriction interactively influence plasma leptin concentration in rats." *Journal of Lipid Research* 39, no. 8 (1998): 1655–60.

Mori, T. A., Bao, D. Q., Burke, V., Puddey, I. B., Watts, G. F., Beilin, L. J. "Dietary fish as a major component of a weight-loss diet: effect on serum lipids, glucose, and insulin metabolism in overweight hypertensive subjects." *American Journal of Clinical Nutrition* 70, no. 5 (1999): 817–25.

Seife, C. "Salmon survey stokes debate about farmed fish." Science 303 (2004): 154–55.

Su, W., Jones, P. J. "Dietary fatty acid composition influences energy accretion in rats." *Journal of Nutrition* 123, no. 12 (1993): 2109–14.

Trichopoulou, A., T. Costacou, C. Bamia, and D. Trichopoulos. "Adherence to a Mediterranean Diet and Survival in a Greek Population." *New England Journal of Medicine* 348, no. 26 (2003):2599–2608

U.S. Food and Drug Administration: Overview of the Draft FDA/EPA methylmercury (MeHg) consumer advisory. Dec. 10–11, 2003. www.fda.gov

Chapter 11

Howard, A. A., Arnsten, J. H., Gourevitch, M. N. "Effect of alcohol consumption on diabetes mellitus: a systematic review." Montefiore Medical Center and Albert Einstein College of Medicine, Bronx, New York 10467, USA. ahoward@montefiore.org

Index

Underscored page references indicate boxed text and tables.